Becoming Vegan

Express Edition: The Everyday Guide To Plant-based Nutrition

Brenda Davis, RD
Vesanto Melina, MS, RD

16pt

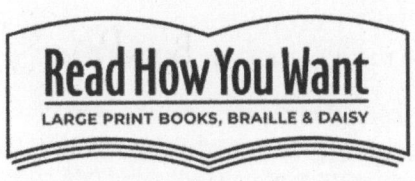

Read How You Want

LARGE PRINT BOOKS, BRAILLE & DAISY

Copyright Page from the Original Book

Library of Congress Cataloging-in-Publication Data

Davis, Brenda, 1959-
  Becoming vegan express edition / Brenda Davis, RD, Vesanto Melina, MS, RD.
    pages cm
  Includes bibliographical references and index.
    ISBN 978-1-57067-295-8 (pbk.) — ISBN 978-1-57067-903-2 (e-book)
  1. Vegetarianism—Health aspects 2. Vegetarianism. 3. Vegetarian cooking. I. Melina, Vesanto, 1942– II. Title.
    RM236.D36 2013
    641.5'636—dc23

                                                    2013023875

To the visionaries before us and beside us, who have dedicated their lives to making this world a kinder, gentler place:

- Donald Watson, Dr. Frey Ellis, and the founders of the vegan movement

- Jay and Freya Dinshah and others who started vegan organizations throughout the world

- Bob and Cynthia Holzapfel and the hundreds of courageous plant-based pioneers at The Farm

- Albert Schweitzer, John Robbins, Jane Goodall, and all those who have guided our paths to compassion

- Michael Klaper, Neal Barnard, Michael Greger, and the many physicians who have dedicated their lives to guiding others toward healthful vegan lifestyles

- Virginia Messina, Reed Mangels, Sue Havala, Jack Norris, George Eisman, and the countless dietitians who laid the foundations of vegan dietary wisdom

Cover art: Julia Ruffles
Cover and interior design: John Wincek

© 2013 Brenda Davis and Vesanto Melina

Printed in Canada

Book Publishing Company
P.O. Box 99
Summertown, TN 38483
888-260-8458
bookpubco.com

ISBN 13: 978-1-57067-295-8

19 18 17 16 15 14 13   1 2 3 4 5 6 7 8 9

BOOK PUBLISHING CO.

TABLE OF CONTENTS

ACKNOWLEDGMENTS i

CHAPTER 1: Widening the Circle of Compassion 1

CHAPTER 2: The Great Vegan Advantage 48

CHAPTER 3: Protein Power from Plants 105

CHAPTER 4: Fat Matters 129

CHAPTER 5: The Two Faces of Carbohydrates 164

CHAPTER 6: Valuing Vitamins 207

CHAPTER 7: Minding Your Minerals 256

CHAPTER 8: Clean Vegan Eating 290

CHAPTER 9: Triumph over Weight 322

CHAPTER 10: Overcoming Underweight 364

CHAPTER 11: From Pregnancy On: Nourishing Strong Children 396

CHAPTER 12: The Prime of Life: Vegan Nutrition for Seniors 462

CHAPTER 13: The Fit Vegan 490

CHAPTER 14: The Vegan Food Guide 530

APPENDIX: Recommended Intakes of Vitamins and Minerals 551

RESOURCES 555

Back Cover Material 561

Index 565

ACKNOWLEDGMENTS

We are most grateful for our brilliant and dedicated colleagues at the Book Publishing Company, including publisher Bob Holzapfel; editors Cynthia Holzapfel, Carol Lorente, and Jasmine Star; and the marketing and support team, Anna Pope, Thomas Hupp, and Liz Murray.

Our deepest thanks go to the insightful vegan professionals who provided invaluable feedback on sections or chapters: Michael Greger, Reed Mangels, Jack Norris, Ginny Messina, Paul Shapiro, Mark Rivkin, Andrea Frisque, Heather Waxman, and James Chicalo.

We are indebted to colleagues and friends who took the time to offer support, inspiration, or thoughtful commentary: Margie Roswell, Carolyn Johnston, Margie Colclough, Daneen Agecoutey, and Angelina Rogon.

We appreciate the supportive energy of our research assistants: Renee Webb-Pelchat, Deanna Ibbitson, Carole Douglas, Katherine Jassman, Hana Tahae, and Cory Davis (Brenda's cherished son).

Many thanks for the time and expertise of our gracious advisors: Dr. Luciana Baroni, Dr. Winston Craig, Dr. Michael Klaper, Dr. Paul Appleby, Dr. Joe Millward, Dr. Melvin H. Williams, Dr. Ricardo Uauy, Dr. Ailsa Welch, Dr. Jagoda Ambroszkiewicz, Dr. Undurti N. Das, John Davis, and Freya Dinshah. We also thank Vesanto's son Xoph Crawford for his insights about food and healing. Thanks to young parents Kavyo Crawford (Vesanto's dear daughter), Stefan Shielke, Stephanie Weisner, Ian Hubbard, Kayla Vierling, and Aimée and Daniel Lindenberger.

Boundless love and gratitude to our partners, Paul Davis and Cam Doré, for their continued dedication and support. Special thanks to Cam for his brilliant and ongoing assistance with technical challenges.

Photographic credits and appreciation to Kevin Trowbridge (kevintrowbridge. com) and his assistant Katherine Trowbridge.

We are also grateful to those who generously shared their excellent products for recipe testing: Kelly Saunderson of Manitoba Harvest (hempseeds), Omega Nutrition (quality oils), Nature's Path Foods, and Adeline Cheong of LeSaffre Yeast Corporation (Red Star Vegetarian Support Formula nutritional yeast). We also thank ESHA Research for their fine nutritional analysis program, the Food Processor.

CHAPTER I

Widening the Circle of Compassion

It takes immense inner strength and courage to oppose the status quo. Yet if people hadn't risen up against social injustice, women wouldn't have the vote, the poor would have remained uneducated, and slavery would be legal. What does social justice have to do with a vegan lifestyle? Nothing, if you regard animals as resources; everything, if you recognize them as sentient beings.

It is possible that the greatest social injustice of our time is committed not against our fellow human beings but against our fellow nonhuman beings. Becoming vegan is about taking a stand against this injustice.

Vegan Awakenings

The seeds of vegan ethics were sown by philosophers and spiritual leaders in the East and spread in the West by the sixth-century Greek philosopher and mathematician Pythagoras, who shunned the consumption of animal flesh and directed his followers to do the same. While many other legendary thinkers, including Plato, Plutarch, Seneca, Ovid, and Socrates, followed suit, it wasn't until the mid-1800s that the moral roots of vegetarianism were firmly established in Western culture. The epicenter was England, and the driving forces were moral leaders of select Christian churches. While the movement was becoming wellgrounded in the West, its influence was limited when contrasted with the practices and teachings of the East, where Buddhism, Jainism, and Hinduism emphasized compassion toward animals and vegetarianism as a part of their core doctrines.

The word *vegetarian* was coined by the founders of the British Vegetarian Society in 1842. The word has nothing to do with vegetables and actually comes from the Latin word *vegetus,* which means "lively, fresh, and vigorous." The ethics of consuming dairy products were hotly debated within the burgeoning UK vegetarian movement, but there is good evidence that the first people to call themselves vegetarians were actually what we now call vegans. Eventually, a small, like-minded group of individuals decided to branch off and promote an entirely new breed of vegetarians, then called nondairy vegetarians.

The father of the contemporary vegan movement, Donald Watson, and his British compatriots recognized that the flesh food industry and dairy product industry were inextricably linked. They contended that the case against the dairy industry rivaled that against the meat industry, and that the use of dairy products was no longer justifiable for ethical vegetarians. Their intent was to eliminate the exploitation of both animals and humans and move closer to a truly humane society. Together, they founded the first vegan society in 1944 with only twenty-five members. Watson coined the word *vegan* (pronounced "VEE-gun") to describe vegetarians who exclude all animal products from their diet and lifestyle. In the 1950s, London physician Frey Ellis joined their ranks, significantly strengthening the scientific understanding of vegan health.

In 1948, Dr. Catherine Nimmo and Rubin Abramowitz established the first vegan society in the United States in Oceano, California. The group continued until 1960, when a national organization, the American Vegan Society (AVS), was founded by H. Jay Dinshah. The society has consistently encouraged the active practice of *ahimsa*—a Sanskrit word meaning "dynamic harmlessness"—as a part of a vegan lifestyle. Ahimsa, which is embraced by AVS as an urgent, worldwide necessity, advocates six pillars, one for each letter of the word:

Abstinence from animal products
Harmlessness, with reverence for life
Integrity of thought, word, and deed
Mastery over oneself
Service to humanity, nature, and creation

Advancement of understanding and truth

In 1987, veganism was catapulted into the mainstream by author John Robbins with the release of his groundbreaking book *Diet for a New America*. Robbins's book provided the first hard-hitting exposé of the consequences of factory farming on food animals, the environment, and human health. Today, vegan groups and societies exist in more than fifty countries.

More Than Diet

Many people believe that being vegan is about eschewing hamburgers and ice cream. It is not. Being vegan is about making an ethical decision to widen your circle of compassion and take a stand against deeply rooted customs and traditions—customs that are often strongly held by people we love, respect, and admire. For most of us, this triggers a long, hard battle with our conscience in which our conscience ultimately prevails.

Being vegan is about including those who are commonly excluded, be they human animals or nonhuman animals. It's about understanding that our choices have consequences for ourselves and beyond ourselves and recognizing that eating animals and animal products is both unnecessary and potentially harmful. Being vegan is about making choices that are a true reflection of our ethical and moral principles.

So how does a philosophy of reverence for life and compassion for all living things translate to diet and lifestyle? In terms of diet, the primary approach is excluding meat, poultry, fish, dairy products, eggs, gelatin, and other foods of animal origin, while allowing all foods of plant origin, including vegetables, fruits, legumes, grains, nuts, and seeds. But a vegan *lifestyle* takes it a few steps further.

A vegan lifestyle also excludes—as far as possible and practical—animal exploitation. A vegan avoids all products derived from animals—not just meat, eggs, and dairy products, but also certain consumer products. A vegan doesn't wear clothing produced from fur, leather, wool, or silk or use personal care or cleaning products that contain animal-derived ingredients. A vegan also avoids products and activities that involve the mistreatment or misuse of animals, including research conducted on animals and entertainment that exploits animals.

There are degrees of veganism. A *pure vegetarian* or *dietary vegan* is someone who consumes a vegan diet but doesn't lead a vegan lifestyle. Pure vegetarians may use animal products, support the use of animals in research, wear leather shoes or wool clothing, or have no objection to the exploitation of animals for entertainment. They are generally motivated by personal health concerns rather than by ethical objections. Some may adopt a more vegan lifestyle as they are exposed to vegan philosophy.

You may wonder how vegan you have to be to call yourself a vegan. Essentially, if you identify as a vegan and strive to avoid animal products and activities that exploit animals, you are vegan, even if you slip on occasion. There are no vegan police scrutinizing your diet and lifestyle habits. Being vegan isn't about personal purity or moral superiority. It's about making a conscious choice to widen your circle of compassion by avoiding animal exploitation as much as possible and practical.

In today's world, it is virtually impossible to be 100 percent cruelty-free. Traces of animal products lurk almost everywhere—as red dye in candy, as filters in the processing of wine, and in phones, matches, sandpaper, theatrical lighting, photographic film, cars, bicycles, planes, computers, and the list goes on. Our efforts to live with compassion far exceed our ability to eliminate the trace amounts of animal products that permeate our marketplace. Besides, there are instances in which the use of a nonvegan product can result in a reduction in animal suffering. Think back to the time before digital cameras. Had we avoided photography because film utilizes animal products, thousands of people moved by graphic images of exploited animals would have continued to exploit them. The vegan lifestyle is a means to an end—which is to reduce animal suffering—and not the end itself.

Their Plight, Our Power

Some people view everything on this planet as a resource that is here for the taking. To them, animals exist only to serve humans. This logic is used to defend the exploitation of animals for fashion, entertainment, experimentation, research, and food. There is often controversy about how animals should be treated in the process, but the actual use of animals is generally not a point of contention for the majority of people in our society.

Perspectives on the appropriate treatment of animals can vary widely from culture to culture. In America, kittens and puppies are beloved pets. In China, they may be skinned and boiled alive for dinner. While the very thought may disgust Americans, they don't give a second thought about dining on lobster. Some people would argue that dogs and cats are more intelligent than lobsters so they deserve to be treated more kindly, yet our treatment of pigs, which are more intelligent than dogs, is arguably worse than our treatment of lobsters.

The industry responsible for the overwhelming majority of animal suffering is the food industry. More than 95 percent of all animals purposefully killed by people are killed to be eaten.

The Making of Meat Machines

Forget the bucolic scenes from your favorite childhood storybooks. The lives of today's farm animals bear no resemblance to those fairy tales.

In 1900, 41 percent of Americans lived on farms; one hundred years later, that figure had dropped to 1.9 percent. With the rising consumption of animal products, how is it possible to supply sufficient meat and milk to satisfy so many people with so few farmers? In a word, agribusiness. In terms of animal products, the goal of agribusiness is to transform animals into production units, generating the greatest amount of meat, milk, or eggs for the least amount of money. The most efficient way to accomplish this is to bring the animals from the fields to factories and do whatever it takes to minimize the time it takes to get them to slaughter.

This quest has become a science in and of itself. Among the most timehonored techniques are keeping animals in small spaces, giving them hormones so they gain more weight more quickly, stimulating their appetite, breeding them for rapid growth, feeding them antibiotics to control disease, and using cheap feed. The result is what the industry terms "concentrated animal feeding operations" (CAFOs), more commonly known as factory farms.

Every year in North America, approximately eleven billion land animals are slaughtered for food. Of these, almost 80 percent of cattle and almost all chickens, laying hens, turkeys, and pigs are raised in factory farms. These animals, so vigilantly hidden from view, endure unspeakable suffering, but the average consumer is so far removed from the animals' lives that they easily forget that the meat at the grocery store is the flesh of an animal.

A PIG'S LIFE

When living in their natural environment, pigs live in groups of six to thirty. They are remarkably clean and particular, having separate sites for eating, sleeping, grooming, and elimination. Pigs are playful and protective and have complex social systems. They love to bathe in water, and while they do roll in mud, this behavior is necessary for temperature regulation since they lack sweat glands and are prone to heat stress. The mud also protects them from insects and sunburn. Pigs have been shown to be more intelligent than dogs or even threeyear-old children. They have remarkably long memories and can learn to play simple games every bit as quickly as primates. They can even be highly skilled at video games, learning to play with a joystick designed for them.

The natural life span of a pig is ten to fifteen years, but pigs raised for food in the United

States live only about six months. Breeder sows live until their reproductive ability wanes, generally three to four years. Most of this time is spent in crates with insufficient room for them to turn around. Although piglets are usually weaned at about fifteen weeks, in intensive farming they are removed from their mothers for fattening after only two to four weeks of nursing, and the sows are then impregnated again.

Weanlings spend the next six weeks in "nurseries," which are generally wire cages stacked one on top of the other. Piglets who don't grow fast enoughare typically "euthanized" by three weeks of age. Although there are a variety of methods for killing them, the most common is blunt trauma to the head, often by picking them up by their hind legs, swinging them, and slamming their heads onto a concrete floor.

Healthy piglets receive medication to prevent the diarrhea that results from eating solid foods, which they are too young to properly digest. Most undergo a variety of mutilations, including castration for males, ear notching, tail docking, and tooth clipping. These agonizing procedures, done primarily to reduce stressrelated behaviors, are performed without painkillers.

The animals destined for meat production are transferred to cramped pens until they reach a slaughter weight of 240 to 300 pounds. The pigs are crammed together in single stalls or groups, with no room for rooting, exploring, nesting, or other natural social behaviors. The floors are commonly metal grid systems that allow urine, feces, and vomit to fall into a huge pit below. The air inside these facilities is riddled with dust, dander, ammonia, and other noxious gases. Not surprisingly, respiratory diseases are endemic. Pig factories are fertile breeding grounds for communicable diseases. In order to ensure the animals' survival until the time of slaughter, antibiotics, hormones, and other drugs are routinely added to their feed.

The only time many of these animals see the light of day is during the trip from their pens to the truck that transports them to the slaughterhouse. It is estimated that one million US pigs die en route to slaughter each year from crushing, freezing, dehydration, or disease. If animals are frightened and resist loading, unloading, or moving forward in slaughterhouse chutes, they are prodded with high-voltage electric rods. Sometimes animals are beaten with metal pipes or kicked by frustrated handlers.

The first step in pig slaughter is stunning the animal with electricity or CO_2 to render it unconscious. The pig is then dragged upside down using chains or ropes around the back feet. Unfortunately, electrical stunning isn't always effective, and reports of animals squealing and kicking wildly are not uncommon. Next comes the "sticker," the person who slits the pig's throat. If the sticker is unsuccessful, the pig continues along the line to the scalding tank, where it is boiled alive to remove its hair. All of this is done quickly, at line speeds of more than one thousand pigs per hour.

Consumers provide a resounding stamp of approval and a financial incentive to continue these practices every time they buy a pound of bacon or a few slices of ham from a grocery store. In the United States, an estimated 110 million pigs were slaughtered for food in 2010. Globally, 1.3 billion pigs per year end up on dinner plates.

LITTLE RED HENS

Chickens are sociable animals that live communally in flocks. Each flock has a well-established "pecking order" in which dominant individuals receive priority in regard to food and nesting areas. Each individual knows its place in the flock and remembers the faces and ranks of up to ninety other birds.

Chickens are far more intelligent than most humans give them credit for. Chicks learn by observation. They can count, and they have self-control and a sense of time and object permanence—a skill human babies don't acquire until they're six or seven months old. Chickens can also anticipate events and predict outcomes. One research team set up a reward system for chickens using colored buttons. If the birds waited two to three seconds to peck on the buttons, they would receive a small amount of food, but if they held out for twenty-two seconds, they were rewarded with a jackpot of food. After learning the rules, more than 90 percent of the time the chickens held out for the jackpot.

More than nine billion chickens, turkeys, ducks, geese, pheasants, quail, and other fowl are slaughtered in North America every year for food, the vast majority being chickens. And more than 95 percent of chickens raised for food in North America are raised in total confinement from birth to death. They are either raised for meat (broilers) or eggs (layers). (For "free-range" conditions, see "The Problem with 'Cruelty-Free.'".)

Broilers

Broiler chickens, also called broiler-fryers, are generally raised on open floors in huge metal sheds that often house 20,000 or more birds per shed, with 150,000 to 300,000 birds per operation. The average space per animal is less than one square foot. This overcrowding causes extreme stress and escalates the risk of injury and disease.

Because of the popularity of breast meat, broilers are selectively bred to have bigger breasts and are almost twice as heavy at slaughter as their ancestors from the 1950s. This selective breeding causes muscle growth to surpass bone growth, resulting in deformities, fractures, tears, and ruptures. Many birds are literally crippled under their own weight. Some starve to death because they can't physically access food or water because of their deformities, and some die of heart attacks or organ failure.

At only six or seven weeks of age, the birds reach market weight. A single catcher will grab the legs of three or four birds per hand and load 1,000 to 1,500 birds per hour into crates for transport to slaughter. The process is highly stressful and commonly associated with serious and sometimes fatal injuries. At the slaughterhouse, chickens are dumped onto conveyor belts and hung upside down on a moving rack. There is no requirement for stunning prior to slaughter because chickens are exempt from the Humane Slaughter Act. Instead, they are subjected to an electric water bath that paralyzes them but doesn't always render them unconscious. If they aren't unconscious, their throats are slit so they can die prior to being plunged into scalding water to loosen their feathers. For some unfortunate birds, this process is also unsuccessful, so they drown in scalding hot water.

Layers

Egg-laying hens are packed into wire battery cages so tightly that they are afforded less than half the space of broilers, only about 67 square inches per bird. This is slightly more than half the size of a standard sheet of paper. For perspective, a hen needs about 72 square inches of space to be able to stand up straight, 178 square inches to preen, and 291 square inches to flap her wings. This degree of overcrowding makes it impossible for the birds to carry out natural behaviors such as nesting, perching, roosting, foraging, taking a dust bath, preening, or exploring. In order to manage the aberrant behavior resulting from these conditions, about one-third to one-half of the beak is seared off with a heated blade to prevent birds from pecking one another to death. This amputation is conducted without anesthetic and causes severe nerve injury and acute and even chronic pain.

Many egg factories also subject their birds to the practice of forced molting in an effort to induce another egg-laying cycle. During this time, food is either completely withheld or restricted for ten to fourteen days, causing weight losses of up to 35 percent of body weight.

The entire system, from feeding and watering to egg collection, is typically fully automated. The cage floors slope forward so that eggs roll onto a conveyor belt that transports them directly to the cleaning stations. Layers are productive for one to two years, after which time egg production drops below the level necessary to provide an economic return. These "spent" hens are genetically selected for efficient egg production, and they don't have much meat on them. Because a great deal of calcium is required for egg production, they also have very fragile bones that break easily during handling. These two factors make these birds of little value to processors. Traditionally, spent hens were used for soup and school lunch programs, but with the large supply of broilers available there is little demand for these smaller birds, so they are gassed to death and then incinerated or ground up and fed to other animals, including other chickens.

Of course, in order to keep the industry going, new layers must constantly be produced. At one day old, chicks are sexed to determine their fate. A total of 260 million male chicks born each year in the United States have no economic value because they can't lay eggs and are poor meat producers, so they are immediately disposed of in several grisly manners: ground up alive, gassed, suffocated, electrocuted, even put through a wood chipper.

CATTLE, DAIRY COWS, AND CALVES

Today's domestic cattle provide humans with about half of their red meat, about 80 percent of their leather, and 95 percent of their milk. Although they are subjected to branding, dehorning, and, for males, castration, all without painkillers, their lives seem rather enviable when compared with pigs or chickens.

Beef Cattle

Beef cattle are among the few food animals that spend their lives outdoors, with their first seven to nine months in pasture. When they reach about 650 pounds, cattle are taken to a feedlot for "finishing." Most finishing facilities house more than 1,000 head of cattle, and larger operations accommodate 30,000 to 150,000 animals. At the feedlot, they receive a high-energy, grain-based diet designed to pack on about 400 pounds in three to four months. Of course, adding about 100 pounds per month by feeding the animals an unnatural diet has consequences for the animals' health. Cattle are perfectly designed to eat a diet that is foraged, extremely high in fiber, and low in starch. A grain-based diet causes a variety of health problems and, in severe cases, can lead to liver abscesses, acidosis, and bloat.

Feed is routinely laced with antibiotics to help promote growth and reduce the risk of diseases induced by these intensive feeding systems. Livestock now receive an estimated 70 percent of all the antibiotics used in the United States, which contributes to the increasing problem of antibiotic-resistant bacteria. But the antibiotics don't seem to be doing the job: One study showed that almost half of 136 samples of meat and poultry taken from twenty-six grocery stores in five US cities tested positive for the disease-causing bacteria *Staphylococcus aureus*. Almost all of the staph bacteria tested were resistant to at least one antibiotic, and at least half were resistant to three or more.

Cattle producers have used growth hormones since the 1950s to make the animals grow larger more quickly on less feed. This reduces cost and produces leaner meat, which is more in line with consumer preferences. Currently, approximately twothirds of all cattle and about 90 percent of feedlot cattle receive growth hormones. In large commercial feedlots, they are used in almost 100 percent of the animals.

Hormone residues that remain in beef may act as endocrine disruptors in humans, interfering with the actions of natural hormones in the body. They may also affect fertility, age of onset of puberty, and the risk of certain cancers in people who eat the meat. In addition, hormones wind up in feedlot waste and often contaminate local water sources.

The final journey for cattle is to the slaughterhouse, where 300 head per hour file one by one up a ramp to be stunned and hoisted into the air, and then have their throats slit and make their way down the disassembly line.

Not surprisingly, slaughterhouses are among the most dangerous workplaces in North America. At one time, most slaughterhouse workers were unionized and had good pay and stable jobs. Line speeds were slower, and the work was relatively safe. Today, most slaughterhouses are nonunionized, the pay is low, and workers are largely immigrants. Line speeds have escalated, and accidents have multiplied. Because meatpacking plants receive fines for high injury rates, plant managers and owners have been caught keeping records that misrepresent the actual occurrence of injury and illness by as much as 1,000 percent.

Dairy Cows and Veal

Some vegetarians believe drinking milk and eating eggs are reasonable choices because the animals don't have to die for us to take their milk or eggs. While animals don't *have* to die to produce these items, they're almost always sent to slaughter once their efficiency wanes. The current intensive methods of milk and egg production result in suffering and death on par with that in meat production, and in the case of eggs, probably more.

In the early 1900s, the average dairy cow produced about 3,000 pounds of milk per year. By 1950, annual milk production per cow had almost doubled, and today each animal produces an astounding 17,000 pounds of milk per year—almost a sixfold increase in milk production in one century.

In the 1950s, most farm families had at least two dairy cows to ensure yearround dairy products for their family. Typical dairy farms had about a dozen cows, and the very largest farms boasted 50 to 100 cows. Today, standard dairy farms exceed 100 cows, with many large facilities housing 700 to 1,000 animals and the largest accommodating several thousand animals.

Every aspect of dairy farming is designed to maximize production and profit. Dairy cows begin their cycle of milk production by being impregnated, generally by artificial insemination, at about thirteen to sixteen months of age. They are then impregnated once a year to ensure a steady production of milk. In most cases, calves are separated from their mothers within a day of birth. Although the separation is extremely traumatic for both mother and calf, allowing more time together would strengthen their bond and increase the stress of separation.

Female calves are raised to replace the "spent" cows, but male calves, of course, are of no use to the dairy industry, except for the few that are used for breeding. Among the remainder, the more fortunate males are funneled into the beef industry. The rest become veal calves. In the United States, this generally means "special-fed veal," also called "white veal" or "milk-fed veal," terms that reflect the market's desire for light-colored meat. This is achieved by feeding the calves an iron-deficient milk replacement, and the tenderness of their flesh is assured by tethering them in small stalls so they can't move and develop their muscles.

Most veal calves are slaughtered at the age of sixteen to eighteen weeks. That may seem young, but the remaining 15 percent of US veal, called "bob veal," comes from calves ranging from two days to three weeks of age.

More than 80 percent of dairy cows are confined in primarily indoor systems, with some having access to barnyards. Fewer than 10 percent are raised on pasture. Some are reared in stalls where they are tethered at the neck, while others are permitted to roam within the barn.

These methods of rearing trigger two key conditions: lameness and mastitis. Lameness occurs in an estimated 14 to 25 percent of cows and is caused primarily by hoof lesions associated with concrete flooring and insufficient physical activity. This painful condition is the leading cause of dairy cow deaths. Extremely high milk production and bacterial infections caused by poor sanitation can trigger a painful swelling and infection of the mammary glands called mastitis, the most common medical condition among dairy cows and the second leading cause of their death. One factor that is strongly associated with both lameness and mastitis is the use of recombinant bovine somatotropin, also known as rBst or recombinant bovine growth hormone (rBGH), a genetically engineered hormone that increases milk yields. By the age of four, most US Holstein cows have produced milk for about 729 days and are no longer of use to the industry, so they are slaughtered. Their natural life span would have been more than twenty years.

SOMETHING FISHY

Until recently, science didn't pay much attention to fish as sentient beings. Few believed that fish had much capacity to think, and even fewer believed that they had the capacity to feel. Since the 1990s, however, a steady stream of studies has forced us to rethink this position. We now know that fish form relationships, recognize other individuals, pass on knowledge and skills, have long-term memory, solve problems, collaborate in hunting, use tools, strategize, experience fear and distress, and avoid risky situations. There is no longer any doubt that fish feel pain, although it is difficult for us to weigh the extent of their suffering against that of mammals because it is expressed differently.

Health authorities advocate eating more fish to reduce the risk of disease, but concerns about exploitation of these creatures and the impacts of fishing practices grow by the year. The commercial fishing industry is divided into two sectors, each harvesting roughly half of the seven billion fish (excluding shellfish) killed per year: commercial, or capture fisheries, and aquaculture, or fish farms.

Capture Fisheries

The consequences of our current fishing practices for marine ecosystems are incalculable. More than half of all monitored fish stocks are now fully exploited, meaning that we have reached our limit for catching this species and capturing any more will threaten its survival. Another quarter is overexploited, depleted, or slowly recovering. More than 90 percent of the global predatory fish population has been wiped out, yet consumers continue to be urged to eat more fish. If current trends in fishing continue, all stocks could collapse by 2048, meaning it would be unlikely that endangered fish species could make a comeback.

Capture fisheries use a wide range of catching techniques, many of them highly malicious, such as dynamiting coral reefs, exceedingly efficient bottom trawling, longlining, gillnetting, and purse seining. In addition, poisons are routinely used to paralyze or stun fish for aquariums or live-fish restaurants, killing reefs in the process. Less ecologically destructive systems are also commonly used. Sharks, for example, are caught using hooks. Their fins are cut off and the living animal is then returned to the ocean, where it slowly suffocates because water must be moving over its gills in order for it to breathe, yet it no longer has fins for swimming—all because shark fins, a delicacy in Asian cuisine, fetch a premium price.

The depths of the oceans are among the most pristine ecosystems remaining on our planet. They are the homes of yet unnamed species that may well become extinct before they have even been identified. It's estimated that 95 percent of damage to these ecosystems results from deep-sea bottom trawling. Huge nets with metal plates at each end and metal wheels along the bottom are dragged along the ocean floor like giant underwater bulldozers, demolishing seafloor ecosystems. This is the underwater equivalent of clear-cutting. As the nets are brought to the surface, fish and sea animals caught in the nets experience extreme decompression, causing vital organs to rupture. Among the worst offenders are shrimp trawlers, which "unintentionally" kill up to 20 pounds of marine life for every pound of shrimp plucked from the net. This "bycatch," as it's known, includes sea turtles, dolphins, sharks, and numerous other fish and nonfish species that are simply tossed overboard.

Longlining uses one or more main lines with short attached lines with hooks at the ends. The main lines can be as long as 75 miles, holding hundreds or thousands of baited hooks. They are set at varying depths in the water depending on the target species. Fish captured by longlines can by dragged behind a boat for hours or even days. The longline industry is notorious for killing millions of marine mammals, including birds, dolphins, sharks, and turtles. It is, however, less destructive to the ocean floor than bottom trawling.

Gillnetting is a method that uses huge nets measuring hundreds of feet to over a mile long to snare target fish. Fish attempt to swim through the openings in the mesh nets, but their gills become trapped, so they can't escape. Other species may be small enough to swim through or large enough that their gills aren't snagged. Gill nets are often left unmonitored for long periods, so the trapped fish slowly suffocate.

Purse seining is another type of fishing that employs large nets. The purse seine gets its name from its structure: a rope passes through a series of rings that run along the bottom of the net, which can be pulled to completely close the net at the bottom, like a giant drawstring bag. Purse seining is the preferred method of capturing fish that congregate in schools near the surface of the water. One of the primary concerns about purse seining is that dolphins are commonly trapped in the nets. Fish are often still alive when they are pulled on deck and are conscious when they are slit and gutted.

Aquaculture

The imminent global collapse of wild fish stocks is driving a massive shift from capture fisheries to fish farming. Aquaculture or aquafarming, popularly called fish farming, is the fastest growing animal-based food sector in the world. In 2008, an estimated 46 percent of fish consumed worldwide were raised on farms, up from only 9 percent in 1980. Some fish farms are based on land, using ponds, pools, tanks, or man-made waterways. Others are created near ocean shorelines, with the fish being held in the water in huge nets, pens, or cages. All are intensive operations, similar to factory farms for land animals.

The goal of fish farming is no different than that of factory farming: to generate the greatest amount of meat for the least amount of money. Fish farms maintain a density of animals that seldom occurs in the wild. As a result, fish can become sick or infected, and the usual response is antibiotics, antimicrobials, and other pharmaceuticals.

The consequences of these intensive operations are widespread and severe, although we can only speculate how severe for the individual animal. Crowding, an inappropriate physical environment, polluted water, and disease outbreaks can cause stress, fear, discomfort, and pain in fish. But the most pressing concerns are the welfare of all sea creatures, the negative effects on the environment, and the toll on wild fish.

Waste, food pellets, and drug residues from fish farms seriously threaten ecologically sensitive areas, such as mangrove swamps, coastal estuaries, and salmon migration routes. Untreated waste goes directly into the ocean, where it affects sea life and water quality. Aquaculture operations also fuel harmful algal blooms, a proliferation of toxin-producing algae that that can cause massive die-offs of fish, shellfish, marine mammals, seabirds, and the animals that consume them.

The strongest argument used to justify fish farming has been that it protects wild fish. Paradoxically, for carnivorous sea animals, fish farming could do the opposite, because a farmed carnivorous fish has to eat 2.5 to 5 pounds of wild fish to produce I pound of flesh. In addition, farmed fish can escape, infecting wild fish with diseases, sea lice, and other parasites. When nonnative species escape into nearby waters, they can devastate native fish populations by competing for food and habitat.

In addition, the fish industry hasn't escaped genetic engineering. While not yet approved for market sales, salmon, prawns, and abalone are currently being genetically altered. Atlantic salmon, for example, have been modified with genes from Chinook salmon so they reach market size in half the time. Genetically modified fish that escape into the wild, as many fish farmed in open systems do, pose a significant threat to related native species if they interbreed.

The Problem with "Cruelty-Free"

People often wonder what could possibly be wrong with eating meat from free-range animals that are raised on organic feed and treated well. This brings up an important distinction in ethical perspectives.

Vegans are ethically opposed to the exploitation of animals. Vegans don't view animals as ours to use and therefore reject the notion that if animals are treated well, we are justified in killing and eating them. While most people agree that animals raised for food should be treated humanely, only a rather small percentage seem to be willing to actually pay more for meat, milk, and eggs from such animals. In addition, consumers who say they prefer products from humanely treated animals often make concessions when eating out or if they can't find those foods at the store.

Although a small percentage of consumers go directly to small local farmers to buy "humane" products, most shop at grocery stores, where consumers must rely on catchphrases on food labels, such as "free-range," "cage-free," "grass-fed," and "humanely raised," to determine whether the product came from an animal treated in an acceptable manner. Unfortunately, there is no independent inspection or verification to ensure that farmers are living up to consumer expectations. These animals are still generally bred by the thousands, kept in crowded conditions, and removed from their mothers shortly after birth. Chickens are usually still debeaked, and the male offspring are still disposed of. Even in facilities that offer "access to the outdoors," the access can be a small opening to an outdoor enclosure that is inaccessible to many of the animals crowded into the building.

Of course, in the end, all food animals meet the same fate, regardless of how they are raised.

While a few are slaughtered on small farms, most are killed in the same facilities that slaughter animals raised on factory farms. The fact that they may have suffered less than most other farm animals doesn't justify their exploitation in the first place.

We have just scratched the surface of the animal rights argument for veganism. We encourage you to dig deeper and learn more about these issues. For a list of recommended books and films, see nutrispeak.com/resources or the resourceslink at brendadavisrd.com.

Paying the Price with Our Planet

The human species is consuming the earth's resources more rapidly than they can be replenished, and our food choices may be the greatest contributor to this depletion. If we all ate the average American diet, it would take 3.74 earths to sustain our current population of about 7 billion people. By 2050, there will be an estimated 9.2 billion people on the planet; at that point, even if every individual minimized their carbon footprint by using 95 percent renewable energy and consumed a plant-rich diet, we would still need the equivalent of 1.3 planets to sustain the population. Celebrated environmentalist Paul Hawken notes that if every single company on earth were to adopt the highest environmental standards and policies, we still couldn't forestall the environmental collapse of our planet.

The earth has a limited capacity to produce precious resources on which our lives depend, from oxygen and algae to soil and trees. When we use more than what is produced and the earth can't keep pace, our manner of living is no longer sustainable for future generations. The global population is growing by a staggering 250,000 people per day, or 166 people per minute. Our fragile planet is ill-equipped to handle an exponentially increasing population of human beings. The ecological crisis we face is a reflection of sheer numbers, and perhaps sheer greed.

Humans have essentially attempted to outwit Mother Nature, but we are slowly coming to realize that the laws of nature are not up for grabs. Our tireless effort to reinvent the natural order to suit our own species only puts us at greater risk. The network of life depends on a complex food web. The lowest level of the food web sustains plants, which in turn sustain animals, with both plants and animals constantly recycling nutrients back into the soil. Humans have altered the food web to such an extent that many species and entire ecosystems must adapt or perish. But eventually the toll will become so great that the entire system will collapse. While some believe that we already are beyond the point of no return, we must do what we can—if not for ourselves, for our children, and if not for our children, then for all other species, whose future we hold in our hands. Our greatest hope lies *within* the laws of Mother Nature. She has beckoned us for years, and we have largely ignored her. Now her patience is wearing thin.

When considering human impacts on the environment, most people focus on the use of fossil fuels, but another activity has an equal impact: raising livestock. Many experts have already suggested that a global shift toward a vegan diet can protect the world from increased hunger and poverty and the worst impacts of climate change. There is no question that intensive animal agriculture is among the most notorious polluters of air, water, and soil, and one of the greatest contributors to deforestation, desertification, and the extinction of species. The shift toward a vegan diet may well be the most powerful step an individual can take toward the preservation of this planet, and at this point, it may be an ecological imperative.

GLOBAL WARMING

These days, when people think about going green with their diet, the focus is usually on eating local. The idea is that fewer miles in transport trucks cuts the use of fossil fuels. They may not realize that the majority of food-related greenhouse gas emissions are due to food *production* rather than food *miles*.

According to a United Nations Food and Agriculture Organization (FAO) report called Livestock's Long Shadow, livestock are responsible for 18 percent of greenhouse gas emissions—more than all forms of transportation combined. Efforts to curb global warming, both nationally and internationally, have concentrated largely on reducing or capping CO_2 emissions. When we clear forests to make room for food animals, run farm machinery, bring in feed, or transport animals, CO_2 is released. Fertilizers generate nitrous oxide, and manure releases methane (as do cow burps and flatulence). One-fifth of human-generated greenhouse gas emissions—9 percent of the CO_2, 37 percent of the methane, and 65 percent of the nitrous oxide—comes from livestock production. When compared to CO_2, the global warming effects of methane are 23 times greater, and those of nitrous oxide are 296 times greater.

Transportation accounts for only 11 percent of food-related greenhouse gas emissions, and final delivery from the producer to retail stores is responsible for one-third of that (4 percent of all emissions). The other two-thirds of transportation-related emissions originate from production (feed for animals, fertilizer for vegetables, resources for processing, and so on). Within the category of food production, 44 percent of greenhouse gases are CO_2, 32 percent are nitrous oxide, 23 percent are methane, and 1 percent are other gases. So the impact of food on climate change is due mainly to greenhouse gases other than CO_2. Nitrous oxide and methane emissions are most strongly linked to the red meat and dairy industries.

The bottom line is that livestock animals consume far more food than they yield. It takes about 15 pounds of feed to make 1 pound of beef, 6 pounds of feed for 1 pound of pork, and 5 pounds of feed for 1 pound of chicken. Consumers are always being told to use alternative energy sources, select fuel-efficient appliances, and drive low-emission vehicles, but how many have heard that they should eat veggie burgers instead of hamburgers? Ultimately, the average consumer could reduce his carbon footprint more effectively by eating 100 percent vegan *one* day a week than by eating 100 percent local *seven* days a week. If everyone in the United States were to do this, the effect would be equivalent to taking 31.5 million cars off the road.

WATER

Water is intrinsically tied to our food supply and to the maintenance of our ecosystems. More than one billion people worldwide are experiencing water shortages, and water pollution affects many more. In addition to threatening human food supplies, water shortages and water pollution severely reduce biodiversity and boost rates of infectious diseases.

In 2009, approximately 45 percent of freshwater in the United States was deemed unfit for drinking or recreational use because of contamination by dangerous microorganisms, pesticides, and fertilizers. A year later, an assessment by the World Wildlife Fund's *Living Planet Report 2010* found that the global freshwater Living Planet Index (LPI), a measure of the earth's biodiversity and a solid indication of humanity's demands on the earth's resources, declined by 35 percent between 1970 and 2007, and the tropical freshwater LPI declined by almost 70 percent.

Animal agriculture is one of the leading threats to our water systems. It takes 43 times more water to produce 1 pound of beef than to produce 1 pound of grain—about 5,160 gallons of water per pound of beef (43,000 per kg) and about 120 gallons per pound (1,000 liters per kg) of grains. According to the US Environmental Protection Agency (EPA), the agricultural industry is "the leading contributor" to the pollution of US waterways. On the global scale, an estimated 70 percent of freshwater consumption is for agricultural production.

In the United States, factory farms produce approximately 500 million tons of raw waste every year, about triple that of the human population. A farm with 2,500 dairy cows produces about the same amount of waste as an entire city of 411,000 people. Human waste must be treated before finding its way into our water systems, yet no such requirements exist for animal waste.

On factory farms, animal manure is stored in open pits or huge holding tanks before being spread on fields as fertilizer. But concrete manure pits can crack, and if laid in sand or gravel, manure can leak out and work its way into groundwater. Tanks can also overflow and pollute nearby surface water. If the waste is applied to fields at a rate greater than the ability of the soil and crops to absorb and utilize it, the excess can release toxic gases into the environment and contaminate waterways with pathogenic bacteria, carbon compounds, nitrates, phosphorous, antibiotics, hormones, sediments, heavy metals, and ammonia. Pathogenic bacteria can end up in nearby rivers and streams, which may in turn be used to irrigate vegetable crops; most vegetable-related food-borne disease outbreaks can be traced back to contamination from nearby factory farms.

Carbon compounds, which are the primary constituents in manure, can contribute to oxygen depletion in water. In addition, water runoff from contaminated farms and fields contains nitrogen and phosphorus—about half to two-thirds of it from poultry farms—which cause dead zones in water systems where algal blooms deplete oxygen from the water and choke out aquatic life.

Antibiotics and both natural and synthetic hormones also make their way into surface water and groundwater when released in manure. According to the EPA, as much as 80 percent of antibiotics administered orally to livestock end up in manure *unchanged.* This poses a significant concern for human health, since the routine use of antibiotics in animals can lead to antibiotic resistance in pathogenic bacteria and reduce the effectiveness of antibiotics in people who become infected with these organisms. There are also serious concerns about the health consequences of hormone use in livestock production, which has been directly linked to increased rates of breast, prostate, and testicular cancer.

LAND

The livestock industry is by far the largest user of land on earth, utilizing 30 percent of the land surface of the planet and 70 percent of all agricultural land. Therefore, it has a massive impact on both the quality and quantity of available soil, generally damaging and depleting it. Plus, intensive farming and monocrop agriculture deplete the soil of nutrients and cause erosion, and overuse of fertilizers and pesticides causes serious contamination.

Every year, US cropland loses soil at a rate thirteen times higher than what is considered sustainable, and ranges and pastures lose soil at a rate six times higher than is sustainable. An estimated 60 percent of US pastureland is overgrazed. In a 2006 report to the US Senate, the Nutrition Security Institute stated that if soil loss continues at present rates, it is estimated that there are only fortyeight years of topsoil left on the planet. By 2054, the earth's farmable topsoil will be gone, as will our ability to provide food to the nine billion people who are expected to occupy this planet. Soil forms at a rate of about 1 inch every 381 to 1,270 years, so waiting for soil regeneration is not an option.

Raising livestock is among the leading causes of deforestation globally, particularly in rain forests such as the Amazon. An estimated 91 percent of these deforested areas are used for livestock production. Deforestation is responsible for 15 percent of annual global CO_2 emissions and also threatens millions of plant and animal species, causing the global loss of an estimated 50,000 species a year or 137 species a day. Many of these species haven't even been identified yet. If we continue to destroy the rain forest, we could eventually reach a point where the entire ecosystem collapses. While the human race can recover within a few generations from economic hardships, natural disasters, and even wars, species extinction is permanent. As the rate of extinction accelerates, our own safety net disappears.

Livestock production also can result in desertification, the conversion of usable, semiarid land into nonproductive deserts. Desertification decimates plant diversity and causes soil erosion. Overgrazing strips away plants that anchor topsoil, leading to irreversible losses of soil, decreased biodiversity, and the invasion of alien species.

AIR

Factory farms stink, both figuratively and literally. While their horrific stench has long been viewed as merely an inconvenience in the eyes of the industry and the courts, evidence suggests that the impact is far more insidious.

The Real Costs

A typical fast-food burger costs about $2, but experts suggest that, in the absence of government subsidies, the real cost would be closer to $200. (If we subsidize anything, it should be kale—that would make sense.) Each passing day brings us a little closer to the realization of an old Cree proverb: "When all the trees have been cut down, when all the animals have been hunted, when all the waters are polluted, when all the air is unsafe to breathe, only then will you discover you cannot eat money."

Whether animal waste is stored or spread on fields, it decomposes, and noxious fumes are released into the air. Odors from factory farms are associated with numerous respiratory and health conditions, including mood disturbances, depression, and severe respiratory problems. Nearly 70 percent of workers employed in concentrated swine facilities report at least one respiratory symptom, and 58 percent have chronic bronchitis. Manure pits are especially problematic, posing confined-space hazards due to oxygen deficiency and toxic gases. Farmworkers are advised to never enter a manure pit without wearing a self-contained breathing apparatus.

Beyond Vegan

Becoming vegan is the biggest step you can take to lighten the ecological footprint of your diet, but it isn't the only step. Here are a few tips for further fine-tuning your planet-friendly habits.

Choose organic food. Organic foods are farmed in a manner that is more ecologically sustainable than conventionally produced food, avoiding the use of synthetic fertilizers, pesticides, and genetically modified organisms. Organic farming preserves the soil, decreases water pollution, and helps store carbon dioxide, minimizing the harm to air, water, and soil. Compared to conventional farming, organic farming has been found to reduce carbon dioxide emissions by 49 to 66 percent.

Opt for local, seasonal plant foods. By some estimates, the average North American meal travels about 1,500 miles (2,400km) from field to plate and contains ingredients from five other countries, beyond the United States. If a typical family bought 100 percent local for a year, their greenhouse gas emissions would be reduced by 4 to 5 percent. Also consider growing your own food, even if it's just a few herbs or tomatoes on your balcony. Purchase directly from farmers or farmers' markets, and frequent stores that feature local products. Buy in season when possible to reduce the energy required for food preservation, storage, and transportation. Also purchase unprocessed or minimally processed food.

Avoid products with excessive packaging. All that plastic, paper, and aluminum contributes to environmental degradation. Besides, foods that are overpackaged tend to be rife with sugar, salt, and fat. Shop in places that don't overpackage food: farms, farmers' markets, produce markets, bulk stores, and food co-ops. Opt for the most reusable or recyclable items available, such as products in glass containers. Join a community-supported agriculture (CSA) enterprise or sign up for regular deliveries of farm-fresh produce and other local goods.

Reduce food waste. Rotting food releases methane and contributes to greenhouse gas emissions. Plus, all of the resources that went into producing the food are wasted. Using food before it goes bad will help the environment—and your pocketbook. Plan your meals in advance, then buy only as much food as you need and prepare only what you'll eat. Store food properly, and keep track of what's in your fridge. Get creative with leftovers. Freeze foods that tend to go rancid or spoil quickly, such as nuts, seeds, and bread. If you do have to throw food away, compost it rather than sending it to a landfill.

Compost your food scraps. Composting not only minimizes the amount of garbage you produce, it also enriches your garden. If you live in an apartment or don't have a yard, consider worm composting, called vermicomposting. It can be done indoors, it's odor-free, and it doesn't take much space. Many cities also offer a compost pickup system; check with your city for details, and if they don't have such a program available, request that they start one.

Walk, bike, or use public transportation. Transportation contributes an estimated 13.5 percent to greenhouse gas emissions. When purchasing food or eating out, try to select markets and restaurants within walking or biking distance. In addition to saving money, you'll also stay fit. If the distance is too long or your cargo too heavy, take public transit, carpool, or limit shopping trips to once a week. If a motorized vehicle is a necessity, consider a motorcycle, scooter, or small fuelefficient car.

BYOB. Bring your own bag, that is. Plastics find their way into oceans, breaking down into tiny suspended particles and acting like sponges for water-borne carcinogens such as PCBs and pesticides. They work their way into the food chain, poisoning fish and killing marine mammals that mistake the plastic for food. In the ocean, plastics and other wastes often become trapped in rotating currents called gyres, forming massive mats of garbage. Opt for reusable cloth bags instead of plastic, and try to use glass storage containers and jars whenever possible.

Vegan Goes Mainstream

Up until the early 1980s, the word *vegan* conjured up images of cultish extremists who were essentially wasting away on diets of roots and shoots. If you inquired about vegan options in a restaurant, you usually received a blank stare in response. The only place the word *vegan* ever appeared on a product label was in a natural food store. If you happened to mention your vegan diet to a doctor or dietitian, they would probably try to "educate" you about the risks of eliminating what were considered two essential food groups: meat and dairy. University textbooks warned soon-to-be doctors and dietitians that vegan diets were downright dangerous. Fortunately, the tables have turned.

In 2010, *BusinessWeek* featured an article called "Power Vegan." The first paragraph completely obliterated the old vegan stereotype: "It used to be easy for moguls to flaunt their power. All they had to do was renovate the chalet in St. Moritz, buy the latest Gulfstream jet, lay off 5,000 employees, or marry a much younger Asian woman. By now, though, they've used up all the easy ways to distinguish themselves from the rest of us—which may be why a growing number of America's most powerful bosses have become vegan. Steve Wynn, Mort Zuckerman, Russell Simmons, and Bill Clinton are now using tempeh to assert their superiority. As are Ford Executive Chairman of the Board Bill Ford, Twitter co-founder Biz Stone, venture capitalist Joi Ito, Whole Foods Market Chief Executive Officer John Mackey, and Mike Tyson. Yes, Mike Tyson, a man who once chewed on human ear, is now vegan."

There is no denying it: vegan is on the radar of mainstream America. It has arrived because of the moguls and other pioneers who have defied the stereotypes and made vegan attractive to the masses. Vegan bodybuilders have won international titles and blown away images of skinny weakling vegans. Elite endurance athletes are gaining a competitive edge by fueling their bodies with plant-based foods. (See chapter 14). Executive chefs are dazzling judges with extraordinarily colorful and creative vegan masterpieces. Movie stars, musicians, and models are strutting their vegan stuff. Doctors and dietitians are endorsing plant-based diets as ideal for the prevention and treatment of lifestyle-induced chronic diseases.

Not surprisingly, the market is responding. Vegan restaurants are popping up everywhere, and conventional restaurants are adding vegan options to their menus. Products featured in mainstream grocery stores are using the word *vegan* on labels as a marketing tool. A proliferation of documentary films with noticeably vegan messages are making a splash at the box office. Vegan lifestyles are topics of conversation on wildly popular talk shows. Vegan books, shoes, cosmetics, and specialty products are proliferating in the marketplace. Peer-reviewed articles examining the therapeutic value of vegan diets are making headlines. Internet sites dedicated to veganism and support services are emerging daily.

In 2011, the Vegetarian Resource Group (VRG) commissioned a Harris Interactive poll to estimate the number of Americans consuming a vegetarian or vegan diet or regularly eating vegetarian meals. An estimated 5 percent of Americans consume a vegetarian diet, and about half of the vegetarians consume a vegan diet. This is almost double the rate reported in a 2009 poll (1 percent vegan and 3 percent vegetarian). About 17 percent of Americans avoid meat, poultry, and fish at up to half of their meals, and 16 percent avoid these foods at more than half of their meals. These numbers suggest that about one-third of Americans are choosing vegetarian meals on a regular basis.

In a National Restaurant Association poll, "What's Hot in 2011," more than half of the 1,500 chefs polled included vegan entrées as a hot trend. Of six hundred participants surveyed in a research report from Context Marketing, 21 percent said vegetarian is important or very important to them, and 14 percent said vegan is important or very important to them. Almost 70 percent said that they would be willing to pay more for food produced using higher ethical standards. Eating mostly vegetarian—now known as flexitarian—was one of the top ten consumer food trends in 2011.

Close to half of the US population is trying to reduce its meat consumption. People are interested in eating foods that are produced sustainably, responsibly, and ethically. They want to buy local, fresh, organic, whole foods, as well as foods with minimal or biodegradable packaging. They are drawn to a way of eating that can reduce obesity, diet-induced diseases, and health care costs. Whereas two or three decades ago, the word *vegan* was associated with dangerous nutritional deficiencies, today it is the one word that's instantly recognized as being consistent with the personal, ethical, and ecological objectives of conscious consumers. The shift in public thinking is palpable, and the future is hopeful.

Of course, challenges remain. Businesses that earn hefty profits from animal exploitation wield a great deal of power. These industries have tremendous influence on government policy and are key recipients of agricultural subsidies. Consumers are constantly bombarded with advertising that makes leather, suede, silk, steak, and lobster seem attractive, sexy, sophisticated, and highly desirable. Fortunately, we have a choice. We can fall into a hypnotic consumer trance, or we can honor our inner moral compass. By doing so, we restore the Golden Rule: "Do unto others as you would have others do unto you."

The Golden Rule has long served as a moral foundation for humanity. Our shared vegan vision is one that would have humankind expand the definition of "others" to include our nonhuman brethren. In July 2012, *Reader's Digest* featured a cover article titled "Why Whales Are People Too." The piece described the work of a group of scientists who presented the "Declaration of Rights for Cetaceans" at the annual meeting of the American Association for the Advancement of Science in Vancouver, British Columbia, in February of 2012. The declaration essentially protects whales and dolphins as nonhuman "persons" and protects their right to life, liberty, and well-being. If the declaration were binding, these animals could not be slaughtered, held in captivity, or owned. The scientists plan to bring the declaration before the United Nations to have it legally endorsed. There is a push to extend this sort of protection to other animals that exhibit "person" traits of self-awareness, creativity, communication, and intentionality.

Perhaps as we gain a greater understanding of nonhuman animals, we will come to the conclusion that simply being a sentient being, able to think, feel, and suffer, is enough to warrant compassion from human animals.

The advantages of being vegan are associated with compassion not only for animals and the earth, but also for ourselves and for our health. Let's learn how a vegan diet can provide everything we need to help lower our risks for disease.

CHAPTER 2
The Great Vegan Advantage

You may have decided to adopt a vegan diet in an effort to lose weight, reduce disease risk, or even reverse an existing condition. Rest assured that you are on the right track. The evidence for the benefits of vegan diets to prevent many chronic conditions is accumulating by the minute. While you may encounter naysayers who warn about malnutrition, in truth, you are more likely to be malnourished on a standard American diet than on a wellplanned vegan diet.

While we generally associate the word malnutrition with undernutrition, or hunger, there are actually more people in the world who suffer from overnutrition, or overconsumption of food, and that too is a form of malnutrition. In the year 2010, for the first time in history the number of people suffering from overnutrition worldwide exceeded the number of people suffering from undernutrition.

Vegan diets rarely lead to undernutrition or overnutrition in adults.

Research has consistently demonstrated a greater prevalence of overnutrition, overweight, and obesity within the general population than within the vegan community. In the U nited States, an estimated 68 percent of the general population suffers from overnutrition and the associated problems of overweight and obesity. This increases the risk of type 2 diabetes, coronary artery disease, stroke, hypertension, and many other serious health conditions.

A third type of malnutrition, called micronutrient deficiency, is common across all dietary groups. It can appear in both vegans and omnivores and in both undernutrition and overnutrition as a result of insufficient access to high-quality food, poor variety in the diet, or an excess of fat and sugar. In vegans, micronutrient deficiencies, especially deficiencies of vitamin B $_{12}$, are more prevalent in those who overly restrict their diets.

Where Do We Stand?

Scientific evidence about vegan diets has been flowing into scientific journals since 1976, thanks in large part to Seventh-day Adventists. Members of this Protestant denomination have adopted healthful lifestyles as part of their faith. Most don't drink alcohol or coffee, and many are vegetarian or vegan. Two key studies have provided a wealth of data: The Adventist Health Study-1, which followed 34,198 members of the church between 1974 and 1988, resulting in dozens of research papers, and the Adventist Health Study-2, which began in 2002, and is ongoing. Of the 96,000 participants in the latter study, 28 percent are vegetarian and 8 percent are vegan.

Another large population study is the European Prospective Investigation into Cancer and Nutrition (EPIC). It is the largest study of the diet and health of a group of people to date, with approximately 520,000 participants from ten European countries. EPIC-Oxford, which is one of twenty-three EPIC centers, purposefully recruited as many vegetarians and vegans as possible. Of the 65,500 people enrolled, approximately 29 percent are vegetarian and 4 percent are vegan. Other smaller but significant studies have also been conducted in the United Kingdom and Germany.

These studies have found that well-planned vegan diets supply adequate nutrition. However, vegans are not a homogeneous group. While they tend to eat more vegetables and fewer processed foods than the general population, there are vegans who live on tea and toast, pasta and bagels, or soda and French fries, and research doesn't always tease out these kinds of crucial diet details. Finally, the methods of obtaining dietary information are far from foolproof. Often, participants are asked to recall their diets or to fill out questionnaires, and these provide only very rough estimates of food intake. In addition, participants may not be followed for a long enough time to obtain sufficient information about changes in their nutritional status.

While properly designed vegan diets provide ample nutrients, poorly planned vegan diets can fall short—as can poorly planned omnivorous diets. When vegan diets are poorly designed, the nutrients most commonly lacking are vitamin B_{12}, calcium, and vitamin D. Other nutrients that are potentially deficient for some vegans are protein, essential fatty acids, riboflavin, zinc, selenium, and iodine. Still, although intake of some of these nutrients may be below recommended levels, in most cases they are close to the recommended amount, and the overall health of vegan subjects is good. Plus, vegans as a group tend to be leaner than people following any other type of diet, and their diets consistently provide better levels of fiber, vitamin C, vitamin E, thiamin, folate, iron, copper, and magnesium.

The nutrition challenges commonly faced by vegans are relatively easy to overcome. In fact, many foods popular with vegans, such as nondairy milks, meat substitutes, and breakfast cereals, are fortified with nutrients such as calcium, vitamin B_{12}, vitamin D, riboflavin, and zinc. The bottom line? You don't need animal products to have a healthful and nutritionally adequate diet.

Vegans on Trial

Prior to the 1990s, chronic diseases such as cardiovascular disease, diabetes, cancer, and lung disease were commonly known as "diseases of affluence" because they occurred among people who had the luxuries of eating too much and exercising too little. The term has since become obsolete as rates of these diseases are rising most rapidly in poorer countries. In 2008, 63 percent of deaths worldwide were due to such conditions. It's estimated that, by 2020, lifestylerelated chronic diseases will be responsible for almost three-quarters of deaths globally. This shift has created a major public health threat with catastrophic implications for struggling economies throughout the world. The four primary causes of this epidemic, according to the World Health Organization, are poor diet, lack of exercise, smoking, and alcohol consumption. Simply put, the majority of deaths globally are self-inflicted.

Governments, health organizations, and nutrition authorities are acutely aware of the connection between diet, lifestyle, and chronic disease, and of the health benefits associated with plant-based diets. Nutrition education materials consistently reflect this knowledge. For instance, in 2010 the Dietary Guidelines Advisory Committee recommended four steps to help reduce the risk of chronic disease. In simple terms, they advised consumers to eat less, exercise more, eat a more plant-based diet, and eat fewer refined grains and foods with added sugar, solid fats, and salt.

The 2010 Dietary Guidelines for Americans state that vegetarian diets are associated with lower levels of obesity, reduced risk of cardiovascular disease, lower blood pressure, and lower total mortality. According to the guidelines, vegetarians typically eat less fat, fewer calories, and more fiber, potassium, and vitamin C than nonvegetarians.

But here's the rub: Although health authorities agree that eating mostly whole plant foods makes good sense, few suggest eating *only* plant foods. Many who urge a shift toward a more plant-centered diet also advocate increases in what are considered "healthful animal products," such as fish and low-fat dairy products. The healthiest, longest-living populations on the planet consume whole-foods, plant-based, or mostly plant-based diets, but none of these groups is entirely vegan. Vegan diets are essentially on trial in the eyes of the world. Fortunately, as the evidence unfolds, vegan diets are not only being vindicated, they are increasingly being recognized as rising stars in the arsenal against many chronic diseases.

Based on current evidence, vegans come closer to meeting recommendations for intake (or avoidance) of total fat, saturated fat, cholesterol, trans-fatty acids, and fiber than people of other dietary persuasions. In addition to being low in saturated fat, free of cholesterol, and high in fiber, well-planned vegan diets provide abundant antioxidants and protective phytochemicals, so they may be useful in the prevention and treatment of numerous chronic diseases, including asthma, cancer, cardiovascular disease, cataracts, diverticular disease, fibromyalgia, gallbladder disease, gastrointestinal disorders, kidney disease, overweight and obesity, rheumatoid arthritis, and type 2 diabetes.

Let's take a look at some of these diseases and see just how helpful a vegan diet can be in preventing or reducing the risk of certain chronic illnesses.

Cardiovascular Disease

Cardiovascular disease (CVD) refers to diseases of the heart and circulatory system, including coronary artery disease, hypertension, congestive heart failure, congenital cardiovascular defects, and cerebrovascular disease, or stroke. As the leading cause of death worldwide, CVD accounted for 30 percent of all deaths in 2005. In the United States the toll is higher: 34.3 percent of all deaths in 2006 were due to CVD—that's one of every three deaths, or about one death every thirty-eight seconds.

Recently, CVD has been increasing in low- and middle-income countries due to increased smoking, decreased physical activity, and increased intake of meat and high-calorie foods laden with fat, oil, sodium, and sugar. In China, for instance, meat consumption jumped 246 percent between 1980 and 2003. This trend has been directly linked to rising cholesterol levels, which one study found to be responsible for 77 percent of the increased risk of CVD.

There is no question that meat eaters have more risk factors for cardiovascular disease than vegans. Unfortunately, few studies have separated out data on vegans because the number of vegan participants in these studies is generally small. In 1978, however, a very preliminary report of the Adventist Mortality Study found that, among vegan men older than thirty-five, death rates due to coronary artery disease were only 14 percent that of the general population. In a 1999 analysis, the death rate for vegans from ischemic heart disease was 26 percent lower than for meat eaters, compared to 34 percent lower for both the vegetarians and the fish eaters. The vegans' risk for stroke was 30 percent lower, compared to 13 percent lower for vegetarians and 4 percent higher for fish eaters, although these findings were not statistically significant.

A 2013 report from EPIC-Oxford found that vegetarians and vegans had a 32 percent lower risk of ischemic heart disease compared to meat eaters and fish eaters. Surprisingly, fish eaters didn't enjoy an advantage over meat eaters. Although the reason for this finding isn't clear, it is possible that fried fish, a favorite in the UK, could have predominated in the fish eaters' diets.

It may seem surprising that vegans don't have a greater advantage where heart disease is concerned than the evidence has shown. This may be because vegan diets favorably affect some CVD risk factors while negatively affecting others. It's important for vegans to be aware of any potential pitfalls that may increase risk and take steps to avoid them, so let's take a look at the CVD risk factors that are potentially affected by a vegan diet.

CHOLESTEROL

Cholesterol is an essential component of cell membranes, but an excess can increase the risk of CVD. Cholesterol is a large, fat-soluble molecule that's carried in the blood by lipoproteins. The two main lipoproteins, low-density lipoprotein (LDL) and high-density lipoprotein (HDL), are essentially cholesterol carriers. Although LDL transports cholesterol to various tissues for cell building, it also dumps excess cholesterol in artery walls, contributing to the formation of plaque, hence its nickname: "bad cholesterol." HDL is referred to as "good cholesterol" because it transports excess cholesterol to the liver for removal.

Elevated LDL is a major risk factor for coronary artery disease. The higher the LDL, the higher the risk. However, the higher the HDL, the lower the risk. Although HDL tends to be slightly lower in vegans, the balance of LDL to HDL is more favorable, and therefore CVD risk is reduced.

In addition to lower cholesterol levels, vegans also appear to be at an advantage when it comes to cholesterol metabolism. A healthy blood cholesterol level is considered to be no higher than 200mg/dl (5.2mmol/l), and based on the results of twenty-four studies of vegan populations over about thirty years, vegan cholesterol levels average about 150mg/dl (3.9mmol/l)—lowest of any dietary group. A cholesterol level of 150mg/dl (3.9mmol/l) is a bit of a magic number in the medical world. People with cholesterol levels lower than that have the lowest risk of heart disease. Indeed, in the first fifty years of the famous Framingham Heart Study, only five patients with cholesterol levels less than 150 developed coronary artery disease.

Vegans have significantly lower LDL levels as well, averaging 85mg/dl (2.2mmol/l), compared to 105mg/dl (2.7mmol/l) for lacto-ovo vegetarians and 119mg/dl (3.1mmol/l) for nonvegetarians. The differences in HDL were small, however: HDL levels of vegans averaged 49mg/dl (1.27mmol/l), compared to 52mg/dl (1.34mmol/l) for lacto-ovo vegetarians and 54mg/dl (1.4mmol/l) for nonvegetarians. It's important to note that the participants in most of these studies—regardless of their dietary group—were from health-conscious populations, so even the nonvegetarians had death rates close to half that of the general population.

Intake levels of saturated fats, trans-fatty acids, and, to a lesser extent, cholesterol are all associated with elevated cholesterol levels. There is good evidence that replacing saturated fat with polyunsaturated fat significantly reduces CVD risk, and that replacing saturated fat with refined carbohydrates—white flour products, white rice, and sugar-sweetened beverages and treats—may actually elevate CVD risk.

Vegans consume no cholesterol and typically have the lowest saturated fat intake of all dietary groups and a lower intake of trans fats. They average 6.3 percent of calories from saturated fat, compared to 10.6 percent for lacto-ovo vegetarians and 12 percent for nonvegetarians. Although only a few studies have assessed trans fat intakes in vegans, they consistently show lower levels compared with lacto-ovo vegetarians and nonvegetarians. Vegans also tend to opt for unrefined carbohydrates rather than refined, and their diets maximize intake of cholesterol-lowering food components, such as soluble fiber, plant proteins, phytosterols (beneficial plant sterols and stanols), polyunsaturated fats, and phytochemicals, all of which are found exclusively or predominately in plant foods.

Research suggests that the most damaging form of cholesterol is oxidized cholesterol, or oxycholesterol. Oxidized cholesterol hastens the formation of plaque and hardening of the arteries, reducing their elasticity and increasing the risk for CVD. Cholesterol can oxidize in the body when people don't eat well, and this is particularly likely to occur with the consumption of fried foods, fast foods, and other processed foods.

Within the body, cholesterol can become oxidized if you eat too much cholesterol and not enough antioxidants, such as vitamins C and E, carotenoids, flavonoids, and polyphenolic compounds. Just as their name implies, antioxidants block oxidation. Since antioxidants come primarily from whole plant foods, vegans tend to eat more of them than typical omnivores do. A vegan or other plant-based diet improves antioxidant intake and decreases cholesterol oxidation.

In addition, high intakes of heme iron—the type from meat, as opposed to nonheme iron from plants—may also increase LDL oxidation and atherosclerosis. Since vegans don't consume heme iron, they may be further protected against CVD.

TRIGLYCERIDES

Triglycerides are a type of fat in your blood synthesized from the food you eat. Elevated triglycerides—considered to be more than 150mg/dl (1.7mmol/l)—can increase your risk for heart disease and for metabolic syndrome, a condition that can lead to diabetes.

If you eat more calories than you need, particularly too much fat, cholesterol, sugar, refined carbohydrates, or alcohol, your liver converts the excess into triglycerides and packages them in a molecule called very low-density lipoprotein (VLDL). VLDL transports triglycerides through the bloodstream to fat tissue, also called adipose tissue, to store it for later use. If you make a habit of eating more than your body uses, your VLDL will increase in order to manage all of the excess triglycerides. After the VLDL dumps its triglyceride load into your fat tissue, it turns into LDL, the bad cholesterol—a lose-lose situation.

One common criticism of plant-based diets has been that they increase triglycerides. This can happen to vegans if they eat too much fat, sugar, or refined carbs, but those who focus on whole, high-fiber foods generally have low triglycerides. Vegans have been shown to have the lowest triglyceride levels of all dietary groups, with an average of 83.5mg/dl (0.94mmol/l), compared to 107mg/dl (1.2mmol/l) for lacto-ovo vegetarians and 95.5mg/dl (1.1mmol/l) for meat eaters.

HIGH BLOOD PRESSURE

Vegans are less likely than other dietary groups to have to worry about high blood pressure. This is probably because vegans are, for the most part, fairly lean, and body mass index (BMI) is a strong indicator of blood pressure. About half of the variations in hypertension between dietary groups can be attributed to BMI, with the remainder being due to differences in fiber, fat, sodium, alcohol intakes, and nondietary factors, such as physical activity.

INFLAMMATION

CVD has been solidly linked to inflammation, from the earliest stages of atherosclerotic plaque formation to the sudden rupture of established plaques and the ensuing heart attack. A widely available lab test called high-sensitivity C-reactive protein (hs-CRP) can predict cardiac risk by measuring levels of C-reactive protein, which is produced in response to inflammation. Generally, lifestyle factors such as smoking, inactivity, being overweight, and poor food choices cause the inflammation that results in elevated CRP levels.

Four of five studies of vegetarians showed significantly lower inflammation levels compared with omnivores. The only study assessing CRP levels in vegans found markedly lower levels of inflammation compared to endurance athletes and people who ate a standard Western diet. In this study, the vegans consumed raw diets.

HOMOCYSTEINE

Homocysteine is a by-product of the metabolism of the essential amino acid methionine. Low levels of vitamins B_{12}, vitamin B_6, and folate can cause homocysteine levels to rise. Elevated homocysteine damages blood vessel walls, triggering oxidation, inflammation, and the formation of blood clots. High homocysteine levels can be predictive of CVD and coronary problems. It is estimated that for every 5mmol/L increase in homocysteine, risk for CVD jumps 20 to 23 percent and risk of death from CVD increases up to 50 percent (or up to 60 percent in people with type 2 diabetes).

Elevated homocysteine is usually treated with folic acid, vitamin B_6, and vitamin B_{12}, which may reduce the risk of stroke. However, this treatment may not reduce heart disease in patients with CVD.

Vegans generally have excellent folate and vitamin B_6 status, but their B_{12} tends to be low, and numerous studies have reported elevated homocysteine in vegans who don't supplement with B_{12}. Poor homocysteine status in vegans may therefore counteract some of the cardioprotective benefits of a vegan diet. While we don't know precisely how low B_{12} levels must go to affect homocysteine, limited evidence suggests that it needs to stay above 300pg/ml, and that 400pg/ml may be better still. If you're concerned about your B_{12} intake, consider having your B_{12} and homocysteine levels tested.

ABNORMAL BLOOD COAGULATION

Many serious cardiovascular events begin with the formation of a blood clot, or thrombus, that blocks the flow of blood in the blood vessels. Heart attacks occur when arteries to the heart are blocked; strokes occur when arteries to the brain are blocked. The initial stage of thrombus formation is when blood platelets clump together, called platelet aggregation. Injuries to the blood vessel walls or rupture of a plaque accelerates platelet aggregation.

Unfortunately, few studies have assessed platelet aggregation in vegans, but those that have been done suggest vegetarians and vegans may actually be at a slight disadvantage compared to nonvegetarians. These negative findings are a surprise, since many dietary factors associated with increased platelet aggregation, such as consumption of saturated fat and cholesterol, are low in most vegetarian and vegan diets. Plus, vegetarians and vegans consume more of the dietary compounds known to diminish platelet aggregation, such as phytochemicals from vegetables, fruits, and herbs. The most likely explanation for the increased platelet aggregation seen in these studies is that the vegetarians and vegans had poor omega-3 fatty acid status. Vegetarians, especially vegans, can usually benefit from boosting intakes of omega-3 fatty acids and improving the balance of omega-3s and omega-6s.

(See section entitled "GETTING ENOUGH OMEGA-3S", for more on omega-3 and omega-6 fatty acids.)

What Does "Percent-Fat Diet" Mean?

Percent fat refers to the percentage of calories in the diet obtained from fat. A 10-percent-fat diet, for example, means that 10 percent of the calories eaten that day were derived from fat. (Also see section entitled "Percent of Calories".)

EMERGING RISK FACTORS

Although research has shown that antioxidants provide some protective benefits, their impact on CVD risk remains unclear. People consuming vegan, raw vegan, and vegetarian diets have better antioxidant status than nonvegetarians, but the associated benefits may be limited. One thing we do know is that obtaining antioxidants from food appears to be more protective than getting them from supplements.

Thicker, stiffer arteries also increase CVD risk, as do diets high in meat and low in fiber, so it's no surprise that vegans, near-vegans, and vegetarians have been shown to have healthier arteries than nonvegetarians and even many endurance athletes.

Low vitamin D status also could be a significant CVD risk factor, and this could be a problem for vegans, who usually have less than optimal vitamin D levels (although this isn't an inevitable result of being vegan).

Vegans who eat a whole-foods diet low in saturated fat and high in fiber, antioxidants, and protective phytochemicals, and who include reliable sources of vitamin B_{12}, vitamin D, and essential fatty acids, have a reduced risk for CVD. But vegans who eat a diet of refined, processed foods may actually increase their risk.

THE VEGAN FIX FOR CVD

Vegan and near-vegan diets have been used in a variety of medical trials to improve blood fat or lipid levels and blood pressure and as a treatment for severe coronary artery disease. Even though lacto-ovo vegetarian diets reduce total lipid and LDL levels by 10 to 15 percent, a vegan diet can do even better, resulting in a 15 to 25 percent decrease in total cholesterol and LDL levels. Vegan diets rich in specific protective components, such as phytosterols, soluble or viscous fiber, soy protein, and nuts, can reduce levels even more: from 20 to 35 percent.

Two researchers have demonstrated that very low-fat vegan or near-vegan diets can effectively reverse established coronary artery disease (CAD): Dean Ornish and Caldwell Esselstyn.

In 1983, Dean Ornish, MD, used a near-vegan diet with only 10 percent of calories from fat, along with exercise, smoking cessation, and stress management, to treat twenty-three CAD patients for twenty-four days. At the end of the trial, patients had better heart muscle function and cholesterol levels and could exercise for longer periods of time, and 91 percent of them had a reduction in angina episodes.

In 1990, Ornish published the results of his landmark study, the Lifestyle Heart Trial. In this study, twenty-eight participants used a lifestyle intervention program similar to his 1983 study, while twenty participants were assigned to a control group. Coronary blockages actually regressed, or became smaller, in 82 percent of the participants in the lifestyle intervention group, compared with 53 percent in the control group. The frequency of angina, in which an inadequate blood supply to the heart causes chest pains, fell 91 percent in the lifestyle intervention group, compared to a 165 percent jump in the control group. LDL levels dropped approximately 37 percent in the lifestyle intervention group compared to 6 percent in the control group. In a five-year follow-up, arterial blockages had regressed even further among those in the lifestyle intervention group, and they had experienced 60 percent fewer cardiac events than the control group.

Caldwell Esselstyn, MD, also used a very low-fat, near-vegan diet, plus cholesterol-lowering medications if necessary, to treat twenty-four patients with severe CAD. Most participants were debilitated by angina and other symptoms of their disease, and several had such advanced heart disease that traditional interventions such as bypass surgery could no longer be offered. Of these, eighteen patients adhered to the program long term.

At the five-year follow-up, none of the participants had experienced a cardiac event. Blockages in eleven of the eighteen participants stopped growing, and in eight of the eleven the blockages had regressed. Interestingly, the six patients who returned to standard care experienced thirteen new cardiac events in the first five years. Twelve years later, the mean total cholesterol of the seventeen remaining patients on Esselstyn's program was 145mg/dl (3.8mmol/l). Not one person who stayed with the program experienced disease progression, a cardiac event, or cardiac interventions.

Although we don't have studies on changes in artery lesions and blockages using higher-fat vegan or near-vegan diets, we have considerable evidence for dramatic lipid reductions and improved cardiovascular markers with higher-fat, whole-food vegan diets. Vegan diets are associated with improvements in blood lipids, blood pressure, blood viscosity, and inflammation, whether low or higher in fat. The bioactive compounds and nutrients in higher-fat vegan foods such as nuts, seeds, and avocados have been shown to favorably affect the markers of cardiovascular disease. While we don't know if higher-fat vegan diets would prove as effective as low-fat vegan diets in improving artery lesions and blockages, we do know that whole-foods vegan diets are powerful allies in the battle against the world's leading killer.

Cancer

Cancer, the most dreaded of all chronic diseases, is currently the secondmost-common cause of death globally, and the incidence is rising. While perhaps less predictable than heart disease or type 2 diabetes, cancer generally isn't an indiscriminate killer. Consider the striking differences in cancer rates between populations throughout the world. For example, the prevalence of colon, breast, and prostate cancers is several times higher in North America and northern Europe than in rural Asia. While it is tempting to assume that rural Asians are genetically protected against these cancers, risk increases tremendously within a generation or two after Asians migrate to the West.

Contrary to what many people believe, only 5 to 10 percent of cancers are determined by genetics. The remaining 90 to 95 percent of cancers are a product of the environment, and what we eat is the linchpin, accounting for an estimated 30 to 35 percent of all cancers. As shown in table 2.1, the impact of diet varies with the type of cancer; it's particularly high in the hormone-related and colorectal cancers that are prevalent among those consuming Western diets.

Beyond diet, an estimated 25 to 30 percent of cancers—and 87 percent of lung cancers—are due to smoking, 15 to 20 percent are linked to infections, 10 to 20 percent are triggered by obesity, and 4 to 6 percent are tied to alcohol. The balance can be attributed to radiation, stress, inadequate physical activity, and environmental contaminants.

DIET AND LIFESTYLE

While only a small percentage of cancers are the result of genetics, gene expression—the process by which genes are turned on or off—is influenced by multiple factors. Diet and lifestyle choices are the factors that cause most of the genetic mutations that lead to cancer. Mutations can occur when normal by-products of metabolism, such as free radicals, damage our genetic material. Our cells may fail to repair the damage if we've been exposed to carcinogens or if we lack certain components needed for DNA synthesis and repair, such as selenium, folate, or coenzyme Q10.

TABLE 2.1. Estimated contribution of diet to cancer deaths

TYPE OF CANCER	PERCENT OF DEATHS LINKED TO DIET
Prostate	75
Colorectal	70
Breast, endometrial, gallbladder, and pancreatic	50
Stomach	35
Lung, larynx, pharynx, esophagus, mouth, and bladder	20
Other	10

Source of data: P. Anand et al., "Cancer is a Preventable Disease that Requires Major Lifestyle Changes," *Pharmaceutical Research*, no. 9 (2008): 2097-116.

The World Cancer Research Fund and the American Institute for Cancer Research convened two expert panels to determine the strength of the evidence linking diet and lifestyle to cancer. The resulting reports are considered the most authoritative and influential in this field to date. They found convincing evidence linking diet and lifestyle to several cancers:

- **Breast cancer.** The reports found that the best lifestyle interventions to reduce risk for breast cancer are to keep a lean body weight, avoid alcohol, and, for mothers, to breast-feed their babies.

- **Colorectal cancer.** Eating foods rich in fiber—in other words, plant foods—and engaging in physical activity can reduce the risk for colorectal cancer, as can eating garlic. Getting sufficient calcium, whether from supplements or dairy products, has also been associated with decreased risk. Eating red meat and processed meat, drinking alcohol (particularly for men), being overweight, and carrying abdominal fat can increase the risk.

- **Esophageal cancer.** Alcohol and body fatness can increase the risk of esophageal cancer. The risk can probably be decreased by eating fruits, nonstarchy vegetables, and foods high in vitamin C.
- **Lung cancer.** Fruits and foods high in carotenoids (see "Vitamin A,") can reduce the risk of lung cancer, but beta-carotene supplements and being overweight may increase the risk.
- **Prostate cancer.** Men who want to lessen their risk for prostate cancer should probably eat more foods containing lycopene and selenium (see for more on selenium) or take selenium supplements. High-calcium diets may increase the risk for prostate cancer, although the evidence against dairy products is still considered to be limited.
- **Stomach cancer.** A diet high in salt and salty foods may increase the risk of stomach cancer, while consuming plenty of fruits and nonstarchy vegetables probably decreases the risk.

THE VEGAN VERDICT ON CANCER

Well-planned vegan diets can provide impressive protection against cancer, especially cancers that are closely tied to dietary choices. While the evidence is just beginning to emerge, results are encouraging.

In 2012, the Adventist Health Study-2 (AHS-2) released results based on almost three thousand cancer cases. Compared to nonvegetarians, overall cancer risk was 16 percent lower among vegans and 8 percent lower among lacto-ovo vegetarians. In terms of female-specific cancers, vegans enjoyed a 34 percent risk reduction compared to nonvegetarians. The authors concluded that vegan diets confer lower risk for cancer overall and for female-specific cancers compared to other dietary patterns.

In the EPIC-Oxford studies, cancer rates among vegetarians and vegans were 89 percent those of health-conscious meat eaters. However, cancer rates were lower still in health-conscious pescatarians (people who are primarily vegetarian but also eat fish), at 83 percent of the rate among health-conscious meat eaters. When compared with the general British population, which is less health-conscious than the meat eaters in the study, the overall cancer rate among vegetarians and vegans was 65 percent of the rate among the general population.

Findings on colon cancer among vegetarians differed significantly in the EPIC-Oxford and AHS-2 studies. While AHS-2 found a 25 percent risk reduction for vegetarians compared to meat eaters, EPIC-Oxford actually reported an increased risk among vegetarians. The reason for this discrepancy is unknown; however, it's possible that the British vegetarians were consuming diets higher in refined carbohydrates and processed fats and lower in whole plant foods. Whatever the reason, switching to a vegetarian diet doesn't automatically guarantee protection from colon cancer—or any other cancer for that matter. As always, the quality of the diet is a key factor.

DOES A RAW VEGAN DIET PROTECT AGAINST CANCER?

It remains unclear what type of plant-based diet affords the greatest protection against cancer, but it does appear that whole plant foods are an important part of an anticancer diet, and that raw vegetables offer several advantages over cooked vegetables.

More than two dozen studies have examined the relationship between raw and cooked vegetables and cancer risk. These studies were not done on people consuming raw vegan diets; rather they focused on the possible advantages of specific foods or components of foods. While most studies have shown that cancer risk decreases as vegetable intake increases, findings have been more consistent for raw vegetables than for cooked vegetables. Studies have also shown that the more raw vegetables you eat, the more benefits you get.

Researchers have suggested several reasons why raw vegetables provide greater protection against cancer:

- Several protective substances, such as vitamin C and phytochemicals, are water-soluble and heat sensitive and can be destroyed or leached out during cooking.
- Cooking disables enzymes that are responsible for converting certain phytochemicals into their active forms, so they can lose their powerful anticancer effects (see "Enzymes,").
- Cooking changes the physical structure of the food and its physiologic effects. For example, it can destroy insoluble fiber, reducing the body's ability to bind and excrete cancer-causing substances.
- Cooking at high temperatures can form compounds that damage DNA.

It's also well established that raw diets can favorably alter intestinal bacteria, which can reduce levels of toxins that may increase cancer risk. In addition, some raw food preparation techniques can enhance the protective substances in food. For example, juicing removes plant cell walls, and with them the phytate compounds that can inhibit the absorption of nutrients and phytochemicals. Sprouting increases the nutrient and phytochemical content of seeds, grains, beans, and nuts.

On the other hand, cooking can kill many potentially harmful organisms, improve the bioavailability of some nutrients, destroy compounds that interfere with nutrient absorption, and improve the digestibility of some foods, such as legumes. To minimize harmful products of oxidation from cooking, use moist preparation methods, such as steaming, stewing, or poaching.

VEGAN TREATMENTS FOR CANCER

There isn't a lot of evidence that a vegan diet helps treat cancer, but in a US study published in 2005, an intervention consisting of vegan diet, exercise, stress management, and group therapy apparently reduced the progression of prostate cancer. After one year on this lifestyle program, the levels of prostate-specific antigen (PSA), a protein that's elevated in prostate cancer, decreased 4 percent in the lifestyle-intervention group but increased 6 percent in the control group. In addition, prostate cancer cell growth was inhibited nearly eight times more in the vegan lifestyle group than in the control group. Further research is needed to see if such interventions could produce similar benefits in patients with other forms of cancer.

Metabolic markers for cancer, such as PSA, are less clear-cut than those for heart disease or diabetes, but they do provide worthwhile information. Vegans tend to show more favorable test results for these markers than vegetarians, nonvegetarians, and even endurance athletes. In several studies, vegans, particularly raw-food vegans, have shown lower levels of tumor promoters, less DNA damage or better protection against damage, and fewer toxins known to promote cancer. Several studies have confirmed the positive effects of a mostly raw vegan diet on intestinal bacteria and other factors that may prove beneficial in cancer risk reduction.

In addition, a number of metabolic changes that occur with vegetarian and vegan diets may provide further protection against cancer:

- **Lower estrogen levels.** A lower lifetime exposure to estrogen is associated with a reduced risk of breast cancer.

- **Fewer bad bacteria.** Vegans and vegetarians apparently have fewer of the intestinal bacteria that convert bile acids into a more carcinogenic form. Plus, they have a less acidic colon, which reduces the activity of the enzymes responsible for this conversion.

- **A healthier gut.** Larger, heavier, softer stools and more frequent bowel movements mean potential carcinogens have less time to harm the intestinal lining. In addition, fecal mutagens—substances that damage DNA—have less opportunity to damage DNA, possibly reducing the risk for colon cancer.

- **More antioxidants and less oxidation.**
  Increased antioxidant intake and the resulting lower levels of oxidation can protect against DNA damage, potentially reducing cancer risk.

THE SOY-CANCER DEBATE

Soybeans are unique among legumes because they contain high levels of isoflavones, a type of phytoestrogen (plant estrogen). These compounds can bind to human estrogen receptor sites, but they are generally much weaker in their activity and more selective than human estrogens in the receptors they bind to. Plus, the type of estrogen receptor they bind to determines whether the isoflavones have weak estrogen-like effects or antiestrogen effects. Also see section entitled "The Final Word on Protein".

Soy intake has been associated with a reduced risk of prostate cancer and reduced prostate cancer cell growth. Recent research suggests that in reproductive cells, such as breast and uterus tissue, isoflavones act more like antiestrogens, while in bone-forming cells they behave as weak estrogens, in both cases with beneficial effects. The evidence to date suggests that lifetime soy consumption may actually help protect against breast cancer and improve breast cancer prognosis. Here are the results of some of the more promising studies:

- Soy consumption during childhood and adolescence reduces lifetime breast cancer risk.

- Among Asian women, the more soy a woman consumes, the lower her risk for breast cancer, but so far this association hasn't been found in Western women. This could be because Asians appear to metabolize isoflavones in a way that produces more of a compound called S-equol, which may provide added protection; however, the research on this topic is limited. Interestingly, one study reported that vegetarians were 4.25 times more likely to produce S-equol than nonvegetarians.

- Most studies show that the risk of recurrence or death from breast cancer is either reduced or unaffected by isoflavones. A pooled analysis of both Chinese and American women found that those with the highest intakes (10mg isoflavones or more) were 17 percent less likely to die from breast cancer and 25 percent less likely to have a recurrence of breast cancer. The protective effect of soyfoods appears to be due to their isoflavone content.

The weight of evidence suggests that soy is protective against breast cancer, breast cancer recurrence, and death due to breast cancer, although some studies suggest that it doesn't affect risk either way. The strongest evidence exists for moderate intake (about two servings a day) of traditional soy foods, such as tofu and soy milk.

ANTICANCER TIPS FOR VEGANS

Based on the evidence currently available, vegans are at an advantage where cancer risk is concerned. Still, there are steps you can take to maximize the benefits of a vegan diet:

- Eat mostly whole plant foods. Choose organic whenever possible. Try to meet most if not all of your nutritional needs through diet rather than through supplements.
- Eat at least nine servings of vegetables and fruits every day. Eat plenty of dark, leafy greens, and select produce in all the colors of the rainbow.
- Aim for at least 35 grams of fiber each day from a variety of plant foods (see Table 5.2).
- Don't eat foods that contain trans-fatty acids.
- Limit your consumption of processed foods, particularly those containing refined carbohydrates and those that are energy dense. (Energy density refers to the number of calories per weight of food.) Processed foods with high energy density are associated with weight gain, which increases cancer risk.

The worst offenders are sugary drinks, fruit juices, fast foods, and processed foods with added fat and sugar.

- Make pure, clean water your beverage of choice. Other healthful beverages include fresh vegetable juices and antioxidant-rich teas, such as green tea.
- Rely on foods such as nuts, seeds, and avocados for most of your fat, and ensure you're obtaining sufficient essential fatty acids (see chapter 4).
- Eat raw foods daily. Eat more sprouted foods.
- If you cook your food, try to stick mainly to moist cooking methods, such as steaming.
- Flavor foods with immune-boosting herbs and spices, such as turmeric, ginger, garlic, basil, oregano, rosemary, and coriander.
- Be lean. Try to keep your body weight at the low end of the normal range for your height and build. Too much body fat can cause insulin resistance and inflammation, which may trigger cancers of the esophagus, colon, rectum, pancreas, breast (postmenopause), kidney, gallbladder, and liver.
- Be physically active. Do moderate exercise—the equivalent of brisk walking—for at least one hour a day, or vigorous exercise for thirty minutes daily. Activity provides protection from colon and endometrial

cancers and, after menopause, breast cancer. Inactivity has been linked to lung and pancreatic cancers.

- Limit your intake of alcohol. Alcohol increases your risk for several cancers, and there is no apparent safe intake level. Two drinks per day for men and one for women is considered the absolute maximum.
- Keep your salt intake to no more than 2,300mg per day, and limit your consumption of smoked, pickled, and salted foods.

Type 2 Diabetes

Diabetes has become a twenty-first-century plague, crippling rich and poor nations alike. In the United States, the rate of diabetes has climbed more than 900 percent in fifty years, from 0.9 percent in the late 1950s to 8.3 percent in 2010. According to the Centers for Disease Control and Prevention, one in ten US adults had diabetes in 2010. If the current trend continues, it's estimated that as many as one in three adults will have diabetes by 2050. Statistically, diabetes is the seventh-leading cause of death in the United States, but this figure belies the fact that most people with diabetes don't die of diabetes; they die of heart disease, kidney failure, and other complications of the disease.

WHAT IS DIABETES?

Glucose is the primary source of energy for the body, and in order for glucose to enter the cells, a "gatekeeper" called insulin must let it in. Diabetes is a metabolic disorder that diminishes the body's ability to move glucose into cells so it can be used for energy. People with diabetes either don't produce insulin, don't produce enough insulin, or have become resistant to the insulin they produce. This means insulin can't do its job, so levels of blood glucose, or blood sugar, rise. When blood glucose is elevated over time, body tissues become awash in it, and health tumbles down a predictable slippery slope.

There are two main types of diabetes. Type 1, previously known as juvenileonset diabetes, occurs suddenly and most often affects children and adolescents. It is characterized by a lack of insulin production by the pancreas and is generally regarded as an autoimmune disease. In type 2 diabetes, once called adult-onset diabetes because it rarely occurred in people younger than fifty, the body continues to produce insulin but the cells have become resistant to the action of this hormone. Insulin resistance causes a rise in blood glucose, so the body responds by pumping out more insulin. Eventually the pancreas can wear out and insulin production declines. Today, type 2 diabetes is seen in young adults, teens, and even children. Untreated or poorly controlled type 2 diabetes is a leading cause of blindness, premature heart attack and stroke, kidney failure, nerve damage, and amputations.

Essentially the product of diet and lifestyle, type 2 diabetes is an insidious disease, often going undetected for many years. Globally, type 2 accounts for more than 90 percent of all diabetes, and the rise in the disease runs roughly parallel with the rise in overweight and obesity. If you're overweight, your risk of developing the disease is double that of a person of normal weight. If you're obese, your risk is tripled.

Although excess body fat plays a strong role in this disease, the way the fat is distributed is perhaps even more significant. Weight concentrated around the abdomen and in the upper part of the body, resulting in an apple shape, increases risk far more than weight that settles around the legs and hips, resulting in a pear shape. Fat that collects in and around vital organs, called visceral fat, is far more damaging than fat that accumulates close to the skin's surface, or subcutaneous fat.

Diabetes is defined as a fasting blood glucose level of at least 126mg/dl (7mmol/l), but problems can begin at lower levels. When fasting blood glucose reaches 100mg/dl (6mmol/l), the condition is called prediabetes or impaired glucose tolerance. Often, prediabetes appears as part of metabolic syndrome, a cluster of risk factors characterized by elevated blood glucose, abdominal fat, elevated blood pressure and triglycerides, and low levels of HDL. These conditions often escalate to full-blown type 2 diabetes.

LUCK OF THE DRAW?

Some people believe that type 2 diabetes is more a matter of bad genes than bad habits. While it is true that some populations have a greater susceptibility to the disease, you might think of genes as a loaded gun. It is almost always diet and lifestyle that pull the trigger. Eating animal products and processed foods—red meat, processed meat, high-fat dairy products, foods containing trans fats, fried foods, soft drinks, and refined carbohydrates, such as white flour and sugar—almost always increases the risk. In contrast, eating a fiber-rich diet of vegetables, fruits, whole grains, and legumes almost always decreases the risk. Lean, physically active people who eat diets consisting primarily of whole plant foods, such as those in poor, rural populations in Africa and Asia, have the lowest rates of type 2 diabetes in the world. However, as soon as people adopt Western eating patterns and become sedentary and overweight, their diabetes rates escalate.

Rates of diabetes among vegans have been reported to be less than 3 percent, compared to about 8 percent for nonvegetarians. A study following sixty thousand Americans reported that vegans developed diabetes about half as often as lacto-ovo vegetarians and 25 percent as often as nonvegetarians. Vegans were only 62 percent as likely to develop diabetes as nonvegetarians.

METABOLIC MARKERS OF DIABETES IN VEGANS

Vegans have fewer metabolic markers for diabetes. They are typically leaner, have lower blood glucose levels, more efficient insulin production, and lower levels of intramyocellular lipids, the fat inside cells that interferes with insulin action.

Research also suggests that blood glucose levels are much less likely to rise quickly after a vegan meal than after a nonvegetarian meal. Finally, a study on raw vegans reported reduced fasting glucose, fasting insulin, insulin resistance, and inflammation compared with endurance athletes or people eating standard Western diets.

TREATING DIABETES

In addition to reducing the risk of diabetes, a vegan diet can also successfully treat and even reverse the disease, as evidenced by several lifestyle programs. Although the vegan programs that have been found effective vary in the amount of starch, fat, and raw food they contain, all are built on whole plant foods. The most effective diets are consistently rich in fiber, phytochemicals, and antioxidants while also being low in saturated fat and free of trans-fatty acids and cholesterol.

Although many programs focus on very low-fat vegan diets, evidence suggests that higher-fat plant foods, especially nuts and seeds, may be beneficial for people with diabetes. In the Nurses' Health Study, the relative risk of developing diabetes dropped 27 percent for those eating five or more servings of nuts per week, compared to those never or almost never eating nuts.

Vegan diets also have been shown to significantly reduce nerve damage, fasting glucose levels, and the need for insulin. One research team showed that people with diabetes could lose weight on low-fat vegan diets without restricting calories or portion sizes. In these studies, people with diabetes improved more dramatically on a vegan diet than on a diet that followed the guidelines of the American Diabetes Association.

A WORD OF CAUTION

Not getting enough vitamin D, vitamin B_{12}, and omega-3 fatty acids can accelerate the progression of diabetes. Recent evidence suggests that many people with diabetes or prediabetes don't get enough vitamin D. Vitamin B_{12} was found to be an effective treatment for diabetic peripheral neuropathy—perhaps even more effective than standard medications. Low levels of omega-3 fatty acids increase the risk of depression in people with diabetes, and preliminary evidence suggests that plant sources of omega-3s may reduce diabetes risk.

THE TAKE-HOME MESSAGE ON DIABETES

Currently, whole-foods vegan diets appear to be more effective than conventional therapy in preventing and treating type 2 diabetes. Well-designed vegan diets can even reverse the disease in some people. But to maximize this potential, the diet must be based on whole plant foods—vegetables, fruits, legumes, nuts, seeds, and whole grains—and it must ensure adequate intakes of all nutrients, especially vitamin D, vitamin B_{12}, and omega-3 fatty acids.

Osteoporosis

To most consumers, the popular advertising slogan "Got Milk?" is synonymous with "Got Bones?" The dairy industry's party line is straightforward: osteoporosis is a calcium-deficiency disease, and dairy products are the best sources of calcium. However, that argument quickly falls apart if you examine global differences in calcium intakes. High dairy consumption doesn't always result in lower rates of osteoporosis. As it turns out, those who consume the most calcium (and also the most dairy products) have *higher*, not lower, rates of osteoporosis than populations that consume far less calcium.

While some consider this proof that dairy products contribute to osteoporosis, the evidence doesn't bear that out either. There are plenty of studies of people who have similar diets and lifestyles but varying dairy intakes. In such cases, those who consume dairy tend to have better bone density than those who don't. So what's going on?

To put it simply, osteoporosis isn't a dairy-deficiency disease; it isn't even a calcium-deficiency disease. It's a disease that involves a complex interplay of factors. While calcium is important to bone health, its impact can be significantly mitigated by other diet and lifestyle choices. No one would argue that cow's milk is a rich source of calcium; it provides about 300mg per cup (250ml). But that doesn't make it any more essential for people than moose or deer milk, which, incidentally, both contain about twice as much calcium as cow milk. It's estimated that during the Paleolithic era, when humans didn't have access to the milk of other mammals, calcium intake averaged 2,000mg per day or more, predominantly from wild leafy greens. Some came from other plants or mineral ash, but none came from dairy.

WHAT IS OSTEOPOROSIS?

Bones are strong, somewhat flexible, living tissues that are constantly being remodeled by tearing down old bone and building up new. Up to the age of about thirty, the balance favors the cells that build bone, and bone density continues to rise until peak bone mass is reached. After age thirty or so, the body is able to balance the two processes for a while, but eventually the demolition crew begins to overtake the builders, and bone mineral density begins to diminish.

In some people, especially those who failed to achieve good peak bone mass during their early years, a condition of weakened bones known as osteopenia results. If the imbalance between bone breakdown and formation further accelerates, it can lead to the more serious osteoporosis, characterized by fragile, porous, and often brittle bones. In medical terms, osteoporosis sets in when 30 to 40 percent of existing bone has demineralized. Many people are unaware that their bones are losing minerals until a relatively minor fall, a bump, a hug, or even a cough causes a fracture.

Approximately 80 percent of osteoporosis occurs in women. Men are also at risk, but they tend to have greater bone mass, and the hormonal changes that negatively affect men's bone density occur almost a decade later than those that affect women. It's estimated that one in four North American women will develop osteoporosis. Postmenopausal women are at the greatest risk because bone is an estrogen-dependent tissue, and estrogen levels decline dramatically at menopause. The key to preventing osteoporosis is to accumulate as much bone as possible before age thirty and then make diet and lifestyle choices that minimize losses thereafter.

DEM VEGAN BONES

When Brenda was in her early forties, her doctor ordered a complete bone mineral density test because he believed she was at high risk for osteoporosis. He went through all of the strikes against her: she was a slim Caucasian female, she had stopped menstruating for two years in her late teens, and her mother was diagnosed with osteoporosis in her fifties. The fact that Brenda hadn't consumed dairy in more than a decade indicated to him that Brenda was at high risk.

As it turned out, he was stunned by the results of her test. It indicated that her bone mineral density was far greater than expected for her age. In fact, her bones were even stronger than what would have been expected at age thirty, when she had reached peak bone mass. Her doctor said, "I don't know what you are doing, but whatever it is, just keep doing it. Your bones are made of steel." The moral of the story is not that a vegan diet guarantees strong bones, but rather that a vegan diet doesn't preclude strong bones. It's possible to maintain excellent bone health without a single drop of cow's milk if your diet is well planned. On the other hand, a poorly planned vegan diet provides no advantage in terms of bone health and could potentially increase your risk.

Research on vegan bone health to date is somewhat limited, and the data isn't particularly encouraging. Although six studies found little or no significant differences in the bone health of vegans compared to other dietary groups, eight others reported that average bone mineral densities of vegans were about 10 to 20 percent lower than those of lacto-ovo vegetarians or nonvegetarians. One study showed increased fracture rates in vegans and one showed increased fracture risk.

No studies have reported significantly better bone health in vegans compared with lacto-ovo vegetarians or nonvegetarians. It is important to note, however, that the bone health of older adults reflects lifelong habits of diet, sun exposure, and exercise. The vegan diets consumed by the participants in these studies generally included few foods fortified with calcium or vitamin D. Today, vegan products fortified with calcium and vitamin D, such as nondairy milks, are far more readily available and most vegans consume them often. This can be expected to improve the results of future studies.

BONE BUDDIES AND BULLIES

Osteoporosis risk is increased by two groups of factors. The first are things we can't change: genetics, family history, advanced age, female gender, and Caucasian or Asian descent. In addition, we have limited ability to change low estrogen levels in women and low testosterone levels in men. The second group includes things we can change: smoking, heavy alcohol use, physical inactivity, minimal sun exposure, and poorly planned diets. All of these choices can have a profound impact on both the quality and the quantity of bone we produce and maintain. Physical activity, particularly weight-bearing exercise, sends a message to the bones to intensify bone-building efforts, helping increase bone density during childhood and adolescence and maintain bone density as we age.

The association between diet and bone health is complex, and research findings are inconsistent. We know that diets that supply sufficient calcium, magnesium, manganese, copper, boron, iron, zinc, fluoride, vitamin D, vitamin K, and vitamin C contribute to bone health, and that fruits, vegetables, and soy inhibit bone breakdown. Phosphorus is an important structural mineral for bones, but too much phosphorus and not enough calcium can weaken bones. While protein has generally been found to be protective and is an important component of bones, eating very high amounts of protein may be detrimental if you're not getting enough calcium.

Other dietary factors that are known to adversely affect bone health include the following:

- **Alcohol.** Chronic, excessive alcohol consumption reduces calcium and vitamin D absorption and can injure the liver, impairing the ability to activate vitamin D. Alcohol also can lower estrogen production, eroding the capacity to build bone.
- **Caffeine.** Caffeine appears to reduce the absorption of calcium; however, the effect is completely mitigated by a small increase in calcium intake. For example, adding milk to coffee compensates for the modest reduction in calcium absorption caused by the caffeine content. Fortified soy milk might be expected to do the same.
- **Sodium.** High sodium intake increases the excretion of calcium through urine and perspiration.
- **Vitamin A.** While preformed vitamin A, or retinol, which is present in animal products and some supplements, is necessary for bone growth, very high intakes can increase bone breakdown and interfere with the efforts of vitamin D to help the body absorb calcium. Carotenoids that can be converted to vitamin

A, such as beta-carotene from plants, don't have this effect.

Numerous dietary factors benefit bone health, and vegan diets provide many of them. Vegans generally don't consume retinol and generally have lower intakes of sodium, alcohol, and caffeine (though not always). On the other hand, vegans tend to have lower intakes of calcium, vitamin D, and protein—nutrients that are critical to bone health—so you need to plan menus with these in mind.

THE CALCIUM CONUNDRUM

There is no controversy regarding the importance of calcium for bone health. Calcium is the structural mineral that predominates in bones, and it's necessary for both building and maintaining bone tissue. However, calcium also plays an important role in the functioning of the heart and nervous system. If dietary calcium is insufficient to maintain the levels necessary in the blood, calcium is quickly drawn from the bones to avert disaster.

A somewhat ambiguous and unpredictable relationship exists between calcium and bone health. While the evidence generally supports a positive association between calcium intake and bone health, some populations who eat less than 400mg of calcium per day have lower rates of osteoporosis than populations who consume more than 1,000mg per day. This is because calcium *balance* is more critical than calcium *intake*.

Calcium balance is determined by a complex interplay of intake, absorption, and excretion. When you retain enough calcium, you don't have to draw upon body reserves; you are in calcium balance. So if you eat foods that compromise calcium absorption and increase calcium excretion, you need to consume more calcium to compensate for the loss. On the other hand, if your diet maximizes calcium absorption and minimizes calcium excretion, your requirements would be considerably lower.

How much calcium do vegans need? It depends on how well designed the diet is and other lifestyle factors, such as physical activity. There is good evidence that intakes less than 525mg per day increase risk. Until more definitive research is released, it's a good idea to make sure you get the recommended amount (1,000mg per day for adults younger than fifty and 1,200mg for those fifty and older). While foods, including those that are fortified with calcium, are the best option, take a supplement if your dietary calcium intake falls short. (For more information on calcium.)

THE VITAMIN D DEBACLE

Vitamin D is no minor player in bone health. When blood levels of calcium begin to drop, the body converts vitamin D into its active form and puts it to work enhancing calcium absorption and reducing losses. Considering how absorption and excretion of calcium are involved in overall calcium balance, it's easy to see why vitamin D is every bit as relevant to bone health as calcium.

The problem for vegans is that they consistently consume less vitamin D than nonvegetarians. The reason is simple. Historically, humans derived vitamin D from sunshine, not food. Apart from fatty fish, very few foods were reliable sources of vitamin D. As humans migrated farther away from the equator, covered themselves in clothing, protected themselves against the elements by staying indoors, and began to live in smog-filled cities, vitamin D deficiency became widespread. Health authorities responded by adding vitamin D to a basic staple: cow's milk. Today, nondairy milks with added vitamin D are also widely available, although few people get enough vitamin D from either dairy or nondairy milk.

As a result of recent research, many experts believe that we should consider getting 25mcg (1,000 IU) or more of vitamin D per day. In view of the reduced vitamin D status of many vegans, it is especially important that they get at least that much vitamin D per day, particularly if their exposure to sunshine is limited. (For more information on vitamin D.)

THE PROTEIN PARADOX

For many years, a common belief among vegans was that avoiding animal protein provided protection from osteoporosis. This belief was supported by the fact that osteoporosis rates are higher in developed nations with high consumption of animal protein, even when intakes of calcium are high.

This theory held that a high intake of animal protein leads to bone loss and osteoporosis. The standard explanation went something like this: Animal protein is rich in amino acids that raise the acidity of the blood. In order to neutralize this acid, the body draws from its huge store of calcium—specifically, the calcium in our bones. Once the calcium does its job, it's excreted in urine. Given this association between animal protein consumption and calcium loss, the thinking was that vegans were protected against osteoporosis and also required less dietary calcium than meat eaters. Although the theory makes logical sense, it hasn't been supported by science. As it turns out, the connection between protein and bone health is a little more complicated than had been thought. In addition, the data on the bone health of vegans isn't as favorable as would be expected if the animal protein hypothesis were true.

Protein is involved in various metabolic activities, and some are beneficial to bone health, whereas others are detrimental. High protein intake causes calcium loss in the urine. However, the loss isn't as great when protein is consumed as part of a whole-foods diet rather than when it's consumed as a protein supplement. Acid-forming diets may also suppress bone-building activity and stimulate bone breakdown. While these activities can be detrimental, protein does have a flattering flip side. It has been shown to increase calcium absorption and enhance bone building.

Considering all of these factors together, it appears that protein generally offers modest protection to bones, particularly if you eat enough calcium and lots of fruits and vegetables. For vegans, getting sufficient protein appears to be an important piece of the bone health puzzle. In one study, vegetarians who ate the most protein-rich plant foods, such as legumes, meat analogs, and nuts, had the lowest risk for wrist fracture. Those who ate fewer than three servings of those foods per week had the highest risk. (For more information on protein, see chapter 3.)

THE TAKE-HOME MESSAGE ON OSTEOPOROSIS

Vegans do need to be concerned about long-term bone health. Although a wellplanned vegan diet can help protect against osteoporosis, one that's poorly planned can compromise bone health. There are several steps you can take to build and maintain strong bones:

- Follow the recommendations in chapter 14, The Vegan Food Guide, to ensure ample intake of calcium, vitamin D, protein, vitamin K, potassium, and other bone-building nutrients.
- Aim for nine or more servings of vegetables and fruits each day.
- Include soy foods such as tofu, tempeh, and soy milk.
- Consume only moderate amounts of alcohol and caffeine or avoid them altogether.
- Don't smoke.
- Keep sodium intake below 2,300mg/day, or 1,500mg/day if you're over fifty, have high blood pressure, or are African-American.
- Aim for an hour of weight-bearing exercise most days.

Other Diseases

Vegan diets have been shown to reduce risk or provide effective treatment for cataracts, diverticular disease, gallstones, kidney disease, and rheumatoid arthritis. The risk of dementia may increase or decrease with vegan diets, depending on several factors. Here are findings from some of the studies on the effects of a vegan diet on disease.

CATARACTS

Vegans may have the lowest incidence of cataracts of all dietary groups. In a large, fifteen-year study, the incidence of cataracts was highest in meat eaters and lowest in vegans, who had a 40 percent reduction in risk for the condition. This study doesn't prove that meat eating causes cataracts, but it certainly suggests an association that warrants further investigation.

DEMENTIA

Poor vitamin B_{12} status is a well-recognized contributor to memory loss and brain dysfunction. (However, supplementing with B_{12} doesn't appear to benefit those who already have dementia or Alzheimer's disease and aren't deficient in vitamin B_{12}.) Vitamin B_{12} in animal products is bound to protein, and as we age, we get less efficient at cleaving the B_{12} off the protein. For this reason, everyone is advised to rely on B_{12} supplements or eat foods fortified with B_{12}. This is especially important for vegans, as B_{12} status is often lower in this population. Then again, there's reasonable evidence to suggest that the risk is actually decreased for vegans who ensure adequate B_{12} intakes, because other components in plantbased diets are protective.

In addition to vitamin B_{12}, folate and vitamin B_6 are important; however, these two nutrients are abundant in most vegan diets. As an added bonus, vegans tend to have high intakes of antioxidants and phytochemicals, which appear to protect brain health. Of course, vegans who are physically active, get sufficient rest, avoid smoking and excessive alcohol, and keep their brains active and challenged further reduce their risk.

DIVERTICULAR DISEASE

Diverticular disease is endemic in the Western world but rare in areas where diets are high in unprocessed high-fiber foods. An impressive body of evidence supports the theory that diverticular disease is essentially a result of fiber deficiency. We know that vegans typically consume twice the fiber of nonvegetarians.

Vegans' risk for diverticular disease is 72 percent lower than that of meat eaters, according to a recent report from Epic-Oxford that included more than forty-seven thousand participants. A high-fiber vegan diet was thought to be largely responsible, but it's possible that the absence of meat also provided protection. This is because meat can negatively affect gut flora, reducing the integrity of the colon wall, and increasing the risk of diverticular disease.

GALLSTONES

To date, no studies have examined rates of gallstone formation in vegans. However, there is good evidence to suggest that vegetarians are at lower risk than nonvegetarians and that the factors that afford this protection may be stronger among vegans. Obesity and overweight are strongly linked to increased risk, and eating sufficient fiber, fruits, vegetables, vegetable protein, and unsaturated fat is related to decreased risk for gallstones. Eating lots of saturated fat, trans-fatty acids, cholesterol, and refined carbohydrates may increase the chance of getting gallstones. Vegans have the lowest risk of overweight and obesity, the lowest intakes of saturated fat and cholesterol, and the highest intakes of fiber, vegetable protein, and fruits and vegetables. Therefore, it would be reasonable to assume that the risk of gallstones in vegans would be even lower than it is among lactoovo vegetarians.

KIDNEY DISEASE

Although excessive consumption of either animal protein or vegetable protein can cause renal injury and accelerate kidney disease, plant-based diets don't promote renal decline to the same extent as diets rich in protein from meat. Experts now believe a vegan diet may be a suitable replacement for the conventional low-protein diets prescribed to patients with mild chronic renal failure. (As a bonus, patients say the vegan diet is cheaper and tastes better.)

RHEUMATOID ARTHRITIS

Vegan diets appear to offer significant benefits for some people suffering from rheumatoid arthritis, a chronic inflammatory disease. Limited evidence suggests that raw or living-food diets can be especially effective. Vegan diets are generally replete with vegetables, fruits, and other whole plant foods, and these are the key sources of protective anti-inflammatory and antioxidant compounds. Vegan diets are also free of animal products, such as red meat and processed meats, and typically are low in processed foods, all of which promote inflammation. Phytochemicals beneficial in the treatment of rheumatoid arthritis have been reported to be ten times more abundant in vegan diets than in nonvegetarian diets. In addition, a vegan diet can reduce gut bacteria that produce harmful byproducts associated with inflammation.

Some experts argue that the benefits conferred by vegan diets are due to the removal of allergenic foods or foods that people tend to be sensitive to. Common triggers for food allergies and sensitivities, such as dairy products and eggs, aren't part of a vegan diet, and some vegan and raw diets often also exclude wheat and other gluten-containing grains.

Our Evolving Concepts

Just a few short decades ago, vegan diets were viewed as downright dangerous. As evidence accumulated, vegan diets were recognized as nutritionally adequate as long as they were well planned. Today, vegan diets are acclaimed for their ability to prevent and even reverse chronic disease. Although this attitude shift is palpable, especially in relation to chronic disease, many people have lingering doubts about the nutritional adequacy of vegan diets. They still question the quality of plant protein and the quantities of vitamins and minerals supplied by plants.

In the next chapters, we address these concerns and provide information to help you construct a diet that provides everything your body needs to achieve optimal health. Let's start with protein.

CHAPTER 3

Protein Power from Plants

If you're already vegan, you've probably been asked, more than once, where you get your protein. If you're contemplating becoming vegan, maybe you're wondering about the very same thing. It is reassuring to know that plant foods can supply both the optimal quantity and quality of protein to meet all of our body's needs.

Most people equate protein with meat, seafood, eggs, and cheese so they assume a vegan diet is bound to be insufficient. That's probably because two-thirds of the protein in diets in North America and in many developed countries comes from animal products, and just 32 percent comes from plant foods. But worldwide, these numbers are quite different: plants contribute 65 percent of the protein in human diets globally, with about 47 percent coming from grains; 8 percent from legumes, nuts, and seeds; 1 percent from fruit; and the remaining 9 percent from vegetables.

These days, many vegans, including some influential speakers and writers, take for granted that protein intake is automatically sufficient on any vegan diet. After all, they reason, every plant contains protein. But this line of reason isn't entirely accurate either. It's true that all vegetables, legumes, seeds, nuts, and grains contain protein, and even fruit has a little. But a vegan diet can be short of protein if people eat mostly fruit (as some people on raw food diets do), if you don't eat enough calories (for weight loss or other reasons), if you eat a lot of junk food, or if you don't eat enough legumes (beans, peas, lentils, or peanuts).

What Is Protein?

Proteins, like carbohydrates and fats, are macronutrients, meaning they can be used as sources of energy for the body, with carbohydrates being the body's preferred source. While protein can be used for energy, it's most important for a variety of other crucial functions. As a component of muscle and bone, protein is essential for the body's structure and movement. We also require protein for protection (as antibodies), to accomplish reactions (as enzymes), for coordinating body functions (as hormones), and as carriers (to move oxygen and electrons).

In addition, we need protein for routine maintenance and the replacement of cells.

How Much Protein Do We Need?

The recommended dietary allowance for protein, meaning the amount a person needs each day, is stated in grams of protein per kilogram (2.2lb) of body weight per day, org/kg/d. Both vegetarians and nonvegetarians are advised to get 0.8g/kg/d, but some studies suggest vegans should aim for at least 0.9g/kg/d, and 1g per kg body weight is a reasonable and simple goal.

Table 3.1 lists the grams of protein needed by adult vegans of various weights, based on 0.9g/kg/d. Note that extra body fat requires little protein, so if you're overweight, base your protein intake on what your ideal or healthy body weight would be.

FACTORS AFFECTING PROTEIN NEEDS

The amount of protein required varies depending on age and physical factors. For example, infants and children, who are building muscle and bone, have high protein needs per kilogram (2.2lb) of body weight. In the first year of life, infants require almost twice as much protein per kilogram (2.2lb) of body weight as adults. To be clear, that doesn't mean they require twice as much protein—only twice as much per kilogram (2.2lb) of body weight. Because their bodies are small, the actual amounts of protein they need are small, typically about 11 grams of protein per day for infants ages six to twelve months and 19 grams per day for children ages four to eight. The amounts of protein required per kilogram (2.2lb) of body weight gradually decrease until adulthood. (Menus that meet and exceed protein requirements during pregnancy, lactation, infancy, and childhood can be found in chapter 11.)

TABLE 3.1. Recommended protein intake for vegan adults

BODY WEIGHT (lb)	BODY WEIGHT (kg)	RECOMMENDED PROTEIN (g)
120	54	49
135	61	55
150	68	61
165	75	68
180	82	74
195	88	79

Sources of data are listed in *Becoming Vegan: Comprehensive Edition*, by Brenda Davis and Vesanto Melina (Book Publishing Company, 2014).

After age sixty, the body's ability to use protein becomes less efficient. Vegan seniors need 1 to 1.1g/kg/d, and getting enough protein can be a challenge without some planning. (For more information, see chapter 12.)

Vegans who are moderately involved in sports and exercise generally don't need more than 0.9g/kg/d. They may need more carbohydrates than sedentary folks, since carbs are the ideal energy source for active people, but not more protein. On the other hand, endurance athletes may need more protein, particularly in the early stages of training and muscle building. Expert opinions vary, with recommended amounts ranging between 1.2 and 1.6g/kg/d. Strength athletes also require extra protein, typically from 1.2 to 2.0g/kg/d. For more on sports nutrition, see chapter 13, and for menus at several calorie levels that provide abundant protein, see chapter 14.

Protein Quality

Two factors determine the quality of a protein: digestibility and amino acid content. Digestibility is a measure of how much protein is absorbed by the body, a process affected by the amount of fiber in the food. Plants contain fiber, and we don't digest some forms of fiber. These forms of fiber pass through the intestinal tract, taking a small amount of protein with them. Animal products contain no fiber. Refined plant foods contain only a fraction of the fiber of the original food, ranking them about even with animal protein in digestibility.

Food preparation methods can also affect protein digestibility. For example, soaking or sprouting legumes, seeds, and grains increases their digestibility. As their cells take up water, some of the proteins fragment, making them easier for the body to absorb. Soaking also may activate plant enzymes that begin the digestion process. Compounds that can inhibit digestion, such as phytates, also are broken down by soaking, which enhances digestibility. As a further benefit, sprouting beans for six days was shown to remove 70 to 100 percent of their oligosaccharides, compounds that sometimes cause flatulence. Note that beans larger than lentils and mung beans should always be cooked after sprouting. Sprouting can further improve protein quality by slightly increasing amounts of amino acids that may be in short supply.

Foods can be rated according to the digestibility of their protein. If we absorb 96 percent of the nitrogen (representing protein) and 4 percent passes out through the intestine, the protein digestibility rating of that food is 96 percent. Overall, protein in the American diet and the Chinese diet is rated as 96 percent digestible; Brazilian and East Indian diets of grains and beans are rated as 78 percent digestible.

TABLE 3.2. Digestibility of protein in various foods

PLANT FOODS	DIGESTIBILITY (%)
Refined white flour or white bread	96
Soy protein isolate	95
Peanut butter	95
Tofu	93
Whole wheat flour or bread	92
Rolled oats	86
Lentils	84
Black, kidney, and pinto beans and chickpeas	72–89
ANIMAL PRODUCTS	
Eggs	97
Milk and cheese	95
Beef and fish	94

Sources of data are listed in: *Becoming Vegan: Comprehensive Edition*, by Brenda Davis and Vesanto Melina (Book Publishing Company, 2014).

Based on a glance at table 3.2, you might assume that you should choose white bread rather than whole wheat bread for your peanut butter sandwich, or highly processed soy protein isolate rather than tofu or cooked beans, due to their highly digestible protein. Yet the choice isn't so simple. While processing foods increases the digestibility of their protein by removing fiber and other materials, it can strip the foods of valuable vitamins, minerals, and phytochemicals. In fact, consuming some refined food can be a wise choice at times to help make a diet less bulky for small children or seniors, or for those with high energy needs.

The second factor that determines the quality of protein is its amino acid content. Amino acids are the building blocks of protein. They are made of carbon, hydrogen, oxygen, and nitrogen. Each protein molecule is an intricate structure that consists of amino acids (typically hundreds of them) in specific sequences and arrangements.

Nine of the twenty amino acids are known as indispensable amino acids, formerly called essential amino acids: phenylalanine, valine, threonine, tryptophan, isoleucine, methionine, leucine, lysine, and histadine. They are called indispensable because we have to get them from food. We can build the other eleven amino acids from them. Fortunately, every one of these indispensable amino acids is present in both plant foods and animal products.

Noteworthy Amino Acids for Vegans

Although all indispensable amino acids are readily available from plant foods, it's important for vegans to eat a wide variety of plant foods to ensure adequate intakes of each (not to be confused with protein complementing, discussed below). In addition, two of these, lysine and tryptophan, are of special interest, as well as one amino acid that has become a popular supplement, carnitine.

LYSINE

The indispensable amino acid lysine is in relatively short supply in many diets worldwide, especially in diets centered on foods such as corn, wheat, rice, and most other grains, which tend to be low in lysine. Lysine is required for growth, and low intakes of calories, protein, and lysine specifically are the reasons for the small stature of some people in regions where dietary choices are limited.

The adult recommended intake for lysine is 38mg/kg/d. Three servings of legumes will generally provide half of the recommended intake of protein and two-thirds of the lysine for the day. Since 1/2 cup (125ml) of cooked legumes is considered a serving, this could be met, for example, with 1/2 cup (125ml) of beans in a salad at lunch, plus I cup (250ml) of lentils in a soup at supper. Or you could start the day with a smoothie that includes pea or soy protein powder or soy milk, snack on peanuts or a peanut butter sandwich, and have beans or tofu at supper. Including beans, peas, and lentils as staples on a daily basis goes a long way toward ensuring an adequate vegan diet. A little dab of hummus on a cracker or a celery stick just won't cut it.

People on raw vegan diets tend to eat few if any beans. If you're in that category, you can get your lysine from fresh green peas or sprouted lentils, peas, and mung beans. As a bonus, sprouting increases lysine content.

TRYPTOPHAN

After the growth spurt of early childhood, we need to turn our attention to another indispensable amino acid, tryptophan, which is important for maintenance. Again, beans, especially soy, and peanuts contain abundant tryptophan. Wheat, oats, millet, and buckwheat provide moderate amounts. Those on raw vegan diets can emphasize spinach, peas, sesame and other seeds, and nuts.

CARNITINE

Carnitine isn't indispensable; our bodies can synthesize it from other amino acids—in this case, lysine or methionine, both of which are present in vegan diets. Carnitine helps the body convert fat into energy by carrying fatty acids into the energy production centers in cells (mitochondria) and removing waste products. It's promoted as a supplement for weight loss and improved sports performance, although research hasn't found evidence that it performs as claimed. In fact, carnitine has been linked to heart disease and prostate cancer, so lower intakes of carnitine by vegans may turn out to be a considerable health advantage. The body typically makes sufficient carnitine to meet the needs of most people, with the exception of preterm infants and people on diets deficient in protein.

Carnitine is found in beef and in lesser amounts in other animal products. It is present in a few plant foods in very small amounts. Whereas 1/2 cup (125ml) of cow's milk provides 4mg of carnitine, 1/2 cup (125ml) of asparagus contains only 0.2mg, and a peanut butter sandwich contains 0.3mg.

Although vegans obviously don't eat beef, they still tend to have normal plasma carnitine levels because their bodies make it from the lysine in legumes and the methionine in grains and vegetables. The synthesis of carnitine is dependent on vitamin C, niacin, vitamin B_6, and iron, all of which are abundant in balanced vegan diets.

A small proportion of people (on any diet, vegan or otherwise) have found that taking supplemental carnitine helped reduce migraine headaches, hypoglycemia, or muscle weakness. Over-the-counter acetyl-L-carnitine supplements in veggie caps, which are vegan, are available in the United States, but in Canada they are only available by prescription. Amounts as high as 500mg per day are generally regarded as safe, though research is limited. Taking larger amounts, such as 4 grams per day, can have side effects, including nausea, diarrhea, and a fishy body odor, and may significantly increase your risk of chronic disease. Don't take carnitine if you're pregnant, have thyroid problems, or have a history of seizures.

Protein Complementing

Plant protein has gotten a bad rap for years. It's been dismissed as "incomplete," and vegans were told to be careful to combine foods at each meal to ensure intake of "complete" protein. This idea stemmed from the belief that many plant foods lacked some of the amino acids or contained very little. Vegans were advised to eat certain plant foods together to get the complete spectrum of indispensable amino acids. We now know that all amino acids are present in every whole plant food, and that eating a variety of healthful vegan foods every day usually provides all the needed amino acids.

The theory does have a grain of truth in it. Different foods and food groups contain different amounts of amino acids. Most legumes and seeds provide abundant lysine but are somewhat short in methionine, whereas grains tend to be good sources of methionine but low in lysine. As a result, eating a mixed diet that includes legumes, seeds, grains, and vegetables within a twenty-four-hour period easily provides adequate amounts of every amino acid that we require.

All over the world, legumes and whole grains provide the optimum mix of amino acids. In Southeast Asia, meals are centered on tofu and rice. In the southern United States, a favorite combination is black-eyed peas and cornbread, or the ubiquitous peanut butter sandwich. Ethiopians appreciate lentils and teff. The Scots have long enjoyed white bean soup and oatcakes. In Egypt, menus feature fava beans and millet. The French and French-Canadians appreciate split pea soup with freshly baked bread, and Boston is known for baked beans and brown bread. Latin Americans enjoy colorful meals of black beans with quinoa, rice, or tortillas made from wheat or corn.

Balancing Macronutrients

For a balanced diet, aim for 10 to 20 percent of calories from protein, 50 to 75 percent of calories from carbohydrate, and 15 to 30 percent of calories from fat.

Percent of Calories

When the body converts fat, protein, and carbohydrate to calories, we derive 9 calories from each gram of fat and 4 calories from each gram of protein or carbohydrate. Table 3.3 lists the amount of protein in foods plus the percentage of calories from protein, fat, and carbohydrates.

Every unrefined or whole plant food supplies small or moderate amounts of protein. Calories from protein in green vegetables and in legumes are typically in the range of 10 to 37 percent. Tofu is somewhat higher in protein, and veggie meats are higher still. Calories from protein in most nuts, seeds, and grains typically range from 9 to 17 percent. Fruits are at the low end of the spectrum, with just 2 to 10 percent of calories coming from protein.

Protein. In your overall diet, you should try to get 10 to 20 percent of your calories from protein. Most people get 10 to 15 percent of calories from protein, and vegan diets typically fall within this range. Those who don't consume many calories, such as the elderly or those who are trying to lose weight, should aim toward the upper end of the 10 to 20 percent range. When people consume insufficient calories, as they intentionally do on a weight-loss diet, the percentage of total calories from protein should be about 15 to 20 percent of calories, otherwise they'll lose not only weight but also muscle mass.

Carbohydrates. Carbohydrates should provide 50 to 75 percent of your calories. Raw vegan diets may provide a little less carbohydrate and still be healthful. (For more on carbohydrates, see chapter 5.)

Fat. Fat should provide 15 to 30 percent of your calories, though people on special therapeutic diets for reversal of chronic diseases such as cardiovascular disease can benefit from a diet with as little as 10 percent of calories from fat. As you can see in table 3.3, lettuce and other leafy greens provide 8 to 13 percent of calories from fat (without a drop of salad dressing). Some raw vegan diets with abundant nuts, seeds, and avocados have a higher proportion of calories from fat but are still considered healthful. (For more on fat, see chapter 4.)

TABLE 3.3. Calories, protein, and percentage of calories from protein, fat, and carbohydrates in selected foods

FOOD	CALORIES	PROTEIN (g)	CALORIES FROM PROTEIN (%)	CALORIES FROM CARBS (%)	CALORIES FROM FAT (%)
LEGUMES					
Adzuki beans, cooked (½ c/115 g)	147	9	23	76	1
Black beans, cooked (½ c/86 g)	114	8	26	70	4
Black-eyed peas, cooked (½ c/86 g)	105	7	26	70	4
Chickpeas, cooked (½ c/82 g)	134	7	21	65	14
Cranberry beans, cooked (½ c/88 g)	120	8	27	70	3
Edamame, cooked (½ c/75 g)	100	10	41	37	22
Falafel, cooked (1.7 oz./51 g)	170	7	16	37	47
Great Northern beans, cooked (½ c/88 g)	104	7	28	69	3
Kidney beans, cooked (½ c/88 g)	112	7	27	70	3
Lentils, brown/green, cooked (½ c/99 g)	115	9	30	67	3
Lentil sprouts, raw (1 c/77 g)	82	7	28	68	4
Lima beans, cooked (½ c/91 g)	115	7	25	72	3
Mung beans, cooked (½ c/94 g)	94	7	28	68	4
Mung bean sprouts, raw (1 c/104 g)	31	3	32	64	4
Navy beans, cooked (½ c/91 g)	127	7	23	73	4
Peanut butter (2 tbsp/32 g)	192	8	16	12	72
Peanuts, raw (¼ c/36 g)	207	9	17	11	72
Peas, fresh (1 c/145 g)	117	8	26	70	4
Peas, split, cooked (½ c/98 g)	116	8	27	70	3
Pea sprouts, raw (1 c/120 g)	154	11	23	73	4
Pinto beans, cooked (½ c/86 g)	122	8	25	71	4
Soybeans, cooked (½ c/86 g)	157	15	36	21	43
Soy milk, "original" (1 c/227–245 g)*	80–140	6–11	21–33	33–53	20–35
Tempeh, raw (¼ c/42 g)*	80	8	35	18	47
Tofu, firm, raw (¼ c/63 g)*	91	10	40	11	49
Vegan burgers (2.5–3.2 oz/70–90 g)*	70–95	10–14	45–61	27–55	0–24
Vegan deli slices (1 oz/30 g)*	33	7	85	14	1
Vegan ground round (1 oz/30 g)*	31–32	5	53–71	27–47	0–7
Vegan hot dog (1.5–2.5 oz/42–70 g)*	45–163	7–14	26–92	5–13	0–67
White beans, cooked (½ c/90 g)	124–127	8–9	25–27	70–71	2–4
NUTS AND SEEDS					
Almond butter (2 tbsp/32 g)	203	5	9	13	78

FOOD	CALORIES	PROTEIN (g)	CALORIES FROM PROTEIN (%)	CALORIES FROM CARBS (%)	CALORIES FROM FAT (%)
Almond milk, original (1 c/227 g)*	60	1	7	55	38
Almonds (¼ c/36 g)	207–213	7–8	13	13	74
Brazil nut, large, each	31	0.7	8	6	86
Brazil nuts (¼ c/35 g)	230	5	8	7	85
Cashew butter (2 tbsp/32 g)	188	6	11	18	71
Cashews (¼ c/34 g)	188	6	12	21	67
Chia seeds (¼ c/40 g)	196	6	12	34	54
Flaxseeds, ground (¼ c/32 g)	144	7	14	23	63
Hazelnuts (¼ c/34 g)	212	5	9	10	81
Hempseed milk (1 c/244 g)*	130	4	13	65	22
Hempseeds (¼ c/40 g)*	227	13	27	28	55
Pecans (¼ c/27 g)	187	2	5	7	88
Pine nuts (¼ c/34 g)	227–229	5–10	8–16	7–9	75–85
Pistachio nuts (¼ c/32 g)	178	7	14	19	67
Poppy seeds (¼ c/34 g)	179	6	13	17	70
Pumpkin seeds (¼ c/32 g)	180	10	17	12	71
Sesame seeds, hulled (¼ c/38 g)	237	8	12	7	81
Sesame seeds, whole (¼ c/36 g)	206	6	12	15	73
Sesame tahini (2 tbsp/30 g)	178	5	11	14	75
Sunflower seed butter (2 tbsp/32 g)	185	6	13	18	69
Sunflower seed kernels (¼ c/36 g)	210	7	13	13	74
Walnuts, black, chopped (¼ c/31 g)	190	8	15	7	78
Walnuts, English, chopped (¼ c/29 g)	194	5	9	8	83
GRAINS					
Amaranth, dry (¼ c/49 g)	182	7	15	70	15
Barley, pearl, dry (¼ c/46 g)	163	6	14	80	6
Barley, unhulled, dry (¼ c/41 g)	125	3	9	87	4
Bread, white (1 oz/30 g)*	67	2	12	76	12
Bread, whole wheat (1 oz/30 g)*	69–70	3–4	15–21	67–71	12–14
Buckwheat groats, dry (¼ c/42 g)	150	5	13	81	6
Buckwheat sprouts, raw (1 c/33 g)	65	2	14	80	6
Cornmeal (¼ c/30 g)	110	2	9	82	9
Corn tortilla, 6-inch (1 oz/30 g)*	70	1	6	81	13
Kamut, cooked (½ c/86 g)	126	6	17	78	5
Millet, cooked (½ c/87 g)	104	3	12	80	8

FOOD	CALORIES	PROTEIN (g)	CALORIES FROM PROTEIN (%)	CALORIES FROM CARBS (%)	CALORIES FROM FAT (%)
Oat groats, dry (¼ c/41–45 g)	153–187	5–6	13–14	71–73	14–15
Oatmeal, cooked (½ c/117 g)	83	3	14	67	19
Quinoa, cooked (½ c/92 g)	111	4	15	71	14
Rice, brown, cooked (½ c/98 g)	109	2	8	85	7
Rice, white, cooked (½ c/102 g)	133	2	8	91	1
Rice milk, "original" (1 c/245–248 g)*	120	0.4–1	1–3	82–84	15
Rye berries, dry (¼ c/42 g)	142	6	16	78	6
Spaghetti, white, cooked (½ c/70 g)	99	3	14	82	4
Spaghetti, whole wheat, cooked (½ c/70 g)	87	4	16	80	4
Spelt, dry (¼ c/44 g)	147	6	16	78	6
Wheat berries, hard red or white, dry (¼ c/48 g)	158–164	5–7	12–18	78–83	4–5
Wheat sprouts, raw (1 c/108 g)	214	8	15	80	5
Wheat tortilla (1 oz/30 g)*	59	2	13	83	4
Wild rice, dry (¼ c/40 g)	143	6	16	81	3
VEGETABLES (RAW UNLESS STATED)					
Asparagus, sliced, cooked (½ c/90 g)	20	2	34	59	7
Avocado, California, each (4.8 oz/136 g)	227	3	4	19	77
Avocado, Florida, each (10.7 oz/304 g)	365	7	7	24	69
Basil, fresh, chopped (½ c/21 g)	5	0.7	44	37	19
Beans, snap green/wax (½ c/55 g)	17	1	20	77	3
Beet greens, chopped (1 c/38 g)	8	0.8	33	63	4
Beet juice (½ c/118 g)	41	1	12	88	0
Beets, sliced, cooked (½ c/68 g)	29	1	14	83	3
Bok choy, sliced (1 c/70 g)	10	1	36	53	11
Broccoli, chopped, cooked (½ c/78 g)	26	2	23	68	9
Brussels sprouts (½ c/78 g)	28	2	24	66	10
Cabbage, green, chopped (1 c/89 g)	22	1	18	79	3
Cabbage, napa, chopped (1 c/76 g)	15	1	30	67	0
Cabbage, red, chopped (1 c/89 g)	28	1	16	80	4
Carrot, chopped, cooked (½ c/78 g)	35	0.9	9	88	3
Carrot, each (2.5 oz/70 g)	30	0.7	8	87	5
Carrot juice (½ c/118 g)	48	1	9	88	3
Cauliflower, chopped, cooked (½ c/62 g)	14	1	26	59	15
Celery, diced (1 c/101 g)	16	0.7	17	74	9

FOOD	CALORIES	PROTEIN (g)	CALORIES FROM PROTEIN (%)	CALORIES FROM CARBS (%)	CALORIES FROM FAT (%)
Celery, stalk, each (2.3 oz/64 g)	10	0.4	17	74	9
Celery root, diced (1 c/156 g)	66	2	13	81	6
Chiles, hot green (½ c/75 g)	32	2	17	79	4
Chiles, hot red (½ c/75 g)	30	1	17	75	8
Collard greens, chopped (1 c/36 g)	11	0.9	27	63	10
Corn, kernels, white/yellow (½ c/77 g)	66	2	13	76	11
Cucumber, unpeeled, sliced (1 c/104 g)	14	0.8	18	74	8
Dandelion greens, chopped (1 c/55 g)	25	1	20	68	12
Eggplant, cubed, cooked (½ c/50 g)	14	0.4	11	83	6
Endive, chopped (1 c/50 g)	8	0.6	25	66	9
Garlic clove, each (0.1 oz/3 g)	3	0.2	16	81	3
Garlic cloves (½ c/68 g)	101	4	16	81	3
Jerusalem artichokes, sliced (½ c/75 g)	55	1	10	90	0
Kale, chopped (1 c/67 g)	34	2	22	67	11
Kale juice (1 c/229 g)**	64	6	39	50	11
Kelp, fresh, chopped (½ c/40 g)	17	0.7	14	76	10
Leeks, chopped (1 c/89 g)	54	1	9	87	4
Lettuce, Bibb, Boston, butterhead, chopped (1 c/54 g)	7	0.7	33	55	12
Lettuce, iceberg, chopped (1 c/55 g)	10	0.6	22	71	8
Lettuce, leaf, chopped (1 c/36 g)	5	0.5	30	62	8
Lettuce, red leaf, chopped (1 c/28 g)	4	0.4	33	55	12
Lettuce, romaine, chopped (1 c/47 g)	8	0.6	24	63	13
Mushrooms, whole (1 c/96 g)	23	3	37	60	3
Mushrooms, shiitake, dried (¼ c/36 g)	121	9	31	62	7
Mustard greens, chopped (1 c/56 g)	15	2	34	60	6
Okra, sliced, cooked (½ c/80 g)	18	2	27	66	7
Olives (10 large/44 g)	51	0.4	4	7	89
Onion, green, each (0.2 oz/5 g)	5	0.3	19	77	4
Onions, green, chopped (1 c/100 g)	32	2	19	77	4
Onions, red/white/yellow, chopped (½ c/80 g)	32	0.9	10	88	2
Parsley, chopped (1 c/64 g)	23	2	27	57	16
Parsnips, sliced, cooked (½ c/78 g)	63	1	6	91	3
Pea pods, snow/edible (1 c/63 g)	26	2	26	70	4
Pepper, bell, green, chopped (1 c/149 g)	30	1	14	79	7

FOOD	CALORIES	PROTEIN (g)	CALORIES FROM PROTEIN (%)	CALORIES FROM CARBS (%)	CALORIES FROM FAT (%)
Pepper, bell, green, each (4.2 oz/119 g)	24	1	14	79	7
Pepper, bell, red, chopped (1 c/149 g)	46	1	13	78	9
Potato, baked, each (6 oz/170 g)	189	4	8	91	1
Potato, cubed, cooked (½ c/75 g)	52	1	10	89	1
Radish, daikon, dried (½ c/58 g)	157	5	11	87	2
Radish, daikon, each (12 oz/340 g)	0.8	0	16	79	5
Radish, each (0.15 oz/4.5 g)	0.8	0	16	79	5
Radishes, sliced (½ c/58 g)	9	0.4	16	79	5
Radish sprouts (1 c/38 g)	16	1	29	28	43
Rutabaga, chopped, cooked (½ c/85 g)	33	1	12	83	5
Spinach, chopped (1 c/30 g)	7	0.9	39	49	12
Spirulina, dried (1 tbsp/7 g)	22	4	58	24	18
Squash, acorn, cubed, baked (½ c/102 g)	57	1	7	91	2
Squash, butternut, cubed, baked (½ c/102 g)	41	1	8	90	2
Squash, crookneck, cubed, cooked (½ c/90 g)	18	0.9	15	73	12
Squash, Hubbard, cubed, baked (½ c/120 g)	60	3	17	74	9
Squash, summer, cubed, cooked (½ c/90 g)	18	0.8	15	73	12
Sweet potato, cooked, mashed (½ c/164 g)	125	2	7	91	2
Tomato, cherry, each (0.6 oz/17 g)	3	0.2	17	74	9
Tomato, red, chopped (1 c/180 g)	32	2	17	74	9
Tomato, red, each (4.3 oz/123 g)	22	1	17	74	9
Tomato, Roma, each (2.2 oz/61 g)	11	0.6	17	74	9
Tomatoes, sun-dried (½ c/27 g)	70	4	18	73	9
Turnip, cooked, mashed (½ c/115 g)	25	0.8	12	85	3
Turnip greens, chopped (1 c/55 g)	18	0.8	16	77	7
Watercress, chopped (1 c/34 g)	4	0.8	60	34	6
Water chestnuts, sliced (¼ c/31 g)	30	0.4	5	94	1
Yam, baked, cubed (½ c/100 g)	90	2	9	90	1
Zucchini, baby, each (0.4 oz/10 g)	2	0.3	40	47	13
Zucchini, cubed (1 c/124 g)	20	2	25	67	8
FRUITS					
Apple, chopped (½ c/62 g)	32	0.2	2	95	3
Apple, each (6.4 oz/182 g)	95	0.5	2	95	3
Apples, dried (¼ c/40 g)	110	1	4	96	0
Apricot, each (1.2 oz/35 g)	17	0.5	10	83	7

FOOD	CALORIES	PROTEIN (g)	CALORIES FROM PROTEIN (%)	CALORIES FROM CARBS (%)	CALORIES FROM FAT (%)
Apricots, dried (¼ c/32 g)	77	1	5	93	2
Apricots, sliced (½ c/82 g)	40	1	10	83	7
Banana, dried (¼ c/25 g)	86	1	4	92	4
Banana, each (4.2 oz/119 g)	105	1	4	93	3
Banana, sliced (½ c/79 g)	71	0.9	4	93	3
Blackberries (½ c/72 g)	31	1	11	80	9
Blueberries (½ c/74 g)	45	0.6	5	90	5
Blueberries, dried (¼ c/40 g)	140	1	3	97	0
Cantaloupe, diced (½ c/82 g)	28	0.7	9	87	4
Cherimoya, chopped (½ c/78 g)	73	1	5	92	3
Coconut, dried, shredded (¼ c/23 g)	116	1	4	13	83
Coconut milk, fresh (½ c/127 g)	292	3	4	9	87
Crabapples, sliced (½ c/55 g)	42	0.2	2	95	3
Currants, fresh (½ c/56 g)	31–35	0.8	8–9	87–88	3–5
Currants, Zante, dried (¼ c/36 g)	103	1	5	94	1
Dates, chopped (¼ c/37 g)	104	0.9	3	96	1
Durian, chopped (½ c/122 g)	179	2	4	66	30
Fig, fresh, each (1.8 oz/50 g)	37	0.4	4	93	3
Figs, dried (¼ c/50 g)	129	2	4	92	4
Gooseberries (½ c/75 g)	33	0.7	7	82	11
Grapefruit, each (8.7 oz/246 g)	103	2	7	90	3
Grapefruit juice (½ c/130 g)	51	0.7	5	93	2
Grapefruit sections (½ c/115 g)	37	0.7	7	90	3
Grape juice, bottled (½ c/126 g)	77	0.7	4	95	1
Grapes (½ c/80 g)	55	0.5	3	93	4
Guava, diced (½ c/82 g)	56	2	13	76	11
Honeydew melon, diced (½ c/85 g)	31	0.5	5	92	3
Kiwifruit, diced (½ c/90 g)	57	2	7	86	7
Kiwifruit, each (69 g)	42	0.8	4	86	10
Loganberries (½ c/72 g)	31	1	11	80	9
Mango, dried (¼ c/30 g)	106	0	0	100	0
Mango, each (7.3 oz/207 g)	135	1	3	94	3
Mango, sliced (½ c/82 g)	54	0.4	3	94	3
Orange, each (4.6 oz/131 g)	62	1	7	91	2
Orange juice (½ c/124 g)	56	0.9	6	90	4

FOOD	CALORIES	PROTEIN (g)	CALORIES FROM PROTEIN (%)	CALORIES FROM CARBS (%)	CALORIES FROM FAT (%)
Orange sections (½ c/90 g)	45	0.9	7	91	2
Papaya, cubed (½ c/70 g)	27	0.4	6	91	3
Peach, dried, each (13 g)	37	0.7	7	93	0
Peach, each (5 oz/150 g)	58	1	6	88	6
Peach, sliced (½ c/77 g)	30	0.7	8	87	5
Pear, each (6.3 oz/178 g)	103	0.7	2	96	2
Pear, sliced (½ c/70 g)	41	0.3	2	96	2
Pear halves, dried (1.2 oz/35 g)	92	0.7	3	95	2
Pineapple, diced (½ c/82 g)	41	0.4	4	94	2
Plum, each (2.6 oz/75 g)	35	0.5	5	86	9
Plums, sliced (½ c/82 g)	45	0.7	5	86	9
Prunes, dried (¼ c/44 g)	104	1	4	95	1
Raisins, packed (¼ c/41 g)	123	1	4	95	1
Raspberries (½ c/62 g)	30	0.6	7	84	9
Strawberries (½ c/74 g)	24	0.5	7	86	7
Strawberries, dried (¼ c/20 g)	75	0.5	3	97	0
Watermelon, diced (½ c/76 g)	23	0.5	7	89	4
OILS AND SWEETENERS					
Flaxseed oil (1 tbsp/14 g)	122	0	0	0	100
Olive oil (1 tbsp/14 g)	119	0	0	0	100
Granulated cane sugar (1 tbsp/12 g)	48	0	0	100	0
Maple syrup (1 tbsp/20 g)	52	0	0	99	1
ANIMAL PRODUCTS					
Beef, ground round, 15% fat (1 oz/30 g)	60	5	36	0	64
Cheddar cheese, medium (1 oz/30 g)*	111	7	24	4	72
Egg, large, each (1.7 oz/50 g)	72	6	33	3	64
Milk, 2% (1 c/244 g)	121	8	27	39	35
Chicken breast with skin (1 oz/30 g)	48	6	50	0	50
Salmon, Atlantic, farmed or wild (1 oz/30 g)	40–51	6	45–58	0	42–55

Sources of data: US Department of Agriculture, Agricultural Research Service, *USDA National Nutrient Database for Standard Reference*, Release 25 (2012), ndb.nal.usda.gov. ESHA Research, The Food Processor software, version 10.12.0.

Key: c = cup; g = gram; oz = ounce; tbsp = tablespoon.

*Check labels for product-specific information.

**Laboratory analysis by Cantest Lab, arranged by authors.

Meat, eggs, and cheese are significant protein sources, with 24 to 36 percent of their calories coming from protein. However, what is truly distinctive about these animal products is their high levels of fat and cholesterol. Meat, eggs, and cheese could be viewed primarily as sources of fat, rather than protein, since 60 to 75 percent of their calories are derived from fat. As you can see in table 3.3, many plant foods provide 25 to 35 percent of calories from protein, and veggie meat analogs go even higher—but without cholesterol, and typically with much less fat.

The Soy Controversy

Soy is well-known for its top-quality protein and the protection it offers against certain chronic diseases. At the same time, there may be more controversy surrounding soy than any other food. The roots of the controversy lie in both good science and bad science, and perhaps in the fact that soy poses a threat to the animal products industry. Also see "The Soy-Cancer Debate".

Research has established that the components in soy known as isoflavones have certain protective effects, including reducing hot flashes and perhaps wrinkles. They bind to estrogen receptors in women and girls, and one or two servings per day over a lifetime can protect women against breast cancer, but that protective effect appears to be linked to consumption of soy in childhood and/or adolescence. For women who have had breast cancer, soy and its isoflavones decrease the risk of recurrence and death from breast cancer. Soy also provides health benefits to men. Among men who regularly consume soy foods risk of prostate cancer is reduced by an estimated 26 percent. In addition, significant evidence indicates that eating one or two servings of soy foods per day can lower levels of LDL (bad cholesterol).

However, people with thyroid problems should limit soy, which can affect the thyroid in people who are subject to hypothyroidism and in those who are deficient in iodine. Solutions involve adjusting the dosage of thyroid hormone for those with hypothyroidism and consuming adequate iodine to avert deficiency. (For more on iodine see chapter 7.) For these individuals, it makes sense to limit soy consumption until the thyroid problem is corrected.

The bottom line is that, although soy isn't an essential part of a vegan diet, including some soy foods in the diet is an excellent and often easy way for adults and particularly for children to achieve recommended intakes of protein. Edamame, or young whole soybeans, are a natural, unprocessed form that's generally easier to digest. Tofu and soy milk are versatile soy foods with proven nutritional and health benefits, as evidenced over centuries of use across Asia. Tempeh is similar, and the fermentation process it undergoes enhances its digestibility and increases the availability of its minerals. Soy protein isolate (aka isolated soy protein) is highly refined but also provides concentrated, high-quality protein in a convenient form as veggie meats or protein powder. Rather than judging one of these forms of soy as better than another, it makes sense to regard them as variations that are suited to various uses, occasions, or dietary preferences. Be sure to choose organic soy foods.

The Final Word on Protein

Getting enough protein is easily accomplished on a plant-based diet, especially once you learn simple and tasty ways to include beans, peas, lentils, and soy foods in your diet. As a bonus, these high-protein ingredients also deliver iron, zinc, lysine, tryptophan, and many other nutrients. They also help stabilize blood sugar levels. For these reasons, this book emphasizes the use of legumes, and its companion volume, *Cooking Vegan,* by V. Melina and J. Forest (Book Publishing Company, 2012), provides recipes for delicious protein-rich dips, spreads, soups, entrées, and desserts. Beyond legumes, many vegetables, seeds, nuts, and grains contain plenty of protein.

An advantage of the many high-protein plant foods is that they tend to be low in fat, and the fat tends to be the kind our bodies need. In the next chapter, we will learn that fat isn't always the pariah that it's made out to be. There's good fat, and then there's bad fat. Know the difference.

CHAPTER 4

Fat Matters

For years, the lack of animal fat and cholesterol was the trump card that set vegan diets apart and attracted people afflicted with chronic diet-related diseases or who wanted to prevent them. Today, however, there's controversy over whether fat is the bogeyman we were led to believe, or whether refined carbohydrates bear more of the responsibility for so many diseases. And if fat is the culprit, are all fats bad? In this chapter, we'll cut through the confusion, starting with some basic definitions.

A Primer in Fats

Fat is one of the three macronutrients. Like protein and carbohydrates, fat provides energy for the body. Fat supplies 9 calories per gram, more than twice the energy of protein or carbohydrate. However calorie for calorie, fat is less filling, which may partially explain the link between high-fat diets and weight gain.

In addition to providing energy, fat is also an essential component of cell membranes and is used to make hormones and hormonelike substances that help control many body systems. In digestion, it aids in the absorption of phytochemicals and some vitamins. In addition, fat provides physical padding and insulation that shields the body from extreme temperatures. It also serves as a shock absorber for vital organs, allowing us to take part in high-impact physical activities. Fat is also important for healthy skin, hair, and bones.

GOOD FATS VERSUS BAD FATS

While fats are essential to life, they are not all equal: some are good, some are bad, and others are downright ugly.

The good fats are those in whole plant foods. They come neatly packaged with protein, unrefined carbohydrate, fiber, phytochemicals, phytosterols, antioxidants, and a variety of vitamins and minerals. All plant foods contain some fat, but the most concentrated fat sources are nuts, seeds, avocados, coconuts, and olives. The fat in plant foods is largely unsaturated, with the exception of coconut and palm oils, which are predominately saturated. Although saturated fats are linked to increased risk of certain diseases, when consumed as a part of a whole-foods, plant-based diet, there is little evidence suggesting adverse effects.

It's best to obtain fat through whole foods, since processing exposes them to oxygen, light, and often heat and harsh chemicals, all of which can damage the fat. Plus, refining removes most of the protective components associated with the whole food. However, if properly stored, unrefined expeller-pressed oils can be a source of healthful fats.

Bad fats are so called because they are strongly linked to increases in cholesterol, insulin resistance, colorectal cancer, and lung cancer. They are found primarily in meat and dairy products and are mostly saturated.

Ugly fats are those that wreak havoc in the body and are implicated in many diseases. Trans-fatty acids and fats damaged by exposure to high heat fall into this category. Trans-fatty acids raise cholesterol levels, trigger inflammation, increase insulin resistance, and compete against essential fatty acids for incorporation into cells. Fats heated to high temperatures can be carcinogenic. Ugly fats are mostly found in deep-fried fast foods and in processed foods. In the latter case, they will be noted in the nutritional information on the package. It's best to avoid them completely.

Of course, the terms "good," "bad," and "ugly" are neither scientific nor precise. So in the sections that follow, we'll define some key terms in regard to fats.

FATTY ACIDS

Fatty acids, also sometimes referred to as lipids, are the basic components of fats and oils.

All foods contain three types of fatty acids in varying amounts: monounsaturated, polyunsaturated, and saturated. Those names refer to the amount of hydrogen attached to the carbon atoms in the fatty acid. The more hydrogen, the more saturated they are.

Monounsaturated fats. In monounsaturated fats, one spot in the carbon chain isn't bound to hydrogen (hence "mono"). Oils rich in monounsaturated fats, such as olive oil, are generally liquid at room temperature but become cloudy and thick when refrigerated. The richest dietary sources of monounsaturated fat are olives, olive oil, canola oil, avocados, and nuts and their oils and butters, with the exception of walnuts, butternuts (also known as white walnuts), and pine nuts. Monounsaturated fat has been shown to have neutral or slightly beneficial effects on health, with modest beneficial effects on cholesterol levels. Replacing saturated fat, trans-fatty acids, or refined carbohydrates with monounsaturated fat reduces total and LDL (bad cholesterol) and slightly increases HDL (good cholesterol).

Polyunsaturated fats. In polyunsaturated fats, more than one spot in the carbon chain isn't bound to hydrogen. Oils high in polyunsaturated fat are liquid when refrigerated. Polyunsaturated fats generally have favorable effects on health and are present in many plant foods, especially vegetable oils, seeds, nuts, grains, and legumes. When it replaces saturated fat, trans-fatty acids, or refined carbohydrates in the diet, total and LDL cholesterol levels decrease and HDL may slightly increase.

Saturated fats. In saturated fats, the carbon chain is completely packed or "saturated" with hydrogen. Saturated fat is generally solid at room temperature, as is the case with butter and other animal fats. Most high-fat plant foods contain much less saturated fat than animal fats with the exception of tropical oils. Coconut fat is close to 90 percent saturated, palm kernel oil about 85 percent saturated, and palm oil is about 50 percent saturated. High intakes of saturated fat have been linked to an increased risk of coronary artery disease and insulin resistance. Despite current controversy as a result of contradictory findings in 2010, most of the scientific studies since the mid-1990s have found an association between saturated fat intake and higher risk for diabetes and cardiovascular disease. But again, when saturated fats are consumed as a part of a whole-foods, plant-based diet, there is little evidence suggesting adverse effects.

Cholesterol. Cholesterol is a type of fat called a sterol. It's necessary to the structure of every cell, but the body makes all the cholesterol it needs, so there's no need to eat foods containing it. Only animal foods contain cholesterol. High intakes may increase the risk of chronic diseases, especially those of the heart and blood vessels.

Phytosterols. Phytosterols, or plant sterols, are healthful fats and help block cholesterol absorption in the gut. All whole plant foods contain small amounts of phytosterols. The most concentrated sources are vegetable oils, seeds, nuts, avocados, wheat germ, legumes, and sprouts.

Trans-fatty acids. You have undoubtedly heard of trans-fatty acids, or trans fats. These are fats formed by partial hydrogenation, an industrial process that converts liquid oil into solid fat by adding hydrogen until the fat is almost, but not completely "saturated." (Trans-fatty acids also are found naturally in some animal products, but only in minute quantities.) Although partially hydrogenated vegetable oils were originally introduced as more healthful substitutes for lard and butter, they have since been found to be even more damaging to human health, strongly increasing the risk of cardiovascular diseases. Although the partially hydrogenated fats found naturally in animal products don't appear to be as damaging to the cardiovascular system, they may increase insulin resistance more than manufactured trans fats. In addition, natural trans-fatty acids reduce levels of HDL cholesterol and markedly increase lipid peroxidation, a process that leads to cell damage. In North America, efforts are underway to remove artificial trans fats from the food supply.

Back to the Essentials

There are two distinct families of polyunsaturated fats: omega-3 fatty acids and omega-6 fatty acids. These fats are required for the synthesis of many compounds that regulate immune and inflammatory responses, are important structural components of cell membranes, and are necessary for nervous system function and vision.

Each of these families contains one essential fatty acid (EFA). They are called essential because the body cannot make them, yet they are necessary for life. The two essential fatty acids are alpha-linolenic acid (ALA), the foundation or parent of the omega-3 family, and linoleic acid (LA), the parent of the omega-6 family. The essential fatty acids can be converted into larger, long-chain fatty acids: ALA to eicosapentaenoic acid (EPA) and docosahexaenoic acid (DHA) and LA to gamma-linolenic acid (GLA) and arachidonic acid (AA). These long-chain fatty acids are used to produce hormonelike compounds that have a significant benefit on many body functions, including blood clotting, blood pressure, immune response, cell division, pain, inflammation, and numerous diseases. Vegans must rely on conversion to produce important long-chain fatty acids, as animal products are the primary dietary sources. While vegans tend to produce plenty of long-chain omega-6 fatty acids, omega-3 conversion can be more precarious. There are several steps vegans can take to maximize conversion, and to ensure good EFA status.

GETTING ENOUGH OMEGA-3S

EPA plays an important role in reducing chronic inflammation and may protect against certain mental disorders. Plus, the body can convert EPA to DHA, which is necessary for the development and maintenance of brain and eye function. On average, vegans' blood levels of EPA and DHA are about half those of omnivores. The breast milk of vegan women contains only about 38 percent of the DHA found in the breast milk of omnivores, according to one study. There's some evidence that low levels of DHA in pregnant and nursing women could lead to less visual acuity, growth, development, and cognition in babies and toddlers. However, research on the growth and development of vegan children has failed to reveal any deficiencies in visual or mental development when mothers get sufficient vitamin B_{12} and enough calories. In any case, it seems prudent for vegans to ensure their omega-3 status is optimal.

Begin by eating a nutritionally adequate diet. By following the food guide in chapter 14, you'll make sure you're getting sufficient protein, vitamins, and minerals to maximize your ability to convert ALA into the more biologically active EPA and DHA. Avoid trans-fatty acids and excess consumption of alcohol or caffeine, since they can reduce your ability to convert ALA.

Include good sources of ALA in your diet. The richest sources are chia seeds, ground flaxseeds, hempseeds, and walnuts. Select oils rich in omega-3s, such as cold-pressed flaxseed oil or hempseed oil, or balanced oils that include plenty of omega-3s, for use in uncooked foods and salad dressings. Try Liquid Gold salad dressing for a boost in omega-3s. See Sources of Essential Fatty Acids for food sources of omega-3 and omega-6 acids; then take a look at table 4.1 for the specific amounts of these fatty acids in a variety of foods.

Sources of Essential Fatty Acids

Getting sufficient essential fatty acids, with a ratio of omega-6s to omega-3s ranging from about 2 to 1 to 4 to 1, is an important step in optimizing conversion of ALA to EPA and DHA. For most people, this means eating more omega-3 fatty acids, and in some cases, cutting back a little on omega-6s. However, as you'll see, many foods, such as soybeans, wheat germ, and walnuts are sources of both. For more precise information, see table 4.3. Also, just for the record, regular eggs contain small amounts of DHA, whereas the eggs from chickens given feed rich in omega-3s are considerably higher.

The following lists of sources of omega-3s and omega-6s can help you make better choices.

SOURCES OF OMEGA-3 FATTY ACIDS

Alpha-linolenic acid (ALA)
Canola oil
Chia seeds and chia oil
Flaxseeds and flaxseed oil
Green leafy land and sea vegetables
Soybeans and soybean oil
Walnuts and walnut oil
Wheat germ and wheat germ oil

Eicosapentaenoic acid (EPA) and decosahexaenoic acid (DHA)
Breast milk
Eggs
Fish and seafood, particularly cold-water, oily fish
Microalgae (not blue-green algae)
Sea vegetables (mostly EPA)

SOURCES OF OMEGA-6 FATTY ACIDS

Linoleic acid (LA):
Corn kernels and corn oil
Grapeseed oil
Hempseeds and hempseed oil
Pine nuts
Pumpkin seeds and pumpkin seed oil
Safflower oil
Sesame seeds and sesame seed oil

Soybeans and soybean oil
Sunflower seeds and sunflower seed oil
Walnuts and walnut oil
Wheat germ and wheat germ oil
Gamma-linolenic acid (GLA)
Black currant oil
Borage oil
Evening primrose oil
Hempseed oil
Spirulina

To ensure sufficient ALA for conversion, most vegans will need to double the RDA. This means at least 3.2 grams of ALA for men and 2.2 grams ALA for women. The higher ALA intakes help to shift the balance of essential fatty acids towards more efficient conversion. If you take daily DHA or EPA supplements, the RDA for ALA is sufficient—at least 1.6 grams per day for men and 1.1 grams for women. Table 4.2 lists the recommended daily intakes for both those who rely solely on ALA and those who also include DHA or EPA supplements. In addition to dietary factors, conversion can be adversely affected by genetics, male gender, advancing age, smoking, and chronic diseases such as diabetes, metabolic syndrome, hypertension, and high cholesterol levels.

TABLE 4.1. Essential fatty acid content of selected plant foods

FOOD	SERVING SIZE	ALA (% OF FATTY ACIDS)	LA (% OF FATTY ACIDS)	RATIO OF OMEGA-6 TO OMEGA-3	ALA (g)
Chia seeds	2 tbsp/30 ml (20 g)	58	20	0.34 to 1	4.0
Flaxseed oil	1 tbsp/15 ml (14 g)	54	14	0.26 to 1	7.3
Flaxseeds, ground	2 tbsp/30 ml (14 g)	54	14	0.26 to 1	3.2
Spinach, raw	1 c/250 ml (50–60 g)	58	11	0.19 to 1	0.04
Hempseed oil	1 tbsp/15 ml (14 g)	18	57	3 to 1	2.5
Hempseeds	2 tbsp/30 ml (20 g)	18	57	3 to 1	1.7
Walnuts, English	¼ c/60 ml (28 g)	14	58	4 to 1	2.6

Sources of data: US Department of Agriculture, Agricultural Research Service, *USDA National Nutrient Database for Standard Reference*, Release 25 (2012), ndb.nal.usda.gov. Sanders, T., and Lewis, F., "Review of Nutritional Attributes of Good Oil (Cold Pressed Hemp Seed Oil)," Nutritional Sciences Division, King's College London (2008), goodwebsite.co.uk/kingsreport.pdf.

Key: c = cup (250 ml); g = gram; ml = milliliter; tbsp = tablespoon.

TABLE 4.2. Adequate intake (AI) of omega-3 fatty acids and suggested intakes for vegans

ADEQUATE INTAKE (AI)	DAILY AI OF ALA	SUGGESTED DAILY INTAKE OF ALA WITHOUT EPA/DHA SOURCES	SUGGESTED DAILY INTAKE OF ALA WITH EPA/DHA SOURCES
Infants 0–12 months	0.5 g	N/A*	Omega-3s from breast milk are adequate. If using formula, select one with DHA.
Children 1–3 years	0.7 g	1.4 g	Breast milk or 0.7 g ALA + 70 mg DHA
Children 4–8 years	0.9 g	1.8 g	0.9 g ALA + 90 mg DHA/EPA
Boys 9–13 years	1.2 g	2.4 g	1.2 g ALA + 120 mg DHA/EPA
Girls 9–13 years	1.0 g	2.0 g	1.0 g ALA + 100 mg DHA/EPA
Males 14+ years	1.6 g	3.2 g	1.6 g ALA + 160 mg DHA/EPA
Females 14+ years	1.1 g	2.2 g	1.1 g ALA + 110 mg DHA/EPA
Pregnancy	1.4 g	2.8 g	1.4 g ALA + 200–300 mg DHA
Lactation	1.3 g	2.6 g	1.3 g ALA + 200–300 mg DHA

Sources of data: National Research Council, *Dietary Reference Intakes for Energy, Carbohydrate, Fiber, Fat, Fatty Acids, Cholesterol, Protein, and Amino Acids (Macronutrients)* (Washington, DC: National Academies Press, 2005). Saunders, A., et al., "Omega-3 Polyunsaturated Fatty Acids and Vegetarian Diets," *MJA Open* 1, no. 2 (2012): 22–25.

Key: g = gram; mg = milligram.

*Not applicable because infants get DHA from breast milk or appropriate commercial formula.

Keep tabs on your omega-6 intake. Too much omega-6 can reduce omega-3 conversion, increasing health risk. For vegans, the ideal ratio of omega-6s to omega-3s ranges between 2 to 1 and 4 to 1. For most people this means an omega-6 intake of about 9 to 13 grams daily. Getting too much omega-6 is easy, especially if you use cooking oils rich in omega-6s, such as sunflower, safflower, corn, grapeseed, or sesame oil. Many processed foods rely on oils that contain a lot of omega-6s, so try to limit those. If you use cooking oils or packaged foods containing oils, look for those that are mainly monounsaturated, such as extra-virgin olive oil, organic canola oil, or high-oleic sunflower or safflower oil. While these oils provide some omega-6s, they are present in much smaller quantities.

While it is possible to push your intake of omega-6s too high even when eating whole foods, this isn't an issue for most people. However, a sure way to keep omega-6 intake under control is to minimize use of oils rich in omega-6s and limit consumption of foods rich in omega-6s, such as pumpkin seeds, sunflower seeds, sesame seeds, and pine nuts, to about 1 ounce (30g) per day in a 2,000-calorie diet.

It's also important to recognize that while the fats from avocados and most nuts are mainly monounsaturated, these foods do contribute omega-6s. Most nuts contain 1 to 3 grams of omega-6s per ounce (30g), and pecans have almost 6 grams, while half an avocado provides less than 2 grams. Grains are also far higher in omega-6s than omega-3s, so including some concentrated omega-3 sources can help bring omega-6s into balance.

Consider including direct sources of DHA and EPA in your diet. While this isn't essential, there's good evidence that doing so will boost your omega-3 status. This is especially important during pregnancy and lactation, and also for people who have diabetes or hypertension, who may have difficulty with conversion.

The only vegan sources of EPA and DHA are microalgae and sea vegetables. Vegan supplements providing DHA or DHA plus EPA are widely available, but they're relatively expensive. For most people, an intake of 100 to 300mg per day is reasonable. (For sources, do an Internet search using "vegan DHA" or "vegan DHA and EPA.") Microalgae-based DHA is also being added to some soy milks, cold-pressed oils, juices, cereals, and other foods, although the amounts are relatively small.

Blue-green algae (spirulina and *Aphanizomenon flos-aquae*) are low in EPA and DHA. Spirulina is rich in GLA, while about 40 to 50 percent of the fat in *Aphanizomenon flos-aquae* is ALA. While blue-green algae isn't a significant source of EPA or DHA, some research indicates that it may promote more efficient omega-3 conversion than what is commonly seen with land plants.

To ensure sufficient omega-3 intake for infants, they should breast-feed for at least two years and beyond if possible, with mothers maintaining their intake of omega-3s. If breast-feeding stops before twelve months of age or formula is used as the primary milk, select a formula with added DHA. Once babies are weaned to fortified, full-fat soy milk (only after one year of age), they may benefit from a supplement providing 70mg of DHA per day. For pregnant and lactating women, DHA intakes of at least 200mg per day are recommended.

How Much Fat Do We Need?

One of the most fiercely debated issues in nutrition is how much fat we should eat. For years, the common belief was the less, the better. But recently the low-fat mantra has fallen out of favor, yielding to a more moderate message, and research is backing the idea that quality seems to trump quantity, particularly when calorie intakes aren't excessive.

Fat intakes vary significantly among healthy populations around the world, and it appears that the percent of total calories from fat is not a critical factor in terms of health and longevity. For example, traditional diets of rural Asians commonly provide about 10 to 15 percent of calories from fat, while those of healthy Mediterranean populations frequently exceed 35 percent of calories from fat. So what do the diets of these people, renowned for longevity, have in common?

First, these populations eat mostly plant foods and seldom consume highly processed fast food and convenience foods. Meat is typically reserved for special occasions, and some people avoid it altogether. Beans, whole grains, and garden vegetables are the foundation of the diet among populations with the greatest longevity.

In some regions, nuts, seeds, soy foods, antioxidant-rich spices, and red wine are also important parts of the diet.

Vegans display a similarly broad range in percent of calories from fat. At one end of the spectrum are adherents of a no-oil, very low-fat approach, and at the other are aficionados of a raw vegan diet, who may get 40 percent or more of their calories from fat because nuts and seeds are their primary sources of protein and they tend to eat fewer starchy foods, such as grains, legumes, and starchy vegetables. Yet somehow, people at both ends of the spectrum are healthy. As to what level of fat intake is best for the garden-variety vegan, it depends on many factors, including stage of life, state of health, metabolism, and the quality and types of fat consumed. The short answer is that a relatively broad range of fat intakes can be healthful, as long as the fat is good fat and calorie intake isn't excessive.

Most major health organizations agree that fat intake should range from a low of 15 to 20 percent of calories to a high of 35 percent of calories. They also agree that saturated fats, trans-fatty acids, and cholesterol should be restricted. There are no separate recommendations for vegans, and there's no reason to assume that their requirements would differ from those of nonvegans. However, limited evidence from studies on people eating a raw vegan diet suggests that higher total fat intakes can be healthful when the fat is from whole plant foods, such as nuts, seeds, and avocados.

If you're very physically active or require a lot of calories to maintain your body weight, you could probably aim toward the higher end of the range: 25 to 35 percent fat. If you're overweight, require fewer calories, or have a chronic disease, such as cardiovascular disease, it might be best to aim toward the lower end: 15 to 20 percent fat. A fat intake below 15 percent of calories can be safe and effective in the treatment and reversal of chronic disease. However, this generally isn't advised for healthy people, and it isn't suitable for children or adolescents.

Let's take a look at what those percentages translate to. Assuming a diet of 2,000 calories per day, at the lower end of the range you could eat 33 to 44 grams of fat per day, and at the higher end you could eat 66 to 77 grams. Most vegans average 30 percent of calories, compared to an average of 36 percent among people eating a standard American diet. While that 6 percent difference is significant, the sources of fat in the vegan diet are more noteworthy. Vegans eat no cholesterol and only about half as much saturated fat as omnivores. Trans-fatty acid intakes vary depending on how many convenience foods and other processed foods the person eats. However, many vegans eat negligible amounts of processed foods.

PROS AND CONS OF A VERY LOW-FAT DIET

Some of the most highly respected vegetarian and vegan health authorities recommend limiting fat in the diet to no more than 10 percent of total calories (22 grams on a diet of 2,000 calories per day) because they believe that this is the best way to protect against chronic disease. While there's little evidence to suggest that lower-fat diets are more protective against chronic disease, very lowfat diets have proven to be an effective therapeutic intervention for thousands of people with life-threatening chronic diseases. Considering the extent to which these diseases afflict Westerners, the value of that dietary approach cannot be ignored. Unfortunately, studies haven't yet compared the disease-fighting power of very low-fat vegan diets with vegan diets that provide more fat in the form of nuts, seeds, and other whole foods.

Low-fat proponents strongly advise against the use of concentrated fats and oils, yet the long-lived populations of the world use some oil in varying amounts. Many very low-fat regimens also minimize higher-fat plant foods, such as nuts, seeds, avocados, and olives, but studies examining the health effects of these foods are overwhelmingly positive. Eliminating or severely restricting higher-fat plant foods may end up being counterproductive. For example, vegan diets with fewer than 10 percent of calories from fat may not provide sufficient essential fatty acids. If you're eating a very low-fat vegan diet, make sure you at least add about 1 ounce (30g) of hempseeds or walnuts per day to ensure you're getting enough. Alternatively, eat a combination of about 1 ounce (30g) of flaxseeds plus pumpkin seeds, or chia seeds plus sunflower seeds.

You need some fat so your body can absorb certain phytochemicals and vitamins, such as A, D, E, and K. These nutrients are essential for health and provide protection against numerous diseases and health conditions. According to the Institute of Medicine, very low-fat diets also have been associated with inadequate intakes of zinc and some B vitamins, nutrients that are most abundant in higher-fat foods such as nuts and seeds.

Very low-fat, high-carbohydrate diets, especially those that rely on refined carbs, can cause a decline in HDL cholesterol and a rise in triglycerides, a situation associated with increased risk for coronary artery disease, metabolic syndrome, and type 2 diabetes. If you adhere to a high-carbohydrate diet, avoid foods made with white flour and sugar, and rely on whole plant foods such as legumes, vegetables, and whole grains to help keep triglyceride levels down.

While very low-fat, whole-foods vegan diets can cause a drop in HDL cholesterol, this is a natural consequence of total cholesterol reduction and may not be a health risk. The primary function of HDL is the removal of excess cholesterol from the bloodstream, so when there's less cholesterol to remove, less HDL is produced. In vegan populations, as well as other populations consuming low-fat plant-based diets, HDL levels are typically slightly lower than in the general population, yet risk for coronary artery disease is low.

Very low-fat, high-fiber diets may not provide enough calories for infants, children, and adults with high energy needs. Studies of malnutrition in vegetarians and vegans have shown that highly restrictive diets don't adequately support children's growth and development. In one study, vegan infants fourteen to sixteen months of age who had been fed diets with 17 percent of calories from fat were malnourished. Low-fat diets can also result in chronic diarrhea in children. Until we know more, vegan parents should make sure their children get enough fat: 55 percent of calories from fat up to six months of age, 30 to 40 percent of calories from fat for children between six months and three years old, and 25 to 35 percent of calories from fat for those between four and eighteen years old.

Don't make avoiding fat the highest priority when selecting foods. A fat-free sugar-based commercial salad dressing may indeed be in line with a low-fat diet, but that doesn't make it healthful. Homemade tahini dressing with lemon juice provides far greater nutritional value. Plant foods with a higher fat content—nuts, seeds, wheat germ, avocados, olives, and soy foods—are the most valuable fat sources for all vegans beyond one year of age. They provide important nutrients, including a variety of antioxidants, trace minerals, and protective phytochemicals.

PROS AND CONS OF A HIGH-FAT DIET

High-fat diets, defined as more than 35 percent of calories from fat, have long been thought to contribute to obesity and a variety of chronic diseases. However, there are some healthy populations who have long consumed diets with more than 35 percent of calories from fat, including some Mediterranean communities and many people on raw diets. Some leading health authorities promote Mediterranean diets as being optimal for health and encourage liberal use of higher-fat foods, especially olive oil.

In 1980, the well-known Seven Countries Study by biologist Ancel Keys showed a strong connection between total fat, saturated fat, and coronary artery disease. As fat intake increased, so did coronary artery disease, with one important exception: residents of the Greek island of Crete, where people averaged 37 percent of calories from fat, had the lowest rates of all the countries studied, including Japan, where average fat intake was only 11 percent of calories.

What seems to separate the people of Crete and other healthy Mediterranean populations from less healthy populations who also eat high-fat diets is the type of fat they consume. The traditional diet of Crete includes abundant plant foods and olive oil and typically includes less than 2 ounces (60g) of meat, poultry, or fish per day. In addition, most Cretans fast during the forty days of Lent, and an unknown number also follow Greek Orthodox dietary doctrines that prescribe almost 180 days of fasting each year, which involves abstention from meat, fish, dairy products, and eggs, and even olive oil. While these practices weren't factored into the results of Keys's study, leading experts from the University of Crete believe that the regular restriction of certain foods, notably those of animal origin, have significant health benefits.

Mediterranean diets provide a compelling argument that the quality of fat trumps the quantity as a predictor of health outcomes—if you don't eat too many calories. However, even good fats may increase the risk of disease when eaten to excess. High-fat diets have been linked to chronic medical conditions, such as cardiovascular diseases, metabolic syndrome, diabetes, gallbladder disease, and some cancers. The fats implicated here are saturated fats and trans-fatty acids, and vegans tend to eat less of these, but evidence still indicates that diets very high in fat (more than 42 percent of calories from fat) can potentially increase risk for heart disease, no matter what the source of the fat.

Another issue is that concentrated fats and oils, including vegetable oils, are packed with calories—about 120 calories per tablespoon—but contribute few vitamins, minerals, and phytochemicals and no fiber. Therefore, a high-fat diet can dilute nutrient density, meaning you get fewer nutrients per calorie consumed. This makes it a challenge to eat enough to achieve sufficient intakes of many nutrients, especially trace minerals such as zinc and selenium. This is particularly problematic when the main sources of fat are concentrated, as in vegetable oils, margarine, mayonnaise-type spreads, coconut oil, and foods prepared or manufactured with these fats, as opposed to whole foods such as nuts, seeds, soybeans, avocados, and olives. Although unrefined expeller-pressed or cold-pressed oils are generally richer sources of essential fatty acids, vitamin E, and phytochemicals, most of the oils on supermarket shelves are highly refined—another reason to get your fats and nutrients from whole foods.

High-fat diets can make you fat. Because fat is a concentrated source of calories, you can get a lot of calories in a very small amount of a high-fat food, which can lead you to consume more calories than your body needs. If you have a tendency toward being overweight, try eating a diet that contains only moderate amounts of fat.

Another problem with a very high-fat diet is that it makes it difficult for the body to convert essential fatty acids to their usable form. This can increase the risk of chronic diseases and adversely affect mood and energy levels, particularly for vegans and others who don't consume direct sources of EPA and DHA. Finally, free radicals—those compounds that cause oxidative damage to body tissues—are more likely to react with the polyunsaturated fats found in oils such as corn, sunflower, safflower, and soybean. Oxidative stress has been linked to increased risk of numerous diseases, including heart disease, cancer, diabetes, arthritis, age-related diseases, and neurological disorders.

Good Vegan Fats

As mentioned, a number of highly respected vegan health advocates have taken a hard-line view against fats of all types. Although there's evidence that very low-fat vegan diets can improve severe coronary artery disease, there's little evidence that such diets are the gold standard for healthy vegans. There are hundreds of scientific studies that have demonstrated that high-fat plant foods not only deserve a place in our diets, but that they deserve a place of honor.

NUTS

People tend to think of nuts in the same vein as potato chips: as high-fat foods that clog the arteries and lead to weight gain. It's time to put that misconception to rest, because eating nuts has consistently been shown to provide health advantages, reducing risk of chronic disease and increasing longevity. Evidence shows that people who eat nuts on a regular basis generally have a lower body mass index (BMI), smaller waist, less hypertension, higher HDL levels, lower fasting blood sugar levels, and significantly less risk for coronary heart disease. According to the Nurses Health Study, replacing dietary carbohydrates with the same amount of calories from nuts reduces the risk of coronary heart disease by about 30 percent, and replacing saturated fat with nuts may reduce the risk by about 45 percent. In addition, regular nut consumption may prevent stroke, type 2 diabetes, dementia, macular degeneration, gallstones, and all by eating just 1 to 2 ounces (30 to 60g) of nuts per day.

Nuts are nutrient-dense foods, brimming with an array of vitamins and minerals. Most of their fat is monounsaturated. They are also rich in compounds that help preserve the elasticity and flexibility of blood vessels, enhancing blood flow. But they're also high in calories, so keep your intake moderate—sprinkle them on foods rather than eating them by the bowlful.

SEEDS

Far less research has been conducted on seeds than on nuts, and their value tends to be underestimated. Seeds are the most plentiful sources of essential fatty acids. Pumpkin seeds, sunflower seeds, poppy seeds, hempseeds, and sesame seeds are rich in omega-6s. Flaxseeds, chia seeds, hempseeds, and canola seeds are rich in omega-3s. Seeds also are among the richest sources of vitamin E and provide an impressive array of other vitamins, minerals, and phytochemicals, along with protein and fiber.

Flaxseeds are a case in point. They have a remarkably high omega-3 content, so adding them to your diet can go a long way toward correcting any imbalance in intake. They are very high in soluble fiber, which lowers cholesterol, and are one of the richest known sources of the trace mineral boron. Flaxseeds can help reduce cholesterol levels and improve a number of other markers of coronary artery disease. They also are the richest known source of lignans (not to be confused with lignins, a type of fiber), which may help reduce the growth of cancer cells. (Be sure to use ground flaxseeds, since the body can't fully digest whole flaxseeds.)

Chia seeds, both whole and sprouted, are rapidly gaining popularity in plantbased diets. They are the only food higher in omega-3s than flaxseeds. They are also packed with antioxidants and other nutrients. A mere 2 tablespoons (30ml) of chia seeds contains 3.3mg of iron and 142mg of calcium.

Hempseeds also have exceptional nutritional value. About 20 percent of their calories come from easily digestible, high-quality protein, and they provide an impressive array of trace minerals, vitamins, and phytochemicals. Hempseed oil has an excellent ratio of omega-6 to omega-3 fatty acids. It is one of the few foods that provides both stearidonic acid (SDA), an omega-3 fatty acid that more readily converts to EPA than does ALA, and GLA, a beneficial omega-6 fatty acid.

AVOCADOS

Like other fat-rich plant foods, avocados offer some pleasant nutritional surprises. In addition to being rich in monounsaturated fatty acids, they possess high levels of nutrients, fiber, phytochemicals, and antioxidants. Avocados are rich in carotenoids, and vitamins C and E and contain more folate per ounce (30g) than any other fruit, 60 percent more potassium than bananas, and 13.5 grams of fiber per average fruit.

Avocados also contain phytosterols that can inhibit cholesterol absorption, help reduce cholesterol levels, and possibly inhibit tumor growth. In one study, people who followed a diet recommended by the American Heart Association to reduce cholesterol were compared with people who ate a diet that derived 20 to 35 percent of their total calories from avocados. Total cholesterol dropped an average of 4.9 percent among those on the Heart Association diet, but total cholesterol dropped 8.2 percent among those eating the avocado-rich diet.

Eating avocados may provide benefits in cancer prevention and treatment, in certain inflammatory diseases, and in lowering the side effects of certain chemotherapy drugs. There also is preliminary evidence that avocado extract is active against *Helicobacter pylori,* the bacteria associated with ulcers and stomach cancer, and that its anti-inflammatory effects may reduce the symptoms of knee and hip osteoarthritis.

OLIVES

Olives are an ancient food and a cherished part of the Mediterranean diet. They are good sources of copper, iron, and vitamin E, and are rich in phytosterols and a host of phytochemicals, particularly polyphenolic compounds. Oleuropein, the major polyphenol in olives, is a potent free radical scavenger, inhibiting oxidative damage and protecting heart tissue. Olives and olive oil also contain compounds with known anticancer and anti-inflammatory effects.

Raw olives are cured in order to leach out an alkaloid that makes them bitter and unpalatable. Various solutions can be used to cure olives, including water, brine, seasoned oil, or lye. Olives can also be dry cured by layering them with dry rock salt. The choice of curing agent affects the nutritional content of the olives and the sodium content.

Extra-virgin olive oil, which is obtained from the first pressing of the olives, is rich in bioactive compounds compared to more refined varieties. While olive oil has the advantage of being much lower in sodium than most types of olives, olives are whole plant foods, so they contain fiber, whereas olive oil doesn't. In addition, olive oil, like all oils, contains 120 calories per tablespoon (15ml), whereas ten large olives contain only 50 calories.

COCONUT

There are few foods that have been simultaneously so maligned and so acclaimed as coconut and coconut oil. Some view coconut oil as a notorious health villain because it's the most concentrated food source of saturated fat—even higher than lard. Not surprisingly, it rests at the very top of the "avoid" column of mainstream heart-healthy food lists. Others view coconut oil as a fountain of youth and the greatest health discovery in decades, claiming that it can provide therapeutic benefits for everything from Alzheimer's disease to thyroid disease.

The main reason that coconut oil is so often blacklisted by nutrition experts is because almost 90 percent of its fat is saturated, and people think of saturated fat as the sole culprit in clogging arteries. However, there are actually several different types of saturated fats, each with its own effects on cholesterol levels and health. The predominant saturated fat in coconut, lauric acid, does raise total cholesterol, but it appears to also raise HDL levels even more than LDL levels, favorably altering the ratio of total cholesterol to HDL—a ratio that is widely considered a more important predictor of coronary artery disease risk than levels of total cholesterol or LDL.

TABLE 4.3. Fatty acid composition of selected foods

FOOD/SERVING SIZE	CALORIES	TOTAL FAT (g)	SATURATED FAT (g)	MONOUN-SATURATED FAT (g)	OMEGA-6S (LA) (g)	OMEGA-3s		
						ALA (g)	EPA (mg)	DHA (mg)
OILS, 1 TBSP (15 ML)								
Canola oil	124	14	1	8.9	2.7	1.3	0	0
Coconut oil	117	13.6	11.8	0.8	0.25	0	0	0
Corn oil	120	13.6	1.7	3.8	7.3	0.16	0	0
Cottonseed oil	120	13.6	3.5	2.4	7	0.03	0	0
Flaxseed oil	120	13.6	1.2	2.5	1.9	7.3	0	0
Grapeseed oil	120	13.6	1.3	2.2	9.5	0.014	0	0
Hempseed oil	126	14	1.5	2	8	2.5	0	0
Olive oil	119	13.5	1.9	9.9	1.3	0.1	0	0
Palm kernel oil	117	13.6	11.1	1.6	0.2	0	0	0
Palm oil	120	13.6	6.7	5	1.2	0.03	0	0
Peanut oil	119	13.5	2.3	6.2	4.3	0	0	0
Safflower oil	120	13.6	0.8	2	10.1	0	0	0
Safflower oil, high-oleic	120	13.6	1	10.2	1.7	0.01	0	0
Sesame oil	120	13.6	1.9	5.4	5.6	0.04	0	0
Soybean oil	120	13.6	2.1	3.1	6.9	0.9	0	0
Sunflower oil	120	13.6	1.4	2.7	8.9	0	0	0
Sunflower oil, high-oleic	124	14	1.4	11.7	0.5	0.03	0	0
Walnut oil	120	13.6	1.2	3.1	7.2	1.4	0	0
NUTS, SEEDS, AND WHEAT GERM, 1 OZ (30 G)								
Almonds	163	14	1.06	8.8	3.4	0	0	0
Butternuts (white walnuts)	174	16	0.37	3	9.5	2.5	0	0
Cashews	157	12.4	2.2	6.7	2.2	0.018	0	0
Chia seeds, 2 tbsp (30 ml)	138	8.7	0.94	0.66	1.7	5.06	0	0
Flaxseeds, ground, 2 tbsp (30 ml)	75	5.9	0.51	1.05	0.8	3.2	0	0
Hazelnuts	178	17.2	1.3	12.9	2.2	0.025	0	0
Hempseeds, 2 tbsp (30 ml)	113	9	1	1	5.3	1.7	0	0
Macadamia nuts	204	21.5	3.4	16.7	0.37	0.06	0	0
Peanuts	161	14	1.9	6.9	4.4	0.001	0	0
Pecans	196	20.4	1.7	11.6	5.8	0.3	0	0
Pine nuts	191	19.4	1.4	5.3	9.4	0.05	0	0
Pistachios	159	12.9	1.6	6.8	3.8	0.073	0	0
Pumpkin seeds	158	13.9	2.5	4.6	5.9	0.034	0	0
Sesame seeds	165	14.3	2	5.4	6.2	0.1	0	0
Sunflower seeds	165	14.1	1.5	2.7	9.3	0.02	0	0
Walnuts	185	18.5	1.7	2.5	10.8	2.6	0	0
Wheat germ, 2 tbsp (30 ml)	52	1.4	0.24	0.20	0.76	0.1	0	0

FOOD/SERVING SIZE	CALORIES	TOTAL FAT (g)	SATURATED FAT (g)	MONOUN-SATURATED FAT (g)	OMEGA-6S (LA) (g)	OMEGA-3s		
						ALA (g)	EPA (mg)	DHA (mg)
SEA VEGETABLES AND MICROALGAE, 3.5 OZ (100 G) FRESH								
Irish moss	49	0.16	0.033	0.015	0.002	0.001	46	0
Kelp	43	0.56	0.25	0.1	0.02	0.004	4	0
Spirulina	26	0.39	0.14	0.03	0.064	0.042	0	0
Wakame	45	0.64	0.13	0.06	0.01	0.002	186	0
FRUITS AND VEGETABLES								
Avocado, medium, 7.4 oz (201 g)	322	29.5	4.3	19.7	3.4	0.25	0	0
Olives, 10 large (44 g)	51	4.7	0.623	3.5	0.37	0.03	0	0
Spinach, raw, 1 c (250 ml)	29	0.12	0.019	0.003	0.008	0.041	0	0
ANIMAL PRODUCTS (FOR COMPARISON)								
Cod, 3 oz (85 g)	89	0.73	0.14	0.11	0.005	0.001	30	131
Egg, 1 large	72	4.8	1.6	1.8	0.8	0.024	0	26
Salmon, wild Atlantic, 3 oz (85 g)	155	6.9	1.1	2.3	0.19	0.321	349	1,215

Sources of data: US Department of Agriculture, Agricultural Research Service, *USDA National Nutrient Database for Standard Reference*, Release 25 (2012), ndb.nal.usda.gov. Manitoba Harvest, manitobaharvest.com (for hempseeds and hempseed oil).

Key: g = gram; mg = milligram; ml = milliliter; oz = ounce; tbsp = tablespoon.

In addition, lauric acid converts into a powerful antiviral, antifungal, and antiseptic compound in the body, and there is also evidence that coconut products have anti-inflammatory and antioxidant powers. While the health effects of coconut and coconut oil remain somewhat uncertain, in many parts of the world where they are principle sources of dietary fat, rates of chronic disease, including coronary artery disease, are low. There is one major caveat in regard to coconut: its benefits seem to occur only when coconut products are consumed as part of a diet that is rich in unprocessed, high-fiber plant foods.

Based on the available science, coconut oil should be regarded like any other concentrated oil: as a food that provides a lot of calories and only limited amounts of other nutrients. It's okay to use a bit of high-quality coconut oil, but as with any other oil, consumption should be minimized. On the other hand, coconut flesh should be treated in much the same way as other high-fat plant foods: enjoyed primarily as a whole food. As such, it is loaded with fiber, vitamin E, and healthful phytochemicals. As a bonus, it has powerful antimicrobial properties.

The Take-Home Message

The science is crystal clear: a wide range of fat intake levels can support and promote excellent health. Here are the key points to keep in mind in regard to fat consumption:

- Don't overeat.
- Eat good fats. The fats in highly processed foods, fast foods, and convenience foods cause health problems, whereas the fats in whole foods, such as nuts, seeds, avocados, and olives, don't, as long as you aren't consuming excess calories.
- Don't assume that very low-fat diets are suitable for all vegans. Optimal fat intake depends on many things. Needs vary among individuals and change throughout the life cycle.
- Very low-fat diets are highly effective in treating certain chronic diseases, particularly cardiovascular disease. If you've adopted a

vegan diet in an effort to treat cardiovascular disease, explore the very low-fat diet, but be sure to consume sufficient essential fatty acids.

- If you're a vegan with a healthy body weight, focus on eating a variety of nourishing plant foods, including nuts, seeds, and avocados. For most people, eating two or three servings of higher-fat plant foods daily is reasonable. One serving is half an avocado or 1 ounce (30g) of nuts or seeds, about 3 or 4 tablespoons (45 to 60ml).

- Limit your use of concentrated oils. To get sufficient high-quality fat without using concentrated fats and oils, eat nuts, seeds, avocados, olives, tofu, soy milk, and lower-fat plant foods such as whole grains and legumes. Be sure to include choices that contribute a healthful balance of essential fatty acids. If you use oils in salad dressings and uncooked foods, stick mainly to highquality oils that provide omega-3s.

- If you're overweight or obese, avoid concentrated fats and oils. However, you need not avoid nuts and seeds; 1 to 2 ounces (30 to 60g) per day probably won't interfere with healthful weight loss.

Simple, complex, refined, whole ... carbohydrates come in several guises. They're the foundation of a healthful vegan

diet, and knowing the difference between good carbs and not-so-good carbs is important. In the next chapter, we sort them all out for you. No worries.

CHAPTER 5

The Two Faces of Carbohydrates

Foods rich in carbohydrates are the human body's most valuable sources of energy. Globally, carbohydrate intake ranges from about 40 to 80 percent of calories, with people in developing countries consuming diets in the higher end of the range and Western diets falling near the lower end.

In obesity-ridden developed countries, advocates of popular low-carb diets urge people to shun carbohydrates in favor of meat-centered, protein-rich fare, claiming that carbohydrates are responsible for the obesity epidemic and chronic disease. For vegans, these allegations are disturbing. After all, plants are where carbohydrates reside. The only foods that are free of carbohydrates are meat, fish, poultry, and oil. While low-carb diets have been shown to be relatively successful in short-term weight loss efforts, they fail over time. They are also a nightmare for animals and for the planet.

This chapter cuts to the heart of carbohydrates, and clarifies what is myth and what is reality. in the process, we will sort through the questions about carbohydrates that tend to be foremost in the minds of those who cast their vote for plant foods.

Carbohydrates 101

Like proteins and fats, carbohydrates are macronutrients—a source of energy for the body. (The only other dietary source of energy is alcohol.) Carbs are the preferred fuel for the brain, red blood cells, and nervous system. Protein can be used as a fuel, but it must first be processed by the liver and kidneys. Plus, protein is essential for building body tissues; for the production of enzymes, hormones, and antibodies; and for the regulation of fluids, electrolytes, and pH balance. To ensure that protein is used for these important tasks rather than as a source of energy, we must eat sufficient carbohydrates.

Fat is also used as a fuel, but it isn't a preferred energy source either. If the body uses fat for energy on an ongoing basis, by-products called ketones can accumulate. In extreme cases, this can cause ketoacidosis, in which the body's pH drops to dangerously low levels. And for the record, alcohol also isn't a desirable fuel source, as it is highly toxic to the body, especially the brain, liver, and pancreas. That leaves us with carbohydrates, which provide an efficient and safe source of energy for the entire body.

Carbohydrates supply approximately 4 calories per gram. Protein also provides 4 calories per gram, and fat supplies 9 calories per gram. In addition to serving as the body's preferred source of calories, carbohydrate-rich whole foods help to maintain blood sugar levels and insulin metabolism, and keep levels of cholesterol and triglycerides in check. These foods also support a healthy gastrointestinal tract by protecting against constipation and intestinal diseases and disorders.

Nutrition experts recommend consuming between 45 and 75 percent of calories from carbohydrates. On a diet of 2,000 calories per day, that would be 900 to 1,500 calories from carbs, or 225 to 375 grams. When carbohydrate intakes fall below 45 percent of energy, fat consumption can become excessive, potentially increasing the risk of chronic diseases. Not more than 10 percent of calories should come from added sugars—concentrated sugars used in processed foods and beverages or added to food at home or in restaurants. Sugars that occur naturally in whole foods such as fruits and vegetables are not added sugars.

Carbohydrate intake in the United States averages 50 percent of calories; vegans usually eat closer to 60 percent, and those on low-fat vegan diets typically get close to 75 percent of their calories from carbs. At the other end of the vegan spectrum, the carb content of a raw vegan diet, with its generous amounts of nuts, seeds, and avocados, commonly dips below 50 percent of calories.

Most of your carbohydrates should come from whole plant foods, such as vegetables, fruits, whole grains, legumes, nuts, and seeds. Animal products, with the exception of dairy products, contain few carbohydrates, if any. (The carbohydrate in dairy products is lactose, or milk sugar.) See figure 5.1 for the average percentage of calories from carbs in various food groups.

CARBOHYDRATE CONFUSION

In populations with high rates of chronic disease, most people eat carbohydrates in their refined and processed forms. What distinguishes the world's healthiest populations—most of whom eat high-carb diets—is that they eat *unrefined* carbohydrates. This is just one among many reasons why health experts now generally agree that processed or refined carbs can be damaging to health. This has initiated a new era in our understanding of carbohydrates, along with a confusing proliferation of terms.

For many years, carbohydrates were divided into two main categories: simple carbohydrates (sugars) and complex carbohydrates (starches). Simple carbohydrates were viewed as bad, and complex carbohydrates were considered good.

As it turns out, this was more than an oversimplification; it was fundamentally inaccurate. Whether carbohydrates are simple or complex is relevant to their structure, but not so relevant to human health. Simple carbohydrates can be healthful when they come from fruits and nonstarchy vegetables, and complex carbohydrates are generally unhealthful when they come from white flour and other refined starches.

FIGURE 5.1. Average percentage of calories from carbohydrates in common foods

Food	Percentage
Fruits:	92%
Vegetables, starchy:	90%
Grains:	75%
Legumes:	70%
Vegetables, nonstarchy:	58%
Milk, 2% fat:	37%
Nuts and seeds:	12%
Eggs:	3%
Meat, poultry, and fish:	0%

Source of data: US Department of Agriculture, Agricultural Research Service, *USDA National Nutrient Database for Standard Reference*, Release 25 (2012), ndb.nal.usda.gov.

What really matters is whether the carbohydrate is in its natural state. When carbohydrates are eaten in the form of vegetables, fruits, legumes, whole grains, nuts, and seeds, they are teamed with vitamins, minerals, protein, antioxidants, phytochemicals, fiber, and essential fatty acids, and these whole plant foods are consistently associated with disease risk reduction. Because so much confusion (and scaremongering) surrounds carbohydrates, we want to make sure you're clear about the distinctions:

- **Simple carbohydrates** are molecules containing one or two units of sugar. They are found in whole foods like fruits and vegetables, in concentrated sweeteners like sugar, and in products made with those sweeteners.

- **Complex carbohydrates** are starches containing three or more units of sugar linked together. They are found in whole foods such as whole grains, starchy vegetables, legumes, nuts, and seeds, as well as flours, starches (cornstarch and potato starch), and products made with these foods.

- **Refined carbohydrates** are carbohydrate-rich foods made from processed grains (white flour), other processed starchy foods (peeled potatoes), or processed sweeteners (white or brown sugar). Refined carbohydrates may contain either complex or simple carbohydrates. Examples of foods that contain a lot of refined complex carbohydrates are white bread and white pasta. Examples of foods that contain a lot of refined simple carbohydrates are soda, candy, and jam.

- **Unrefined carbohydrates** are naturally present in whole plant foods such as vegetables, fruits, legumes, whole grains, nuts, and seeds. Unrefined carbohydrate foods may contain mainly complex or simple carbohydrates. Examples of foods that provide mainly complex carbohydrates in unrefined form are barley, quinoa, sweet potatoes, and beans. Examples of foods providing mainly simple carbohydrates in unrefined form are fruit and nonstarchy vegetables, such as cucumbers, peppers, and tomatoes.

REFINING

Why would anybody pay four dollars for a bag of potato chips when they could pay a quarter for a potato? It comes down to taste and convenience. So how does the food industry turn a twenty-five-cent commodity into a four-dollar temptress? They strip away everything that might curb its appeal; flavor it with salt, sugar, and fat; package it persuasively; and advertise it relentlessly. Unfortunately, the true cost of these "foods" far exceeds the price tag when you factor in their impact on health.

When wheat berries (and other grains) are refined into white flour, the germ and bran are removed, leaving only the endosperm, which is mainly starch and some protein. Unfortunately, the germ and bran contain about 80 percent of the vitamins, minerals, and fiber and the vast majority of the phytochemicals. (Figure 5.2 shows the amount of fiber and key nutrients that are lost when wheat berries are processed into white flour.)

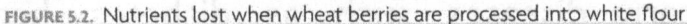
FIGURE 5.2. Nutrients lost when wheat berries are processed into white flour

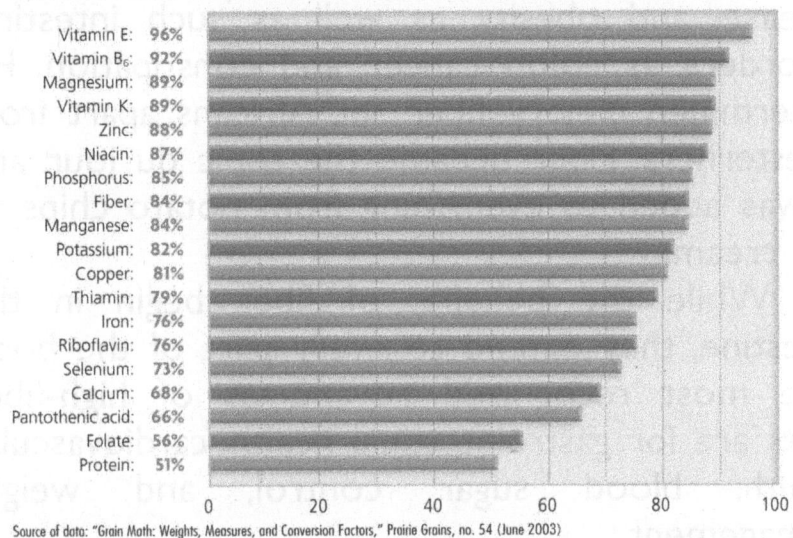

Nutrient	%
Vitamin E:	96%
Vitamin B₆:	92%
Magnesium:	89%
Vitamin K:	89%
Zinc:	88%
Niacin:	87%
Phosphorus:	85%
Fiber:	84%
Manganese:	84%
Potassium:	82%
Copper:	81%
Thiamin:	79%
Iron:	76%
Riboflavin:	76%
Selenium:	73%
Calcium:	68%
Pantothenic acid:	66%
Folate:	56%
Protein:	51%

Source of data: "Grain Math: Weights, Measures, and Conversion Factors," Prairie Grains, no. 54 (June 2003)

Granted, some of the lost nutrients are added back in the process called enrichment. For example, when wheat or rice is refined, it is commonly enriched with iron and four B vitamins (thiamin, riboflavin, niacin, and folic acid). However, not all of the vitamins and minerals that were removed are added back, nor are any of the phytochemicals or the fiber.

Fiber: Just Passing Through?

Everyone knows that fiber is good for you. It is viewed as nature's broom—the part of plants that keeps things moving smoothly and efficiently through the intestinal tract. The benefits of fiber have been universally recognized since the 1970s, when researcher Denis Burkitt discovered that people in rural Africa were free of Western diseases such as diabetes, heart disease, and obesity, as well as such intestinal disorders as colon cancer and constipation. He determined dietary fiber set Africans apart from Westerners. Fiber became the topic du jour, and it was added to everything from potato chips to ice cream.

While the benefits of fiber begin in the intestine, they extend to every part of the body. The most recognized advantages of high-fiber diets are for gastrointestinal health, cardiovascular health, blood sugar control, and weight management.

Fiber has traditionally been divided into two categories: soluble and insoluble. Soluble fiber is the type that dissolves in water; insoluble does not. For many years, experts believed soluble fiber helped improve blood sugar and cholesterol levels, and that insoluble fiber was associated with bowel regularity. More recent research suggests that the effects of soluble and insoluble fibers are more variable. The health benefits of fiber appear to be related more to the viscosity and fermentability of the fiber than to its solubility. As a result, health authorities are phasing out the terms "soluble" and "insoluble" and referring to fiber as "viscous" or "nonviscous," and "fermentable" or "nonfermentable."

Part of the confusion surrounding fiber stems from the fact that much of our fiber research has been conducted on isolated fibers rather than whole foods. While the terms "soluble" and "insoluble" are useful when referring to isolated types of specific fibers, they are less useful when talking about food, because all high-fiber foods contain a variety of both soluble and insoluble fibers. Gums, mucilages, and pectins are all soluble fibers, while celluloses and lignins are insoluble. Hemicelluloses and beta-glucans can be either or both.

Viscous fiber becomes gel-like, or thick and gummy, when mixed with water. Nonviscous fiber may absorb water, but it doesn't become thick or gummy. Viscosity is thought to be responsible for some of fiber's greatest health advantages. It helps delay stomach emptying and increase feelings of fullness after eating. It can stabilize blood sugar levels and reduce cholesterol. Examples of viscous fiber include guar gum, mucilages, and pectins. Examples of nonviscous fiber include celluloses and lignins. As is the case for these types of fiber, most viscous fiber is also soluble and most nonviscous fiber insoluble, although there are exceptions. Hemicelluloses and beta-glucans can fall into either category, although most hemicelluloses are nonviscous and most beta-glucans are highly viscous.

Fiber also serves as food for intestinal bacteria, which are able to extract energy by fermenting fiber. The types of fiber that are the most fermentable by intestinal bacteria include beta-glucans, guar gum, hemicelluloses, pectins, and oligosaccharides—small chains of carbohydrates that the body can't break down. Gums and mucilages are the most slowly fermented, while oligosaccharides are the most rapidly fermented. Less fermentable types of fiber, such as celluloses, resistant starches, and lignins, contribute to stool bulk and improve laxation. Wheat bran is an excellent example of a food rich in these less fermentable fibers. Table 5.1 lists the major types of fiber, their health effects, and food sources.

KEY HEALTH BENEFITS OF FIBER

Clearly, fiber has many health benefits—too many to discuss them all in detail. In the following sections, we'll briefly discuss some of the most significant findings.

Gastrointestinal health. The most obvious benefits of fiber are gastrointestinal. Fiber helps prevent constipation, hemorrhoids, and diverticulosis (small sacs in the wall of the intestines). It may also protect against colorectal cancer, gallstones, and inflammatory bowel diseases such as ulcerative colitis. A high-fiber diet makes stools softer and heavier, helping them pass out of the colon more easily and rapidly. While insoluble, nonviscous, nonfermentable fibers, such as celluloses and lignins, are particularly helpful in this regard, fiber that is fermented in the colon also contributes to stool softening and bulk. Many fermentable carbohydrates serve as prebiotics, stimulating the growth of friendly bacteria. Fermentation generates by-products that can inhibit harmful substances, enhance mineral absorption, reduce food sensitivities and allergies, disable carcinogens, attack cancer cells, and favorably affect the metabolism of fats and sugars.

TABLE 5.1. Types of plant fiber, health effects, and common sources

TYPE OF FIBER	HEALTH EFFECTS	COMMON SOURCES
Beta-glucans	Improve blood sugar and cholesterol levels. Soften stools, add bulk, and improve laxation, especially if insoluble.	Oats, barley, and mushrooms
Celluloses	Increase stool bulk and improve laxation.	Grains, fruits, vegetables, legumes, nuts, and seeds
Gums and mucilages	Improve blood sugar and cholesterol levels. Soften stools; smaller effect on stool bulk and laxation.	Psyllium seeds, guar gum, and sea vegetable extracts (carageenans and alginates)
Hemicelluloses	May improve blood sugar or cholesterol levels, if viscous. Increase stool bulk and improve laxation, especially if nonfermentable.	Fruits, grains (especially outer husks), legumes, nuts, seeds, and vegetables
Lignins	Increase stool bulk and improve laxation.	Stringy vegetables and the outer layer of cereal grains
Nondigestible oligosaccharides	Soften stools, increase bulk, and improve laxation. May act as prebiotics, stimulating the growth and activity of friendly bacteria in the colon.	Fruits, grains, legumes, and vegetables
Pectins	Improve blood sugar and cholesterol levels. Soften stools; smaller effect on stool bulk and laxation.	Berries and fruits, especially apples and citrus fruits
Resistant starches	Improve insulin sensitivity and blood sugar and cholesterol levels. Some increase in stool bulk and laxation.	Legumes, raw potatoes, and underripe bananas

Sources of data are listed in *Becoming Vegan: Comprehensive Edition,* by Brenda Davis and Vesanto Melina (Book Publishing Company, 2014).

Cardiovascular health. Diets rich in fiber have been associated with a reduced risk of cardiovascular disease. Every 10 grams of fiber added to the diet has been associated with a 14 percent decrease in risk for a coronary event and a 27 percent decrease in risk for coronary death. One study of more than forty thousand male health professionals reported that those consuming the most fiber had a 40 percent reduction in risk for coronary heart disease compared with those consuming the least fiber. One popular theory is that soluble, viscous fiber binds with cholesterol-containing bile acids to carry them out of the body. Another possibility is that people who eat lots of fiber eat fewer calories because they feel full sooner. Fiber can also reduce blood pressure, help remove blood clots, and enhance insulin sensitivity.

Diabetes and metabolic syndrome. Eating a high-fiber diet reduces risk for metabolic syndrome and type 2 diabetes. Soluble viscous fiber delays the absorption of fats and carbohydrates from the small intestine, which improves insulin sensitivity and blood sugar levels and helps curb appetite, possibly reducing overeating and weight gain.

Weight. High-fiber foods are associated with healthier body weight. Generally, high-fiber foods take more space on your plate and in your stomach, and they require more chewing time, so you may eat less. Many high-fiber foods are also less energy dense, meaning they have fewer calories for a specific volume of food. All of these factors contribute to satiety, or feelings of fullness.

IDEAL FIBER INTAKE

How much fiber do we need in a day? The Adequate Intake is 14 grams of fiber per 1,000 calories for everyone older than one year. For men, that's a daily intake of about 38 grams between the ages of nineteen and fifty, and 30 grams after age fifty. For women, it's about 25 grams between the ages of nineteen and fifty, and 21 grams after age fifty. If you are consuming the recommended amount but still struggling with constipation, you may need to eat up to 45 grams per day or more.

Western diets typically provide only about 15 to 17 grams of fiber daily, just half the recommended intake. Vegans, on the other hand, consume 35 to 50 grams per day on average. (The menus in chapter 14 provide 48 or more grams of fiber per day.)

Switching to a whole-foods vegan diet usually solves any problems with constipation. If it doesn't do the trick for you, here are some steps you can take to get things moving along:

- Eat at least 1/2 to 1 cup (125 to 250ml) of legumes per day.
- Aim for nine or more servings of vegetables and fruits each day, with an emphasis on higher-fiber options. (For details on serving sizes, see table 14.1, and for the approximate fiber content of various foods, see table 5.2.) To boost fiber even more, eat the edible

peels and consume a good portion of these foods raw. Enjoy a large raw salad every day, and if you cook your vegetables, minimize cooking time.

- When eating grains, opt for intact whole grains most of the time. Processing grains and grinding break down fiber, and the smaller particles generally contribute less to stool bulk. It's best to rely on whole grains rather than adding bran, because too much bran can inhibit the body's absorption of minerals.

- If you use processed grain products, select whole-grain options. Aim for at least 2.5 grams of fiber in a serving of bread or pasta and 5 grams from a serving of breakfast cereal.

- Seeds can be very helpful in increasing stool bulk, particularly whole flaxseeds and psyllium seeds.

- Opt for baked goods, such as bread, muffins, cookies, and crackers with high-fiber ingredients such as whole or sprouted grains, wheat germ, oat bran, flaxseeds, other nuts and seeds, and dried, fresh, or cooked fruits (applesauce, mashed bananas, prunes, dates, and raisins).

- Select high-fiber snacks, such as raw fruits and vegetables, trail mixes, popcorn, stuffed dates, and other raw treats.

- Drink at least 8 cups (2 liters) of fluid each day.
- Get your daily dose of exercise. Whether it's a brisk walk or jog, an aerobics class or yoga, swimming or a game of tennis—any physical activity will help keep your intestines working well.

DEALING WITH GAS

Gas results when bacteria ferment carbohydrates in the intestine, and also from swallowing air. Gas is actually a good thing—at least for your body—because it protects the colon against damage that can lead to cancer, dilutes carcinogens, stimulates beneficial bacterial growth, and keeps the gut at the proper pH.

On average, people pass gas twelve to twenty-five times a day. Of course, there is a point at which passing gas becomes a social liability. Some people limit their consumption of beans and high-fiber foods to help prevent the embarrassment caused by flatulence. However, these foods are extremely healthful, so we'll provide some tips on how to keep gas production tolerable:

- Eat more slowly, with your mouth closed.
- Chew your food really well.
- Avoid carbonated beverages, chewing gum, and sucking on candies.

- Eat smaller meals; stop eating when you are 80 percent full.
- Cook with asafetida, black pepper, cinnamon, cloves, garlic, ginger, and turmeric. Epazote and kombu also are commonly added to foods to neutralize gas-producing compounds.
- Take probiotic supplements or use probiotic powders or rejuvelac (a cultured grain beverage).
- Limit foods rich in added fructose or sugar alcohols (sweeteners such as mannitol, sorbitol, and xylitol). When these sugars aren't completely absorbed, they're fermented by bacteria in the colon. Even fructose from fruits can be a problem when they're eaten in excess or in certain combinations.
- Take activated charcoal right before eating problematic foods. It may reduce both the quantity and the odor of intestinal gas.
- If you wear dentures, make sure they fit properly.
- If all else fails, take a supplement containing the enzyme alpha-galactosidase, which breaks down certain gas-producing components in food that the body can't digest.

THE MUSICAL FRUIT

About one hundred varieties of legumes (beans, peas, lentils, peanuts) are commonly cultivated globally. In South America, Africa, China, the Middle East, and India, legumes have served as dietary staples for centuries; per capita consumption can top 88 pounds (40kg) per year. Americans only consume about 6.5 pounds (3kg) of legumes per person per year, although dietary guidelines strongly promote more.

Legumes provide many of the key nutrients found in meat, such as protein, iron, and zinc, along with protective compounds largely absent from meat, such as fiber, phytosterols, antioxidants, phytochemicals, and often other minerals, including calcium. The iron from legumes is easily absorbed by the body and may have advantages over the iron in meat. (For more on iron see chapter 7.) Most legumes are low in fat and very low in saturated fat, and all are cholesterol-free. Small red beans, red kidney beans, and pinto beans are loaded with antioxidants. It's not stretching it to say that if you want to live longer, you should eat beans regularly. Research shows that risk of death drops 7 to 8 percent for every 0.7-ounce (20g) increase in daily bean intake, probably because they can reduce the risk of diseases such as cancer, cardiovascular diseases, and diabetes, and because of their favorable effects on body weight.

As mentioned, some folks avoid eating beans because of the gas issue. Beans are among the most notorious flatulence producers because they contain nondigestible oligosaccharides, which arrive in the colon relatively unscathed and are finally broken down by bacterial fermentation, resulting in intestinal gas. But as it turns out, oligosaccharides are responsible for many of the health benefits associated with beans, in part because they act as prebiotics, promoting healthy gut flora. And again, we do have some tips to help minimize the undesirable effects associated with the "musical fruit":

- Start with small servings and gradually increase your portion size over two or three weeks. A gradual increase will give the bacteria in your body time to increase their population to digest a normal serving. Begin by adding a small amount of beans to soups, stews, and salads for a couple of weeks before digging into chili or baked beans.

- Soak beans for at least twelve hours or overnight. Then discard the soaking water, and rinse well before cooking them in fresh water. Better yet, soak them overnight, drain, add fresh water, and soak another night. Then drain and cook in fresh water. If you don't have time to soak them, boil the beans briefly in enough water to cover them. Turn off the heat and let them sit in the water for an hour or two, then drain, rinse well, and cook in fresh water.

- Cook beans thoroughly. You should be able to easily crush one between your tongue and the roof of your mouth. Undercooked beans are more difficult to digest.

- Sprout beans. Sprouting converts the oligosaccharides in beans into more easily digested sugars. To sprout beans, soak them in water for at least twelve hours, then drain them and put them in a sprouting jar or sprouter. Rinse every twelve hours until a small sprout appears. This can take three to five days for many legumes. The beans are ready to cook when they have a tiny sprout. Sprouted beans cook in half the time. Sprouted mung beans, lentils, and peas can be eaten raw. Other legumes should be cooked after sprouting.
- Use fresh beans instead of dried beans; their oligosaccharide content is much lower.
- If using canned beans, drain and rinse well before adding to recipes or eating.
- Select smaller beans, such as adzuki, lentils, split peas, and split mung beans. Generally, smaller beans are easier to digest than large beans, such as lima or kidney beans.
- Buy only as many dried beans as you will use within a few months. The longer beans are stored, the more oligosaccharides they develop.

- Use tofu and tempeh. The fermentation process used to make tempeh enhances digestibility and reduces gas.

SOURCES OF DIETARY FIBER

All whole plant foods provide fiber; it's fundamental to their structure. Animal products don't contain fiber; bones give animals their structure. Table 5.2 outlines the approximate fiber content of various foods.

TOO MUCH FIBER?

While it's possible to eat too much fiber, it's unlikely if you are consuming whole plant foods and drinking sufficient fluids. During Paleolithic times, it's estimated that humans consumed more than 100 grams of fiber per day. Excessive fiber is more of an issue for people who consume concentrated fiber sources, such as wheat bran, in large amounts. Very high-fiber diets can be too bulky for small children and some seniors, leading them to eat insufficient calories, but this is seldom a concern in healthy adults.

TABLE 5.2. Fiber content of selected whole plant foods

AMOUNT OF FIBER PER SERVING	FOOD AND SERVING SIZE
Very high-fiber foods 10 to 19.9 grams	Legumes (all varieties), cooked, 1 c (250 ml)
	Avocado (1 medium), 6.7 oz (200 g)
	High-fiber bran cereal, ½ c (125 ml)
	Artichoke (1 medium), 4 oz (120 g)
High-fiber foods 5 to 9.9 grams	Some berries (raspberries, blackberries), fresh, 1 c (250 ml)
	Some fruits (Asian pear, papaya, pear), 1 medium
	Dried fruit (apricots, figs, peaches, pears, prunes, raisins), ½ c (125 ml)
	Coconut, fresh, shredded, ½ c (125 ml)
	Flaxseeds, 2 tbsp (30 ml)
	Most whole grains, cooked, 1 c (250 ml)
	Potatoes, regular or sweet, baked (1 large), 7–10 oz (210–300 g)
	Pasta, whole wheat, cooked, 1 c (250 ml)
Moderate-fiber foods 2 to 4.9 grams	Some berries (blueberries, strawberries), fresh, 1 c (250 ml)
	Most fruits (1 medium or 2 small), 1 c (250 ml)
	Most vegetables: raw, 2 c (500 ml); cooked 1 c (250 ml)
	Most nuts and seeds, ¼ c (60 ml)
	Some whole grains (brown rice, millet, oats), cooked, 1 c (250 ml)
	Many whole-grain breads, 2 slices
	Pasta, white, cooked, 1 c (250 ml)
	Popcorn, 3 c (750 ml)
Lower-fiber foods 1.9 grams or less	Melon, 1 c (250 ml)
	Fruit or vegetable juice (all varieties), 1 c (250 ml)
	Sprouts (all varieties), 1 c (250 ml)
	Lettuce, all types, 2 c (500 ml)
	Cucumber (1 medium), 8 inch (20 cm)
	Most refined grains, (white rice, Cream of Wheat), cooked, ½ c (125 ml)
	Refined cold cereals, 1 oz (30 g)

Source of data: US Department of Agriculture, Agricultural Research Service, USDA National Nutrient Database for Standard Reference, Release 25 (2012), ndb.nal.usda.gov.

Key: c = cup; cm = centimeter; g = gram; ml = milliliters; oz = ounce; tbsp = tablespoon.

Fiber can reduce absorption of calcium, iron, and zinc, although fermentation in the large intestine can release them. In addition, when compared to refined foods, high-fiber whole foods generally provide enough extra minerals to compensate for reduced absorption. That's one reason why it's best to avoid concentrated fiber, such as wheat bran or fiber supplements, and get fiber from food instead. Athletes and others who require very high caloric intakes may want to eat some foods in a refined form; their fiber intake will still be ample.

The Goods on Grains

Grains, or, more precisely, cereal grains, are the edible seeds of grasses. These include wheat, oats, rye, barley, Kamut, spelt, rice, millet, triticale, teff, and corn. Seeds of nongrass plants that are used as grains are more accurately called pseudograins or pseudocereals. However, they are commonly included as grains in the popular press and tend to be used in the same ways, so in this book we include them when referring to grains. Examples include amaranth, quinoa, and buckwheat.

Grains are key sources of calories and protein for the majority of humans and significant sources of fiber, B vitamins, several trace minerals, phytosterols, and phytochemicals. They typically make a significant contribution to total nutrient intakes while providing little fat, no cholesterol, and plenty of fiber. In addition to being very affordable and versatile, whole grains help keep blood sugar levels stable. All of that said, they tend to be less nutrient-dense than other plant foods, so one way of approaching grains is to eat your quota of other plant foods—vegetables, fruits, legumes, nuts, and seeds—and vary your grain intake based on your energy needs. If your energy needs are moderate to high, eat more grains; if low, eat less.

There is widespread agreement that excessive consumption of refined grains contributes to overweight, obesity, and chronic disease, yet an estimated 90 percent of the grains in the typical American diet are refined. Here are just a few of the potential adverse health consequences:

- **Elevated triglycerides and decreased HDL.** Both increase the risk of cardiovascular disease and metabolic syndrome, a prediabetic condition.

- **An increase in blood pressure.** This occurs even when sodium consumption is moderate.

- **Overeating.** Refined carbohydrates are less filling than their whole-food counterparts, which can lead to eating too much.

- **Large fluctuations in blood sugar levels.** Refined carbohydrates are released into the bloodstream more rapidly after eating.

- **Increased gastrointestinal disturbances.** Refined carbohydrates contain little fiber compared to the whole foods from which they were obtained.

- **Increased risk of cancer, especially colorectal cancer.** Sugars and starches contain few of the plant nutrients and phytochemicals that protect against cancer. Refined carbs may increase the risk of colorectal and stomach cancers and possibly cancer of the pancreas.

- **Micronutrient deficiencies.** Refined carbohydrates are generally poor sources of vitamins and minerals. When these are staples of your diet, it can be a challenge to get all of the other nutrients you need.
- **Increased inflammation and oxidative stress.** Refining foods dramatically reduces their quantities of antioxidants and phytochemicals, which protect against inflammatory diseases and oxidative stress.

While there is no doubt that consumption of refined grains should be limited, these foods aren't poison. Eating a piece of pizza or a pasta dish won't sabotage your diet. It isn't a sin to throw a little sugar into your Christmas cookies. Indeed, these departures from a predominantly whole-food diet can make eating more enjoyable and sometimes easier to share with nonvegan friends. Just try to make whole grains your daily fare.

THE WHOLE-GRAIN HIERARCHY

Even within the realm of whole-grain food products, some aren't the best choices for health. For example, you might eat flaked whole-grain cereal in the morning, whole-grain bread at lunch, whole wheat pasta at dinner, and brown rice cakes as a snack. All of these products are made from whole grains, but they are still processed.

The more processed a whole grain is, the lower its nutritional value. The most nutritious form is the intact whole grain as it comes from the plant. You can further enhance your intake of nutrients and phytochemicals from intact whole grains by soaking and sprouting them. Figure 5.3 shows the whole grain hierarchy, with examples of the most healthful at the top and the least nutritious at the bottom.

Components of whole grains, such as oat bran, wheat germ, and wheat bran, aren't technically whole grains. However, they can play a useful role in the diet. For example, wheat germ can add nutritional value to baked goods made with whole wheat flour, and oat bran can provide extra viscous fiber and help control blood sugar levels or reduce cholesterol levels. (And there are times when less processed grains can be helpful to the diet, particularly for children and seniors. See chapters 11 and 12.)

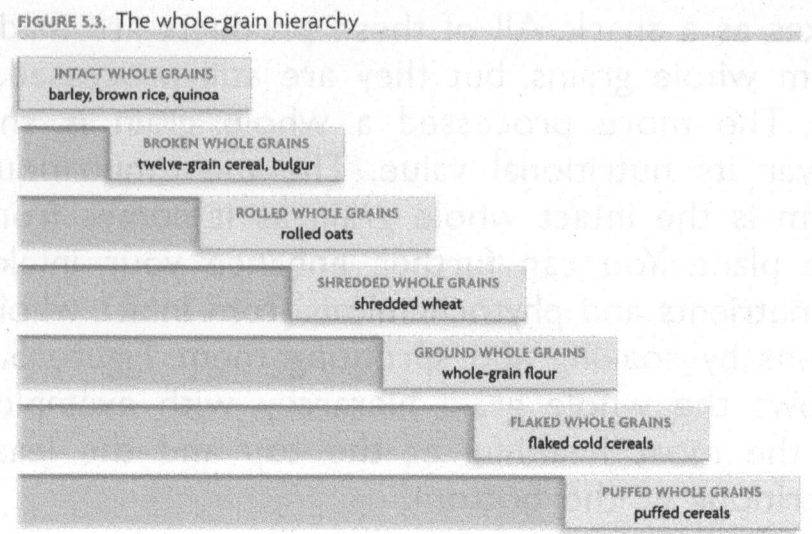

FIGURE 5.3. The whole-grain hierarchy

INTACT WHOLE GRAINS
barley, brown rice, quinoa

BROKEN WHOLE GRAINS
twelve-grain cereal, bulgur

ROLLED WHOLE GRAINS
rolled oats

SHREDDED WHOLE GRAINS
shredded wheat

GROUND WHOLE GRAINS
whole-grain flour

FLAKED WHOLE GRAINS
flaked cold cereals

PUFFED WHOLE GRAINS
puffed cereals

GLUTEN

Many people have difficulty tolerating gluten, a protein that's present in several grains, including wheat, spelt, Kamut, rye, barley, and triticale. About 1 percent of the population has an extreme reaction to gluten due to celiac disease. An estimated 10 percent have a less severe reaction, known as gluten sensitivity. People with celiac disease must eliminate all traces of gluten from their diets. People with gluten sensitivity may have to avoid gluten completely or may be able to eat minimal amounts without symptoms.

In either case, symptoms often affect the gastrointestinal system, causing abdominal pain, cramping, bloating, diarrhea, and constipation. However, adverse reactions to gluten can show up in any body system. Behavioral issues (such as depression, foggy mind, hyperactivity, and autism), iron-deficiency anemia (which causes fatigue, weakness, and lack of concentration), dementia, infertility, joint pain, muscle disorders, osteoporosis, leg numbness, migraines, and sinus problems also are commonly reported.

Celiac disease has increased fourfold in the past forty years, yet humans have been eating grains for centuries. In the August-September 2011 issue of *Living Well,* Alessio Fasano, MD, a world-renowned expert on celiac disease, said the reasons for this surge are twofold: "First, the grains we're eating have changed dramatically. In our great-grandparents' era, wheat contained very low amounts of gluten and it was harvested once a year. Now we've engineered our grains to substantially increase yields and contain characteristics, like more elasticity, that we like. We're susceptible to the consequences of these extremely rich, gluten-containing grains. Second is the upward trend we're seeing in all autoimmune diseases. We're changing our environment faster than our bodies can adapt to it."

If you think you might be sensitive to gluten, it's important to rule out celiac disease and wheat allergy. If these tests are negative, you can still go on a glutenfree diet for two to four weeks to see if your symptoms improve. If they do, that's a strong indicator of gluten sensitivity. To double check, try eating foods that contain gluten for a day and see if your symptoms return.

Sprouting significantly reduces gluten content but doesn't eliminate it. Your sensitivity might be such that sprouting allows you to eat some grains that would normally be troublesome.

Oats may or may not be a problem. They contain a gluten-like protein that most people with celiac disease or gluten sensitivity can tolerate. However, many oats sold in North America are processed on machinery that also handles grains containing gluten, so the oats may become contaminated.

Even if gluten isn't much of an issue for you, it's wise to vary the grains you eat. Whole grains differ in their content of fiber, vitamins, minerals, and phytochemicals, so consuming a variety of grains ensures a better balance. Definitely include pseudograins such as quinoa, amaranth, and buckwheat in the mix. All are protein powerhouses, and they're also gluten-free and more concentrated in vitamins and minerals.

The Sour Side of Sugar

Humans have a soft spot for sweets. We're born that way, and for good reason. In foods found in nature, sweetness generally signals safety, while bitterness serves as a warning flag. The sugar in plants provides a reasonable concentration of glucose to keep the human body running smoothly. It would be difficult to consume excessive sugar when eating a variety of vegetables, fruits, legumes, grains, nuts, and seeds. Unfortunately, when we process foods and concentrate their sugars, our hardwired attraction to sweets begins to work against us.

Prior to the 1500s, concentrated sweeteners were less common, with the exception of honey, for those who had access to it. It wasn't until the mid-1800s that sugar became a common part of everyday diets. By 1900, per capita annual sugar consumption in the United States averaged about 64 pounds (29kg), one of the highest levels globally.

The use of added sugars increased more than 200 percent between 1900 and 2005, and by 19 percent between 1970 and 2005. Americans consumed an average of 30 teaspoons (126g) of added sugars per day in 2005. That amounts to 488 calories, or almost 25 percent of your calories if you're eating 2,000 calories per day. Soft drinks and other sweetened beverages account for close to half of the added sugars Americans consume. Between 1970 and 2000, consumption of sugar-laden soft drinks increased from less than 8 fluid ounces (250ml) per day to almost 16 fluid ounces (500ml).

Between 1970 and 1995, the most notable change was not in the amount of sugar consumed, but the type. While the consumption of table sugar (sucrose) declined by 38 percent, intake of corn sweeteners—mainly high-fructose corn syrup—almost quadrupled. In 2007, 45 percent of all added sugars were sucrose, 41 percent were high-fructose corn syrup, and 14 percent were glucose syrup, pure glucose, and honey.

HOW BAD IS SUGAR?

Sugar isn't inherently harmful. In fact, when it's part of a whole plant food, it's a valuable and healthful source of energy. The human body prefers sugar as a fuel source and can handle it fairly well—in reasonable doses, such as the amounts naturally present in fruits and vegetables. Excess sugar is the issue, particularly when it comes from concentrated sweeteners. The adverse health effects of sugar are similar to those of refined carbs, discussed earlier in this chapter. In addition, high-sugar diets have the following adverse impacts on health:

- They increase levels of triglycerides, the fatty acids implicated in cardiovascular disease, especially when simple sugars exceed 20 percent of energy (as they typically do in Western diets).
- They raise blood sugar levels and increase insulin output and insulin resistance, which can contribute to metabolic syndrome, prediabetes, and type 2 diabetes.
- They cause cavities and impaired dental health.

- They result in nonalcoholic fatty liver disease, which increases risk of atherosclerosis and cardiovascular diseases.
- They adversely affect immunity and increase susceptibility to infection.

HOW MUCH SUGAR IS OKAY?

Clearly, sugar can be toxic when consumed in excess. The million-dollar question is how much is too much. The World Health Organization suggests a maximum of 10 percent of calories from added sugars, or no more than about 12 1/2 teaspoons (53g) per day in a 2,000-calorie diet. There is no question that less is better, but the upper limit suggested by World Health Organization is a reasonable maximum for most people.

Learn to read labels. Manufacturers must list total sugar (sugar naturally present in foods plus any added sugar) per serving, but they aren't required to separate out added sugars. If the food has no naturally occurring sugars, then the sugar listed is all added sugar.

If there are natural sugars from fruits, dried fruits, or vegetables such as tomatoes, then further detective work is called for. Scrutinize the ingredient list. Ingredients are listed in descending order by weight. If sugar is high on the list, this is a good clue that added sugars are high. However, if several different sweeteners have been used in the product, each will be listed separately; they may appear lower in the list, yet their cumulative amount may be substantial. You may not even recognize some of them as sugar. Any of the following ingredients are simply different forms of sugar: agave nectar, barley malt syrup, blackstrap molasses, brown rice syrup, brown sugar, cane sugar, corn syrup, crystalline fructose, dextrose, dried cane juice, evaporated cane juice, fructose, fruit juice concentrate, glucose, high-fructose corn syrup, honey, invert sugar, lactose, maltodextrin, maltose, malt syrup, maple syrup, molasses, raw sugar, rice syrup, Sucanat, sucrose, sugar, syrup, and turbinado sugar.

Also note the serving size; servings are often smaller than you might imagine. Look for the number of grams of sugar per serving. There are approximately 4.2 grams in 1 level teaspoon (5ml) of sugar, so, if a product contains 12 grams of sugar, that's about 3 teaspoons. Table 5.3 lists the sugar content of some common vegan foods.

MORE HEALTHFUL SWEETENERS

Most sugars provide about the same number of calories and are essentially glucose, fructose, or a combination. Glucose tends to raise blood sugar more readily than fructose, but fructose has been implicated in many health conditions. The take-home message is simple: sugar is sugar is sugar, and consumption should be limited regardless of the variety used.

Although a few sweeteners contain tiny amounts of nutrients, you would have to eat far more than you should for them to make a significant contribution to your nutritional needs. One notable exception is blackstrap molasses, which is a significant source of minerals because it contains the minerals stripped away in the process of refining sugar. For example, 2 tablespoons (30ml) of blackstrap molasses provides 344mg of calcium, 7mg of iron, and 996mg of potassium. That's more calcium than I cup (250ml) of milk, more iron than an 8-ounce (240g) steak, and more potassium than two large bananas. (Choose organic molasses, or you'll also have a significant source of pesticides.)

TABLE 5.3. Sugar content of common vegan foods

FOOD	SERVING SIZE	SUGAR (g)	SUGAR (tsp)
Almond milk (Silk, True Almond, original)	1 c (250 ml)	7	1.7
Almond milk (Silk, True Almond, vanilla)	1 c (250 ml)	15	3.6
Chocolate bar, 70% cacao (Greens and Black)	1.7 oz (50 g)	12.5	3
Chocolate bar, rice milk (Terra Nostra)	1.7 oz (50 g)	27.5	6.5
Coconut yogurt (So Delicious, blueberry)	6 oz (170 g)	20	4.8
Granola bar (Nature's Path, all flavors)	1.2 oz (35 g)	10–11	2.4–2.6
Granola, premium (Nature's Path, all flavors)	½ c (125 ml)	12	2.9
Granola, regular (Nature's Path, all flavors)	½ c (125 ml)	7–9	1.7–2.1
Organic soda (Blue Sky)	12 fl oz (375 ml)	37–44	8.8–10.5
Salad dressing (Annie's Raspberry Balsamic Vinaigrette)	2 tbsp (30 ml)	7	1.7
Soy ice cream (So Delicious, all flavors)	½ c (125 ml)	15–27	3.6–6.4
Soy milk (Silk, original)	1 c (250 ml)	6	1.4
Soy milk (Silk, vanilla)	1 c (250 ml)	8	1.9
Tomato sauce (Newman's Own Organic Traditional Herb)	½ c (125 ml)	9	2.1

Sources of data are listed in *Becoming Vegan: Comprehensive Edition*, by Brenda Davis and Vesanto Melina (Book Publishing Company, 2014).

Key: fl oz = fluid ounce; g = gram; ml = milliliter; oz = ounce; tbsp = tablespoon.

Date sugar (dried and ground dates) and coconut sugar (dried nectar from the flowers of coconut palms) also contain more nutrients than many other sugars because they are derived from whole foods. Of course, the most nutritious sweeteners are fresh or dried fruits, which can be used to make fabulous desserts without adding any concentrated sugar or other sweetener.

FRUCTOSE: THE SUGAR VILLAIN

Based on scientific research to date, fructose has damaging effects on the body, particularly when consumed in excess. The body can handle small amounts of fructose, such as those that naturally occur in whole foods. However, regular consumption of significant amounts of concentrated sources of fructose—no matter the source—can quickly exceed the body's capacity to handle it.

Every cell in the human body can use glucose for energy, but fructose immediately goes to the liver, where it is rapidly converted to fatty acids. Some of the fatty acids stay in the liver, and the remainder enter the bloodstream as triglycerides. Many of the adverse effects associated with concentrated sweeteners—such as nonalcoholic fatty liver disease, high triglycerides, increased LDL cholesterol, insulin resistance, visceral fat accumulation, and elevated blood pressure—are even more pronounced with fructose. Remember, it is the dose that makes the poison. The fructose content of a serving of fruit is 2 to 8 grams, whereas the fructose content of a 12-fluid-ounce (375ml) soda is about 25 grams—regardless of whether it is sweetened with high-fructose corn syrup or sucrose.

Are Sugar Substitutes Safe?

There are essentially two classes of sugar substitutes: sugar alcohols and noncaloric sweeteners (also called nonnutritive sweeteners). In small amounts, sugar alcohols, such as mannitol, sorbitol, and xylitol, are relatively benign, although they can cause gastrointestinal distress if you eat too much. They do raise blood sugar levels, but not as much as other carbohydrates.

Noncaloric sweeteners (also called nonnutritive sweeteners) can be further divided into two categories: artificial sweeteners and natural noncaloric sweeteners. In the United States, five artificial sweeteners are approved for use: acesulfame K, aspartame, neotame, saccharin, and sucralose. Natural noncaloric sweeteners include stevia and rebaudioside A, both of which are derived from the stevia plant.

Generally, it's best to minimize your use of sugar substitutes or avoid them. They can have negative effects on health

and provide few, if any, benefits. If you must use these products, stick to sugar alcohols or natural noncaloric sweeteners.

The Glycemic Index

The glycemic index (GI) is a measure of the effect of 50 grams of carbohydrates from a specific food on blood sugar levels. Carbohydrates that are quickly digested and release their sugars into the bloodstream rapidly have a high GI. They usually trigger an exaggerated insulin response, which adversely affects long-term blood sugar control, elevates triglyceride levels, and decreases HDL levels. Carbohydrates that are slowly digested and release their sugars into the bloodstream gradually have a low GI and may have positive effects on insulin response and triglyceride and HDL levels.

The glycemic index uses a scale of 0 to 100, with foods that cause a rapid rise in blood sugar levels having higher values. Pure glucose serves as a reference point and has a GI of 100. White bread has a GI of 75, which means the blood sugar response to the carbohydrate in white bread is 75 percent that of the response to the pure glucose. By comparison, barley has a GI of 28. A low GI is between 0 and 55, a moderate GI is between 56 and 69, and a high GI is above 69.

The GI gives us a ballpark idea of how a 50-gram serving of carbohydrates affects blood sugar levels. But we don't always eat exactly 50 grams of carbohydrate from a food. This is where the glycemic load (GL) comes in. Glycemic load factors in the serving size of the food and the actual amount of carbohydrate consumed. Foods that have a high GI aren't necessarily problematic if they don't contain much carbohydrate and have a low GL.

The GL of a food is calculated by multiplying the GI by the grams of carbohydrate in a *serving* of the food and dividing the total by 100. So although watermelon has a GI of 72, a 120-gram (4oz) serving of watermelon provides only 6 grams of carbohydrate and therefore has a GL of 4, which is low. (Note that this calculation is done using the weight of carbs in a serving, not the weight of the serving.) The important point is that the total amount of carbohydrate in a food is just as important as its GI in determining its impact on blood sugar. A low GL is between 0 and 10, a moderate GL is between 11 and 19, and a high GL is above 19. Table 5.4 lists some common foods and their GI and GL.

TABLE 5.4. Glycemic index (GI) and glycemic load (GL) of selected foods

FOOD	GI	SERVING SIZE	GL
GRAINS			
Barley, cooked	28	5 oz (150 g)	12
Bread, white	75	1 oz (30 g)	11
Bread, whole wheat	74	1 oz (30 g)	9
Buckwheat, cooked	54	5 oz (150 g)	16
Bulgur wheat, cooked	48	5 oz (150 g)	13
Cornflakes	81	1 oz (30 g)	20
Corn tortilla	46	5 oz (150 g)	4
Millet, cooked	71	5 oz (150 g)	26
Oatmeal, instant	79	8 oz (250 g)	21
Oatmeal, made from rolled oats	55	8 oz (250 g)	13
Quinoa, cooked	53	5 oz (150 g)	13
Rice, brown, cooked	50–87	5 oz (150 g)	16–33
Rice, white, cooked	43–109	5 oz (150 g)	15–46
Rice cakes, plain	82	0.9 oz (25 g)	17
Rice crackers, plain	91	1 oz (30 g)	23
Rye crispbread	64	0.9 oz (25 g)	10
Shredded wheat cereal	67	1 oz (30 g)	13
Rye bread (pumpernickel)	53	1 oz (30 g)	6
Spaghetti, white, cooked	49	6 oz (180 g)	24
Spaghetti, whole wheat, cooked	44	6 oz (180 g)	18
LEGUMES			
Baked beans, canned, vegetarian	48	5 oz (150 g)	7
Chickpeas, cooked	28	5 oz (150 g)	8

FOOD	GI	SERVING SIZE	GL
Kidney beans, cooked	28	5 oz (150 g)	7
Lentils, cooked	29	5 oz (150 g)	5
Mung beans, sprouted, raw	25	5 oz (150 g)	4
Navy beans, cooked	38	5 oz (150 g)	12
Peas, split, yellow	32	5 oz (150 g)	6
Soybeans, cooked	18	5 oz (150 g)	1
NUTS			
Cashews	22	1.7 oz (50 g)	3
Mixed nuts	24	1.7 oz (50 g)	4
Peanuts	14	1.7 oz (50 g)	1
VEGETABLES			
Beet	64	2.7 oz (80 g)	5
Carrot, raw and boiled	47	2.7 oz (80 g)	3
Corn, boiled	52	2.7 oz (80 g)	9
Parsnip, boiled	52	2.7 oz (80 g)	4
Peas, frozen, boiled	51	2.7 oz (80 g)	4
Potato, baked	86	5 oz (150 g)	22
Potato, boiled	82	5 oz (150 g)	21
Potatoes, new, boiled	76	5 oz (150 g)	16
Pumpkin, boiled	64	2.7 oz (80 g)	6
Sweet potato, raw and cooked	70	5 oz (150 g)	22
Yam, steamed and boiled	54	5 oz (150 g)	20
FRUITS			
Apple	38	4 oz (120 g)	6
Apricot	34	4 oz (120 g)	3
Apricots, dried	31	2 oz (60 g)	7
Banana	52	4 oz (120 g)	13
Cantaloupe	65	4 oz (120 g)	4
Cherries	22	4 oz (120 g)	3
Grapes	46	4 oz (120 g)	8
Kiwi	53	4 oz (120 g)	6
Mango	51	4 oz (120 g)	9
Orange	42	4 oz (120 g)	5
Papaya	59	4 oz (120 g)	10
Peach	42	4 oz (120 g)	5
Pear	38	4 oz (120 g)	4
Pineapple	59	4 oz (120 g)	8
Plum	39	4 oz (120 g)	5

FOOD	GI	SERVING SIZE	GL
Strawberries	40	4 oz (120 g)	1
Watermelon	72	4 oz (115 g)	4
MILKS			
Cow's milk	31	1 c (250 ml)	4
Rice milk, "original"	86	1 c (250 ml)	23
Soy milk, "original"	34	1 c (250 ml)	5
SNACK FOODS			
Chocolate, dark	23	1.7 oz (50 g)	6
Chocolate, milk	43	1.7 oz (50 g)	12
Dates	42	2 oz (60 g)	18
Ice cream, French vanilla, (16% fat)	38	1.7 oz (50 g)	3
Popcorn	72	0.7 oz (20 g)	8
Potato chips	54	1.7 oz (50 g)	11
Pretzels	84	1 oz (30 g)	17
SUGARS			
Agave syrup	13	0.3 oz (10 g)	1
Fructose	15	0.3 oz (10 g)	2
Glucose	103	0.3 oz (10 g)	10
Golden syrup	63	0.9 oz (25 g)	13
Honey	61	0.9 oz (25 g)	12
Maple syrup	54	0.3 oz (10 g)	10
Sucrose	65	0.3 oz (10 g)	7

Source of data: F. S. Atkinson et al., "International Tables of Glycemic Index and Glycemic Load Values: 2008," *Diabetes Care* 31, no. 12 (2008):2281–2283.

GI - low: less than 55; medium: 55-69; high: 70 or more

GL - low: less than 10; medium: 11-19; high: 20 or more

Key: c = cup; g = gram; ml = milliliter; oz = ounce.

THE LIMITATIONS OF GI AND GL

The GI and GL are sometimes seen as a key way to judge a food's healthfulness. This is a serious error. These tools determine the effect of carbohydrates on blood sugar levels, but they don't tell us anything else about the food and aren't designed to be used as the sole criteria for food selection.

First, foods that contain little if any carbohydrate have a very low GI, and a negligible GL. For example, meat has a small impact on blood sugar, but this doesn't qualify it as a healthy or "free food" for people with diabetes. The GI of potato chips is lower than that of baked potatoes, but adding salt and fat doesn't make potatoes more healthful. Other unhealthful snacks, such as candy bars, cupcakes, and ice cream, also frequently fall within the low GI range because of their high fat content. In contrast, plenty of nutritious, higher-carbohydrate whole foods, such as some fruits, starchy vegetables, and whole grains, have relatively high GIs or GLs, but that doesn't mean you should avoid them.

Despite these limitations, GI and GL can be helpful when used appropriately. Among the best ways to use these tools is to compare similar foods or foods in the same category. For instance, in table 5.4 you might compare corn tortillas with corn flakes; barley with millet (both intact grains); or soy milk with rice milk. It's also helpful to recognize that foods with higher GIs and GLs can serve as valuable fuel sources during demanding physical activity, when you need carbohydrate that's readily available.

Vegans don't necessarily have to worry about GI and GL, because vegan diets have a low overall GI compared with nonvegetarian diets and a low to moderate GL. One study examining the GI and GL of vegan diets reported an average GI of 51 and an average GL of 144—the sum of all the foods eaten during the day—which is considered low to moderate. This could provide a health advantage for vegans in terms of risks for both diabetes and cardiovascular diseases. Both the GI and GL of vegan diets compare very favorably to those of nonvegetarian diets. This could help to explain the health advantages for vegans in terms of risks for both diabetes and cardiovascular diseases.

GI and GL can be useful tools for determining the impact of food on blood sugar levels, but they don't determine the food's nutritional value. For that, we need a more complete picture. Let's start with vitamins.

CHAPTER 6

Valuing Vitamins

Our knowledge of specific vitamins is just a century old, with vitamin A, first in the lineup, not identified until 1913. Yet the awareness that certain foods held mysterious properties that could cure illnesses such as scurvy and rickets goes back thousands of years.

Vitamins are complex molecules that contain carbon along with other elements, including hydrogen, oxygen, and sometimes nitrogen. They have far-reaching effects in the body, governing certain aspects of growth, regulating the metabolism of minerals, protecting us from free radical damage, turning the food we eat into usable energy, and more. The list of their functions is long and impressive. Yet the total amount of vitamins we need is tiny—only about 0.5 gram per day, equal in weight to about one-sixth of a garlic clove.

Vitamins are essential to life, and the body cannot synthesize them—we have to get them from the food we eat. Vegan diets deliver most vitamins in abundance.

The exceptions are vitamins B $_{12}$ and D, but those are easily added.

In this chapter, we examine the roles of vitamins and explore the options for meeting recommended intakes. L et's begin with the two of greatest interest in vegan diets: vitamins B $_{12}$ and D.

Vitamin B^12 (Cobalamin, Cyanocobalamin)

Throughout history, vitamin B_{12} was primarily available from animal products. In the past, when vegans had far less access to plant-based foods fortified with vitamin B_{12}, the average intakes of American vegans were only about one-quarter of the recommended amount. However, shortfalls are easily averted with supplements and the B_{12}-fortified plant foods that have proliferated in recent decades. Fortunately, responsible vegetarian societies and raw-food groups have encouraged vegans to make sure they have a reliable source of this essential nutrient.

Details, Details

For detailed information on vitamins, recommended intakes throughout every stage of life, and food sources of vitamins, see table 6.1, table 6.2, and the appendix.

Vitamin B_{12} is part of a team of nutrients that converts carbohydrates, fat, and protein into usable energy. It helps build DNA and red blood cells, particularly during times of rapid growth, and it maintains the protective sheaths around nerve fibers. In addition, it helps rid the body of homocysteine, a potentially damaging substance that can injure the delicate inner lining of artery walls and trigger heart disease. A deficiency of B_{12} can have severe consequences, such as gastrointestinal problems, nerve damage, and megaloblastic anemia.

Vegans who don't include a reliable source of vitamin B_{12} will eventually become deficient. For some, this will happen in a matter of months; for others, it could take years. The consequences of the deficiency will depend on how soon the symptoms are recognized and how quickly you begin to make up for it. The longer it takes to recognize the problem, the greater the risk of permanent damage. If you have symptoms of fatigue, weakness, mood changes, shortness of breath, or palpitations or have other reasons to suspect a B_{12} deficiency, arrange a lab test through your doctor. Supplementation usually works quickly to improve the deficiency conditions if the damage hasn't gone too far.

RECOMMENDED INTAKES OF VITAMIN B^12

The recommended intake for adults is 2.4mcg, spread over the day, however many experts suggest 4 to 8mcg. When vitamin B_{12} is taken in a single dose, a smaller amount of that dose is absorbed than if you took the same dose in divided portions. If you take a single daily supplement, the suggested intake is 25 to 100mcg per day. Another option is to take 1,000mcg twice a week.

Pregnancy, Lactation, and Infancy

Taking a reliable supplementary source of vitamin B_{12} is especially important for mother and child during pregnancy and breast-feeding. The recommended intake of vitamin B_{12} for pregnant women is 2.6mcg, and for nursing moms it's 2.8mcg. Again, many experts recommend more, with options shown in table 6.1.

It is essential that babies who have not yet built up their reserves of this nutrient get adequate dietary vitamin B_{12}. Without it, an infant can develop irreversible brain damage in a few months. Fortunately, when a breast-feeding mother is getting sufficient B_{12}, her baby gets enough through her milk. As babies are weaned from breast milk or infant formula, they should be given vitamin B_{12} drops.

TABLE 6.1. Options for meeting the recommended dietary allowance (RDA) for vitamin B_{12}

AGE	RDA (mcg)	RECOMMENDED INTAKE FROM TWO FORTIFIED FOODS DURING THE DAY, EACH SERVING	RECOMMENDED INTAKE FROM A SINGLE DAILY SUPPLEMENT	RECOMMENDED INTAKE FROM A BI-WEEKLY SUPPLEMENT
0–5 months	0.4	–	–	–
6–11 months	0.4	0.4–1.0	5–20	200
1–3 years	0.9	0.8–1.5	10–40	375
4–8 years	1.2	1.0–2.0	13–50	500
9–13 years	1.8	1.5–2.5	20–75	750
14+ years	2.4	2.0–3.5	25–100	1,000
Pregnancy	2.6	2.5–4.0	25–100	1,000
Lactation	2.8	2.5–4.0	30–100	1,000

Sources of data are listed in *Becoming Vegan: Comprehensive Edition*, by Brenda Davis and Vesanto Melina (Book Publishing Company, 2014).

Seniors

Vitamin B_{12} can help treat cognitive impairment and dementia in the small number of cases where B_{12} deficiency exists. Vitamin B_{12} deficiency may also be related to depression in later life.

Seniors on any type of diet should have their B_{12} status tested every five years starting at age fifty. With age, the body's ability to absorb the form of vitamin B_{12} found in animal products diminishes. In animal products, vitamin B_{12} is attached to a protein, and as people get older, they start to lose the ability to cleave the B_{12} from the protein. The form of B_{12} in fortified plant foods or supplements isn't attached to protein, so they are good sources even as we age. People older than fifty, regardless of diet, should take B_{12} supplements or eat B_{12}-fortified foods to meet most or all of the recommended intakes based on the amounts for adults in table 6.1, above. Vegan seniors are likely to have an advantage over nonvegetarian seniors if they've already developed the habit of taking a B_{12} supplement.

Some older adults (regardless of diet) also don't produce enough intrinsic factor, a compound necessary for B_{12} absorption. In such cases, monthly B_{12} injections or relatively large oral doses, such as 2,000mcg followed by 1,000mcg per day, have proven to be effective.

GETTING ENOUGH VITAMIN B^12

There are several ways to get enough vitamin B_{12}. You can use one or a combination of the following approaches.

Take a B^12 Supplement Daily

Choose a vitamin or multivitamin-mineral supplement that includes 25 to 100mcg of vitamin B_{12} (cyanocobalamin, the form used in most research). For optimal absorption, chew your B_{12} supplement. Methylcobalamin is advised for smokers and those with kidney problems; 1000mcg daily may be needed for this form.

Take a Larger B^12 Supplement Twice a Week

Because the body retains only a small portion of vitamin B_{12} when a large amount is consumed, you can take a very large amount twice a week instead of a smaller daily supplement and still ensure you're absorbing the correct amount. If you go with this option, take 1,000mcg of cyanocobalamin two or three times per week; chew for optimal absorption.

Get Vitamin B^12 from Fortified Foods Daily

Each day, eat two servings of B_{12}-fortified foods, such as nondairy milks, vegetarian meat analogs, breakfast cereals, and nutrition bars. Check labels to make sure each serving provides 2mcg or more, or at least 50 percent of the actual daily value per serving. Food labels use 6mcg as 100 percent. This means a food labeled as containing 50 percent of the daily value would provide 3mcg per serving.

Fortified foods aren't as reliable a source for vitamin B_{12} as supplements, because even though adequate amounts of the vitamin are added during production, amounts can vary considerably from one sample to another. If you rely on fortified foods for your B_{12} intake, consider including a 1,000mcg supplement once a week to ensure optimal B_{12} status.

Unreliable B_{12} sources include fermented foods, mushrooms, sea vegetables (nori and dulse), spirulina, sprouts, and raw plant foods. Chlorella and AFA (Aphanizomenon flos-aquae), two species of algae, have not yet proven to be reliable sources.

Use Nutritional Yeast

Nutritional yeast is grown on a vitamin B_{12}-enriched medium, and 2 tablespoons (30ml or 8g) may provide 2.4mcg, but the B_{12} content can vary from batch to batch, so it's best to also take a supplement from time to time. Each day, sprinkle 2 tablespoons (30ml or 8g) of Red Star Vegetarian Support Formula nutritional yeast on food or use it as an ingredient in salad dressings and vegan cheeses. (For delicious recipes featuring nutritional yeast, see *Cooking Vegan,* by V. Melina and J. Forest, and *The Nutritional Yeast Cookbook* by Jo Stepaniak.)

For additional information, see "Vitamin B_{12}: Are You Getting It?" by Jack Norris, registered dietitian and coauthor of *Vegan for Life,* available online at veganhealth.org/articles/vitaminb12.

Vitamin D (Calciferol)

For centuries, the puzzling and crippling disease known as rickets prevented children's bones from hardening enough to hold up the weight of their growing bodies. The first scientific description of rickets was written around 1650, shortly after soft coal had been introduced as an energy source in England. The use of coal spread through northern European cities, accompanied by a pall of coal smoke that polluted the air and blocked out the sun. Rickets became known as the disease of the Industrial Revolution since its incidence increased when families left farms to move to smoky, smoggy, sunless cities in the United Kingdom, northern Europe, and the northern United States. By 1900, an estimated 80 percent of the children in Boston, New York, and some other industrialized cities of the northeastern United States and northern Europe had rickets.

Liquid Gold Dressing

Makes 1 1/2 cups (375ml)
We developed this dressing for use on salads, baked potatoes, rice, steamed broccoli, and other vegetables and gave it the name Liquid Gold because of its nutritional wealth. Just 3 tablespoons (45ml) can provide half of your daily B $_{12}$ requirement and a day's supply of omega-3 fatty acids. It's also packed with other B vitamins, and, best of all, it's very tasty.

1/2 cup (125ml) flaxseed oil
1/2 cup (125ml) water
1/3 cup (90ml) freshly squeezed lemon juice
1 tablespoon (15ml) cider, balsamic, or raspberry vinegar
2 tablespoons (30ml) tamari or Bragg Liquid Aminos
1/2 cup (125ml) Red Star Vegetarian Support Formula nutritional yeast
1 tablespoon (15ml) ground flaxseeds
2 teaspoons (10ml) Dijon mustard
1 teaspoon (5ml) ground cumin, turmeric, or a combination

Put all the ingredients in a blender and process until smooth. Stored in a covered jar in the refrigerator, Liquid Gold Dressing will keep for 2 weeks.

Shortly after World War I, scientists had closed in on two effective ways to prevent rickets: ultraviolet radiation from the sun or a lamp, and a substance derived from cod liver oil that became known as vitamin D. In succeeding decades, researchers demonstrated how vitamin D could be produced in human skin when exposed to sunlight. They also learned that one of the forms of vitamin D (vitamin D2) could be produced when mushrooms, yeasts, alfalfa, or lichens were exposed to sunlight or ultraviolet light, and that the human body can convert vitamin D2 to the active form that the body uses. Identification of the vitamin prompted the fortification of cow's milk and then infant formula with vitamin D to reliably provide this nutrient to most infants and children. As a result, rickets was almost eradicated in regions that adopted fortification. Starting in the 1990s, nondairy beverages, such as soy milk, also were fortified.

Vitamin D has many important functions, including helping with the absorption of calcium and phosphorus, maintenance of critical blood levels of calcium, and limiting calcium losses through the urine. This vitamin is important at all ages, including for seniors, who tend to be at risk for osteoporosis. (For more on vitamin D and osteoporosis, see section entitled "CALCIUM AND VITAMIN D" and section entitled "Osteoporosis".) It's also important in the functioning of the muscles, heart, brain, pancreas, and thyroid. Vitamin D controls the growth and maturation of cells, including those in bone and the immune system. Through its impact on the immune system, it helps fight infectious diseases and reduce the risk of Crohn's disease, multiple sclerosis, and rheumatoid arthritis. It regulates insulin production in the pancreas and can protect against diabetes. Due to its active role in blood vessels, it helps regulate blood pressure and prevent cardiovascular disease and stroke. Low vitamin D intakes and serum vitamin D levels are associated with increased risk for colon cancer and other cancers, whereas adequate vitamin D seems to protect against the recurrence of breast cancer. Vitamin D also helps preserve cognitive function as we age, and plays a role in the functioning of the reproductive system.

Those at greatest risk for vitamin D deficiency are breast-fed infants whose mothers are low in vitamin D, people with dark skin living far from the equator, adults older than fifty (whose vitamin D production is diminished), and those who are obese, with a BMI greater than 30. (See table 9.2, Body Mass Index).

HOW VITAMIN D WORKS

Sun shining on human skin stimulates a substance called dehydrocholesterol to become vitamin D_3. Vitamin D_3 enters the bloodstream and is carried to the liver, where it is converted into calcidiol, which is transported to the kidneys, where it is finally converted to its active form: calcitriol. From there, calcitriol moves to other locations in the body, including the intestine, where it stimulates calcium absorption and performs its many other functions.

The amount of vitamin D humans can produce from sunlight depends on many variables: geographic location, time of year, time of day, cloud cover, skin color, age, body weight, how much skin is exposed, length of exposure, and use of sunscreen and UVB light. For example, people who live between latitudes 37 degrees north and 37 degrees south get more of the right kind of rays. People with lighter skin need less sun than people with darker skin. Obese people need more than normal-weight people, since they are less able to produce vitamin D than leaner people. Younger people are far more efficient at vitamin D production than seniors.

Because of all these variables, it's difficult to pinpoint just how much sun will produce enough vitamin D for any given individual, and recommended intake is currently the subject of lively debate among experts. Since vegans don't use fortified cow's milk, they get less than other dietary groups unless they regularly use vitamin D supplements or consume nondairy beverages or other foods fortified with vitamin D. Vegans tend to get only a little more than half the recommended level; however, international studies have found that many adults have low intakes and low blood levels of vitamin D, so this problem isn't specific to a vegan diet. Food fortification policies are changing, and this may help the situation.

In general, if you are in the northern hemisphere, below latitude 37—a horizontal line that divides the United States in half, roughly following the southern borders of Utah, Colorado, Kentucky, and Virginia—you can expect to make sufficient vitamin D throughout the year through sun exposure. To do so, if you're light skinned, spend ten to twenty minutes outdoors (without sunscreen) daily, getting sun on your face, arms, and legs. If you're dark skinned or elderly, you'll need to spend significantly more time in the sun.

If you live north of that latitude, you probably need to take a vitamin D supplement and eat fortified foods in the winter, in addition to spending time outdoors on sunny days in summer. To make sure you're meeting your vitamin D requirements, ask your doctor to check your blood levels of vitamin D, or use a self-testing kit. They're widely available, including through the Vitamin D Council (vitamindcouncil.

zrtlab.com). By the way, the body self-regulates theproduction of vitamin D, so even if you spend a lot of time outdoors, you can'tproduce too much vitamin D.

VITAMINS D^2 AND D^3

Vitamin D is commonly taken in single-vitamin supplements, in multivitaminmineral supplements, and in supplements that contain vitamin D plus calcium and perhaps magnesium. Vitamin D_2 (ergocalciferol) is vegan, and vitamin D_3 (cholecalciferol) is commonly of animal origin but is now available in vegan form, made from lichen. (To find a vegan vitamin D_3 supplement, do an Internet search for "vegan vitamin D_3.")

Research comparing the effectiveness of vitamin D_2 and D_3 offers a variety of perspectives and some lively controversy. The bottom line is that both forms are effective, though it can take a little more vitamin D_2 to achieve optimal vitamin D levels.

RECOMMENDED INTAKES OF VITAMIN D

The recommended vitamin D intake from birth to one year is 10mcg (400 IU) per day; for ages one to seventy it's 15mcg (600 IU) per day; and for ages seventyone and older it's 20mcg (800 IU) per day. However, many experts suggest

25 to 50mcg (1,000 to 2,000 IU) daily for adults. Others advise even higher intakes of up to 100mcg (4,000 IU), though this is the upper limit a person should take without medical supervision. The tolerable upper limits are lower for younger children. Obese people may have somewhat higher requirements for vitamin D because fat can absorb this vitamin D, making it unavailable to the rest of the body.

Pregnancy, Lactation, and Infancy

Breast-fed babies whose moms are low in vitamin D are among those at the greatest risk for vitamin D deficiency and rickets, particularly if they don't receive a vitamin D supplement and live outside of the zone from latitude 37 north to latitude 37 south. The American Academy of Pediatrics recommends a daily intake of 10mcg (400 IU) of vitamin D starting from the first few days of life. Ask your pediatrician about a suitable intake for your baby, and avoid giving the baby more than the doctor suggests, as too much may cause your child's bones to harden too soon.

Seniors

The body's ability to produce vitamin D diminishes with age. For example, the skin of someone who is sixty five or older can synthesize only about 25 percent as much vitamin D as that of a young person. This has potentially severe consequences for older people, who are generally more susceptible to falls, as vitamin D deficiency is linked to muscle weakness. Research has shown that supplementation with 20mcg (800 IU) of vitamin D reduced falls in institutionalized older patients by more than 20 percent.

SOURCES OF VITAMIN D

Few foods, whether of plant or animal origin, naturally contain vitamin D, but a growing number of vegan foods fortified with vitamin D are becoming available, including nondairy milks, juices, and breakfast cereals. Typically, 1 cup (250ml) of soy or rice milk contains 2.5 to 3mcg (100 to 120 IU) of vitamin D; 1 teaspoon (5ml) of margarine contains 0.5mcg (20 IU), and one serving of breakfast cereal contains 1mcg (40 IU). Check food labels for exact amounts.

Mushrooms contain a compound that can be converted to vitamin D_2 when they are exposed to UVB rays. Under these conditions, they can be a good source of vitamin D. Such mushrooms are becoming available in markets and are advertised as vitamin D sources. Most commercial mushrooms are grown indoors, so are not sources of vitamin D. Only wild edible mushrooms and cultivated mushrooms grown with light exposure may be reliable sources.

The ACE Antioxidant Team

Just as oxygen can make food turn brown and metal rust, oxidation in the body can also lead to damage. When oxygen joins with certain molecules, oxidation occurs, causing chain reactions of rampaging molecules called free radicals. Free radicals damage cells and DNA, effectively aging our bodies and increasing our risk for diseases including cancer, cardiovascular disease, cataracts, macular degeneration, diseases of the nervous system (such as Alzheimer's and Parkinson's), and premature aging of skin. The body also produces free radicals during normal metabolism, but if you smoke, drink alcohol, or are exposed to pollutants or radiation, including too many UV rays from the sun, free radicals can multiply rapidly. This chain reaction can only be stopped by substances that intervene and deactivate the process. These substances are called antioxidants.

An important group of antioxidants consists of vitamin A, which the body can make from the carotenoid known as beta-carotene, and vitamins C and E. These antioxidants are team players. Each helps the others function, so we need a regular supply of all three to help prevent cell damage and disease.

DIET AND DETOX

The liver may be the busiest hub of activity in the body. One of its functions is to detoxify the body, ridding it of substances that are potentially damaging, such as caffeine, medications and other drugs, paint and exhaust fumes, pesticides, and tobacco smoke. The liver recognizes dangerous molecules and transforms them into harmless forms and then facilitates their elimination.

Liver detoxification occurs in two phases. The activities of these two phases must be well coordinated because intermediary compounds that form during phase I can be even more toxic than the original substance. If these intermediary compounds aren't quickly processed in phase II, damage such as cell injury or cancer can ensue, particularly if you smoke, drink, or eat barbecued foods, since all of these can increase the damage. This is where the teamwork of vitamins A, C, and E comes in. Other substances, such as phytochemicals, selenium, certain B vitamins, and dietary fiber also are involved in detoxification.

The important thing to know here is that individual antioxidants in pill form don't provide the same protection as the same substances in food. Diet clearly has a major impact on potential damage to cells and protection from that damage. The nutrient teamwork that's involved helps explain why a varied diet of plant foods goes far beyond supplements in keeping people healthy. In the sections that follow, we'll discuss each of the antioxidant team members in detail.

Vitamin A (and Beta-carotene)

There are two forms of vitamin A in food: provitamin A carotenoids from plants, and preformed vitamin A from animal products. The body converts certain carotenoids, such as beta-carotene, to the active form of vitamin A, called retinol. The carotenoids provide many of the beautiful orange, red, and yellow colors in fruits and vegetables. Carotenoids are present in green vegetables too, but the color is masked by the green of chlorophyll. Other carotenoids, such as lycopene, lutein, and zeaxanthin, aren't converted to vitamin A, but they do have powerful health benefits.

Vitamin A plays an important role in cell differentiation, the process that creates different kinds of cells to carry out specific tasks. In the eye, vitamin A or certain carotenoids help us see at night, prevent cataracts and macular degeneration, and keep the cornea healthy. Vitamin A is required for immune system function and to build and preserve the integrity of the skin and mucous membranes so they can act as protective barriers against bacteria and viruses. Many carotenoids help protect us against cancer and heart disease. Vitamin A is needed for the growth of bones and teeth, for reproduction, and for the production and regulation of hormones.

RECOMMENDED INTAKES OF VITAMIN A

Vitamin A is measured both in retinol activity equivalents (RAE) and in international units (IU). Women need 700mcg RAE (2,333 IU) of the active form of vitamin A daily, and men need 900mcg RAE (3,000 IU) daily.

Vegan diets, with their abundance of colorful fruits and veggies, can easily provide more than enough vitamin A. Vegan vitamin A intake has been estimated at 1,500mcg RAE (4,950 IU) for women and 1,200 RAE (3,960 IU) mcg for men per day. The key is to include lots of yellow, orange, red, and green vegetables and fruits. Consuming these with foods that are rich in plant oils, such as olives, avocados, nuts, and seeds, or with oil-based salad dressings, increases carotenoid absorption.

SOURCES OF VITAMIN A

Carotenoids are present in apricot, broccoli, cantaloupe, carrot, leafy greens, mango, nectarine, papaya, peppers (bell and chile), persimmon, plantain, prunes, pumpkin, sea vegetables, squash, sweet potato, tomato, and turnip.

You can get your recommended daily intake from 1/2 cup (125ml) of carrot juice, baked sweet potato, or canned pumpkin, or from 1/4 cup (60ml) of cooked kale. We derive about

470mcg RAE from 1/2 cup (125ml) of cooked spinach or butternut squash or from 1/2 cantaloupe.

Cooking seems to increase the absorption of some carotenoids, as does including a little fat as part of the meal. Juicing provides even greater carotenoid absorption than cooking. We recommend eating some of these colorful vegetables cooked and others raw.

Supplements can be tremendously helpful for those who are deficient. For example, vitamin A supplements can prevent blindness in children who have little access to carotenoid-rich vegetables or fruits. However, the preferred form of this vitamin is from food. Long-term high intakes of vitamin A from supplements have been linked to hip fracture and should generally be avoided. If you take vitamin A supplements, be sure they provide amounts that are within the recommended range. Avoid high intakes without medical supervision.

Vitamin C (Ascorbic Acid)

Scurvy was the scourge of the seas for hundreds of years. After sailing vessels developed the capability for long voyages away from land, many crew members on extended voyages became weak and developed painful joints, swollen gums, and loose teeth. Eating became impossible, and the devastated sailors could barely move. Death typically followed soon thereafter.

For centuries, Native Americans had used herbs and cranberries to cure scurvy. And although some early explorers, including Vasco de Gama's crew in 1499, discovered that citrus fruits could alleviate the condition, it took hundreds of years for European doctors to connect the dots between the disease that had killed thousands and the simple lack of fruits and vegetables. Scientists identified vitamin C in 1912, proved its relationship to scurvy in 1932, and synthesized the vitamin in 1935.

Vitamin C's role in preventing and curing scurvy is due to its ability to build collagen, an essential component of blood vessel walls, scar tissue, tendons, ligaments, cartilage, and bone. Without vitamin C, the gums and other collagen-containing tissues break down. In addition, vitamin C helps metabolize the amino acid that transports fat to the cells for energy.

Vitamin C is a highly effective antioxidant; it helps regenerate vitamin E, another antioxidant, and even small amounts can protect cells from damage. Vitamin C supports the immune system, boosting resistance to infection when under stress, and aids in the production of thyroid hormone. Vitamin C from the copious amounts of fruits and vegetables found in typical vegan diets appears to protect the body from chronic diseases, including heart disease. Vitamin C helps the body absorb iron from plant foods (see "Iron Absorption,", for more information). It also aids in the synthesis of norepinephrine, a neurotransmitter and stress hormone essential for brain function and mood regulation.

RECOMMENDED INTAKES OF VITAMIN C

The recommended intake of vitamin C is 75mg daily for women, 90mg daily for men. Smokers are advised to get an additional 35mg per day (or, better yet, quit smoking). Vegetarians tend to get about 150mg per day—50 percent more than nonvegetarians—and vegans get even more, 138 to 584mg per day. Five servings of fruits and vegetables per day typically provide about 200mg of vitamin C. Organic produce has been shown to provide significantly more vitamin C than conventionally grown fruits and vegetables.

SOURCES OF VITAMIN C

Good sources of vitamin C include blackberries, broccoli, Brussels sprouts, cabbage, cantaloupe, citrus fruits, green peas, guava, kiwifruit, leafy greens, mango, papaya, pineapple, raspberries, red peppers (bell and chile), strawberries, sweet potato, tomato, and vegetables in the cabbage family.

Vitamin E (Alpha-tocopherol)

Vitamin E, the third member of the ACE antioxidant team, is actually a family of related compounds with alpha-tocopherol being the form with the greatest antioxidant activity. Vitamin E's job is to protect vitamin A, polyunsaturated fatty acids, and other fats from free radical damage. Vitamin E stabilizes cell membranes and prevents them from breaking. Through these protective actions, vitamin E plays a role in the prevention of many diseases. When vitamin E neutralizes a free radical, it loses its antioxidant function. Fortunately, vitamin C can come to the rescue and regenerate vitamin E so that it becomes an antioxidant once again.

Vitamin E is found in plant oils. It was discovered in 1922 in spinach, yet it wasn't recognized as essential until 1968. Though we might not think of leafy greens as significant sources of fat, in fact about 10 percent of the calories we derive from these greens are from oils. Since a typical serving of spinach or other greens contains few calories, this proportion of fat has little significance for people who consume greens in only limited quantities. But for many vegans, including those on raw diets, big salads are an important source of vitamin E. You can get one-third of your day's supply of vitamin E from 8 cups (2L) of raw spinach. If you add half an avocado and 3 tablespoons (45ml) of sunflower seeds, the salad contains 15mg (22.5 IU) of vitamin E, which is the recommended daily intake for adults. Steamed spinach cooks down to a small volume, yet it retains this vitamin;

therefore, I cup (250ml) of cooked spinach provides close to 4mg (6 IU) of vitamin E.

Most people in the United States get far less vitamin E than they need for optimal health, averaging only 6.9mg (10.4 IU) per day. These low levels are linked with higher risk of heart disease, and possibly with the development of cataracts and other conditions. Studies indicate that vitamin E from food offers us greater protection than that from supplements.

The natural form of alpha-tocopherol, called d-alpha-tocopherol, comes from plants and is the ideal form to use. Synthetic dl-alpha-tocopherol is also available, but you need approximately 50 percent more IU of the synthetic form from dietary supplements and fortified foods to obtain the same amount you would get from the natural form in plants. The synthetic form isn't as well utilized by the body, and it can even cause health problems in high doses.

RECOMMENDED INTAKES OF VITAMIN E

Adults need 15mg (22.5 IU) of vitamin E per day. Vegan intakes are usually between 14 and 33mg (21 and 49.5 IU) per day.

People on very low-fat diets who get less than 15 percent of their calories from fat tend to consume insufficient amounts of vitamin E. However, a serving of fortified cereal (check the label for serving size and vitamin E content), 1/4 cup (60ml) of sunflower seeds, or 1 ounce (30g) of almonds supplies about half of the day's recommended intake of vitamin E. Alternatively, 1 cup (250ml) of canned, pureed tomatoes provides one-third of your vitamin E for the day, and 1 cup (250ml) of cooked spinach provides one-quarter of the amount needed. You might also want to top off your intake with a supplement that includes natural vitamin E, such as a multivitamin listing d-alpha-tocopherol.

SOURCES OF VITAMIN E

Vitamin E can be found in almonds and other nuts, avocado, broccoli, carrot, kiwifruit, leafy green vegetables, peanuts, sunflower seeds and other seeds, wheat germ, and whole grains. The process of refining vegetable oil destroys vitamin E, so to maximize vitamin E intake, it's best to use unrefined oils.

The Energetic B Vitamins

The body uses carbohydrates, fat, and protein as fuel, and the B vitamins play essential roles in that process. In complex sequences that resemble busy factory production lines, each of the nine B vitamins assists specific enzymes. These enzymes can't function without their particular vitamin assistant, or coenzyme.

For energy production, the body requires dietary sources of thiamin, riboflavin, niacin, pantothenic acid, vitamin B_6, and biotin. Folate, vitamin B_{12}, and choline are crucial to the formation of cells that deliver oxygen and nutrients so the energy production line can function. The B vitamins also help build genetic material, nerve impulse transmitters, certain hormones, and the fats needed in cell membranes. In the sections that follow, we'll discuss the B vitamins in detail, with the exception of vitamin B_{12}, which we covered earlier in the chapter.

Thiamin (Vitamin B^1)

Thiamin is sometimes called the carb burner because it helps convert carbohydrates to usable energy. Thiamin deficiency results in beriberi, a disease characterized by extreme weakness and dysfunction of various physiological systems, including the nervous system. It was described as early as 2600 BC in China, where it got its name, which roughly translates to "weak, weak" or "I cannot, I cannot," clearly reflecting the feeling of weakness that results.

Beriberi was a cause of death among the poor in Asia during the 1800s when polished white rice was introduced to the diets of those who had limited access to thiamin-rich foods. Polishing removes the outer bran layer of the rice, which contains thiamin. Wealthier people tended to include other sources of thiamin in their diets, but rice was a dietary staple among the poor. At that time such diseases were thought to be linked to infection or other causes, but three physicians, one of them Japanese and two Dutch, traced the weakness and nerve disorders in beriberi to a deficient diet. Their insights played a key role in the discovery of vitamins. Now, thiamin, iron, and sometimes several other B vitamins are added to white rice.

RECOMMENDED INTAKES OF THIAMIN

Women need 1.1mg of thiamin per day, and men need 1.2mg per day. Thiamin requirements are linked with calorie intake, so active, high-energy people require more. Studies show that vegans generally meet recommended intakes or exceed them by 50 to 100 percent.

SOURCES OF THIAMIN

Thiamin is found in moderate amounts in many plant foods: whole and enriched grains, whole-grain products, legumes, nuts, seeds, and nutritional yeast. It is also present in avocado, carrot juice, corn, dried fruit, peas, and squash.

Riboflavin (Vitamin B^2)

While the rest of the B vitamins are busy converting carbs, fats, and protein into energy, riboflavin is busy interacting with them, providing support and protection against free radicals and toxins. Deficiency symptoms include cracks at the corners of the mouth and inflammation and redness of the tongue.

RECOMMENDED INTAKE OF RIBOFLAVIN

Women need 1.1mg of riboflavin per day, and men need 1.3mg per day. As with thiamin, the requirement is linked to caloric intake and activity level. Studies show that vegans usually meet the recommended intakes.

SOURCES OF RIBOFLAVIN

Just 1 1/2 teaspoons (7ml) of nutritional yeast provides a day's recommended intake of riboflavin. (The ultraviolet rays of the sun or fluorescent light can destroy riboflavin, so keep nutritional yeast in an opaque container in a dark place.) Soy foods, fortified cereals, and Marmite yeast extract are excellent sources. Moderately good sources include almonds, avocado, banana, broccoli, buckwheat, cashews, enriched wheat flour, green beans, leafy greens, peas, quinoa, sea vegetables, seeds, sweet potato, and whole grains. Sprouting has been shown to increase the riboflavin content of alfalfa seeds and mung beans.

Niacin (Vitamin B^3)

Niacin assists hundreds of enzymes in producing energy and supporting the health of the skin, digestive tract, and nervous system. Niacin-deficiency disease is called *pellagra,* an Italian word meaning "sour skin," and its symptoms are dermatitis, diarrhea, dementia, and death. Deficiency can occur in people whose diets are very low in calories and variety because if we don't get enough riboflavin, vitamin B_6, or iron, we can't convert the amino acid tryptophan to niacin.

Niacin deficiency was first recorded in areas of the world where poorer people subsisted mainly on corn, or maize, a food that's low in both niacin and tryptophan. Yet at the same time, it was also recognized that people in Mexico and Central and South America, who typically relied on corn as a dietary staple, didn't get pellagra. As it turned out, the niacin in corn is in bound form, meaning the body can't absorb it unless the corn is treated with an alkali, which is exactly what cooks do in the traditional cuisines of Mexico and many other Central and South American cuisines: they treat corn with lime before cooking. (Here, lime refers to calcium hydroxide, not the fruit.) This treatment releases the bound niacin, making it easier for the body to absorb. Unfortunately, it wasn't until the early 1900s that niacin deficiency was understood to be the cause of pellagra.

RECOMMENDED INTAKES OF NIACIN

Women need 14mg per day, and men should get 16mg. Studies show that most vegans meet the recommended intakes. In supplements, the maximum upper intake level recommended is 35mg. Pharmacological preparations of niacin use higher dosages as cholesterol-lowering agents in treating heart disease and may lead to side effects such as flushing of the face, chest, and arms.

SOURCES OF NIACIN

Excellent sources of niacin include many foods that are rich in protein: edamame, soybeans, peanuts, peanut butter, peas, tempeh, tofu, and other legumes. Other good sources are avocado, buckwheat, cherimoya, dried fruit, durian, enriched and whole grains, fortified cereals, Marmite yeast extract, mushrooms, nutritional yeast, nuts, quinoa, sea vegetables, seeds, tahini, and wild rice. Good sources of tryptophan include green vegetables, seeds, nuts, and legumes. The great agricultural chemist George Washington Carver's emphasis on the importance of peanuts as a good source of niacin did much to improve the diets of Southerners.

Pantothenic Acid (Vitamin B^5)

The name of pantothenic acid comes from the Greek *pantothen,* meaning "from everywhere." It is present in all whole plant foods, so it's not likely to be lacking in vegan diets unless they are particularly low in calories.

As a coenzyme found in all living cells, pantothenic acid plays a central role in releasing energy from food. It also helps build fats, including any cholesterol that we need, steroid hormones, and other essential compounds. In addition, it supports communication between cells so they work together to our benefit.

RECOMMENDED INTAKES OF PANTOTHENIC ACID

The recommended intake for adults is 5mg per day. Research shows that most vegans meet or exceed recommended levels.

SOURCES OF PANTOTHENIC ACID

All whole plant foods contribute pantothenic acid, at least in small amounts. Certain foods are particularly good sources: Avocado, broccoli, legumes, mushrooms, nutritional yeast, nuts, seeds, sweet potato, and whole grains. It is also possible that we absorb some of the pantothenic acid produced by intestinal bacteria.

Vitamin B^6 (Pyridoxine)

There are many stories about the powers of vitamin B_6. Some are quite mysterious, and not all are substantiated by science. However, there is research showing that vitamin B_6 helps improve morning sickness and could help alleviate depression in cases where the condition is linked to high levels of homocysteine.

Vitamin B_6 is needed to help convert amino acids to energy and for building amino acids, fatty acids, and neurotransmitters. As one of its many functions, vitamin B_6 helps the body get rid of homocysteine, a troublesome compound created during certain metabolic processes. Folate and vitamins B_6 and B_{12} convert homocysteine to two amino acids that the body can use in building protein. When these three B vitamins are in short supply, homocysteine levels rise, which may lead to damage of arterial walls and the formation of blood clots, increasing the risk of heart disease. Vitamin B_6 also helps the body access glycogen, the storage form of glucose, from the liver when energy is needed. In addition, it supports the immune system and many other essential physiological processes.

RECOMMENDED INTAKES OF VITAMIN B^6

The adult recommended intake for vitamin B$_6$ is 1.3mg to age fifty; after fifty, it increases to 1.5mg for women and 1.7mg for men. Studies show that most vegans meet the recommended intakes.

SOURCES OF VITAMIN B^6

Vitamin B$_6$ is widely distributed among plant foods, especially fruit. For example, you can get your day's supply from three bananas. Vegan diets generally include plenty of foods rich in vitamin B$_6$, such as avocado, legumes, nutritional yeast, nuts, seeds, spinach, whole grains, and fortified breakfast cereals.

Biotin (Vitamin B^7)

Along with other B vitamins, biotin is involved in the metabolism of amino acids, fats, and carbohydrates. This vitamin doesn't hit the headlines because deficiencies are rare. Although research is limited, most people on plant-based diets seem to get sufficient biotin. Your intake of biotin is likely to be fine unless you're not eating enough calories.

RECOMMENDED INTAKES OF BIOTIN

Adults are advised to get 30mcg of biotin per day. One study of Seventh-day Adventists found plasma levels of biotin to be higher in vegans than in lacto-ovo vegetarians and nonvegetarians.

SOURCES OF BIOTIN

The many sources of biotin include almonds, avocado, banana, carrot, cauliflower, corn, hazelnuts, legumes, nutritional yeast, peanut butter, raspberries, oatmeal, onion, tomato, walnuts, and whole grains.

Folate (Vitamin B^9, Folic Acid)

Folate helps build DNA and protect it from changes that may lead to cancer. In pregnancy, adequate folate is important for proper growth of the fetus; a deficiency can cause neural tube defects and other types of birth defects. Folate can help prevent heart disease by lowering elevated levels of homocysteine. It supports fertility, and for men it's required to make healthy sperm.

High blood levels of homocysteine may indicate deficiencies of either folate (less likely in vegans) or vitamin B_{12} (likely in vegans who don't take B_{12} supplements or consume enough B_{12}-fortified foods). Lack of these two B vitamins can also cause red blood cells to fail to mature properly, increasing in size until they're big enough to divide, but failing to divide properly and being unable to perform their oxygen-carrying function. This condition is known as macrocytic anemia, or big cell anemia. People with this condition are often weak, tired, and short of breath.

The word *folate* has the same Latin root as *foliage,* so you can probably guess that leafy greens are important sources of this vitamin. In 1945, folate was first isolated; the source was spinach. Since that time, numerous other green vegetables have been added to the list of excellent sources.

Folate is the form of vitamin B_9 that occurs in food. The form in supplements, folic acid, is somewhat different chemically, and scientists are still exploring the similarities and differences of the two forms. Although natural folate in foods is protective against cancer, folic acid supplements in high doses may actually increase risk of asthma and various types of cancer, including breast, prostate, and colorectal, although more research is needed.

RECOMMENDED INTAKES OF FOLATE AND FOLIC ACID

The recommended intake for adults is 400mcg per day. We don't need higher levels than these recommended intakes. It's safest to get this vitamin from food. In order to absorb folate, the body requires adequate intakes of vitamin C and iron. Studies have shown that vegan intakes of folate generally meet or exceed recommended levels.

Large amounts of folic acid can mask a B_{12} deficiency. Therefore, you shouldn't take more than 1,000mcg of folic acid per day. High intakes of folic acid may also provoke seizures in people taking anticonvulsant medications. While many experts suggest that taking less than 1,000mcg of folic acid per day is safe, others recommend getting most or all of your recommended intake for this vitamin in the form of folate from food.

Pregnancy and Lactation

Women capable of becoming pregnant are advised to consume 400mcg of folic acid daily in order to protect against neural tube defects, which can occur in the fetus before a woman knows she is pregnant. Women who are pregnant are advised to take 600mcg daily throughout pregnancy.

SOURCES OF FOLATE AND FOLIC ACID

Excellent sources of folate include almonds, asparagus, avocado, beet, cashews, fortified breakfast cereals, kelp, kiwifruit, legumes, mung bean sprouts, nutritional yeast, oranges, quinoa, spinach, sprouted lentils, sunflower seeds, and yeasts. Folic acid is added to enriched flour, rice, and pasta, and this policy has been credited with greatly reducing the incidence of neural tube defects in North America since 1998.

Sprouting has been shown to more than double the folate content of seeds. Folate is easily destroyed by boiling, whereas steaming has been shown to cause little or no loss of folate from broccoli or spinach.

Choline

Choline has hopped back and forth across the line between vitamin—and therefore essential—and nonvitamin. That's because the body can produce sufficient choline unless a person's diet is short on folate, vitamin B_{12}, and the amino acid methionine. People seem to need significantly different amounts depending on genetics and diet. Choline is present in all cell membranes of plants and animals, and in the brain as part of a fatty mixture of molecules known as lecithin. In cell membranes, choline helps transport fats and other nutrients into and out of cells. In the brain, it helps build important neurotransmitters, making it crucial for the transmission of nerve impulses. Choline also helps clear fat and cholesterol from the liver.

By the way, lecithin is a food additive that acts as an emulsifier. It may be added to a chocolate bar to keep the cocoa and cocoa butter from separating. It's also used in vegetable oil sprays. Most lecithin is derived from soy or sunflower oil and is vegan. However, it may be derived from eggs. Sometimes the source will be included on labels as, for example, "soy lecithin."

RECOMMENDED INTAKES OF CHOLINE

Women should get 425mg of choline per day, and men should get 500mg per day.

SOURCES OF CHOLINE

There are plenty of good sources of choline. A few that are particularly rich are beans, broccoli, peas, quinoa, and soy foods.

Vitamin K (Phylloquinone and Menaquinone)

Vitamin K is a relative newcomer to the vitamin hall of fame. It wasn't recognized until

1974, and its functions are still being investigated. The K is derived from the German word *koagulation* and is related to the vitamin's sential role in helping blood clot. The form of vitamin K that was first discovered, vitamin K_1, or phylloquinone, is widely available in plant foods, especially greens. In addition, intestinal bacteria synthesize forms of this vitamin known collectively as vitamin K_2, or the menaquinones. Vitamin K_2 also is present in meat and in a fermented Japanese soy food called natto. Infants are given a vitamin K shot at birth because their intestinal production of vitamin K doesn't get rolling for a few days. Symptoms of vitamin K deficiency include defective blood clotting and hemorrhaging. There also is a synthetic form, known as vitamin K_3, or menadione.

If You Take Blood Thinners

In the past, doctors often advised their patients who take anticoagulants, or blood thinners, to avoid eating greens, since vitamin K acts as a coagulant. Today, most physicians recommend that people eat about the same amount of greens from week to week. Medication is adjusted to factor in the effects of vitamin K from the vegetables. If you are taking these drugs and have questions about whether you should be eating foods rich in vitamin K, consult your doctor.

Vitamin K regulates calcium levels in the blood and plays a role in bone growth and maintaining bone mineral density. Data from the 1998 Nurses' Health Study showed that those who ate lettuce at least once a day had a significantly lower risk of hip fracture than those who ate lettuce once a week or less. Since then, studies have shown that 200mg of vitamin K, the amount present in 1 1/2 cups (375ml) of raw spinach or 1/2 cup (125ml) of raw or cooked kale, can reduce the risk of bone fracture.

RECOMMENDED INTAKES OF VITAMIN K

Women should get 90mcg of vitamin K per day, and men are advised to get 120mcg. The average intake of the US population has been estimated to be 300 to 500mcg per day, and most vegans probably get more. A study of vegans' bloodclotting rate, an indicator of vitamin K status, indicated that intakes of vitamin K were sufficient.

If you follow popular lay health gurus on the Internet, you may wonder if you need supplemental vitamin K_2, since little of this form is present in a vegan diet. At this time, there is no scientific evidence to suggest that vegans need to worry about supplementing with vitamin K_2.

SOURCES OF VITAMIN K

Leafy green vegetables are vitamin K superstars. You can get your recommended daily intake from 2 tablespoons (30ml) of parsley or kale or 2 cups (500ml) of romaine lettuce. If you put a little dressing (not fat-free) on your salad, the oil increases absorption of this fat-soluble vitamin.

Other excellent sources are asparagus, avocado, broccoli, Brussels sprouts, cabbage, cauliflower, grapes, kiwifruit, lentils, peas, pumpkin, sea vegetables, and soybean oil. It is best not to overcook foods to help minimize losses. Natto, a fermented, bacteria-rich soy food from Japan, is a unique and concentrated source of vitamin K_2.

Vitamins in Vegan Foods

Table 6.2 shows the vitamin content in a typical portion of a variety of vegan foods. You can also find nutrient data on a variety of foods at the US Department of Agriculture website: n db.nal.usda.gov.

TABLE 6.2. Vitamins in vegan foods

FOOD	VITAMIN (unit)	A (mcg)	C (mg)	E (mg)	K (mcg)	THIA-MIN (mg)	RIBO-FLAVIN (mg)	NIACIN (mg)	B₆ (mg)	FOLATE (mcg)	PANTO-THENIC ACID (mg)	BIOTIN (mcg)
Recommended intake for a woman*		700	75	15	90	1.1	1.1	14	1.3–1.5	400	5	30
Recommended intake for a man*		900	90	15	120	1.2	1.3	16	1.3–1.7	400	5	30
FRUITS												
Apple, medium, each		4	6	0.2	3	0.02	0.04	0.1	0.06	4	0.1	2
Apples, dried (1 c/86 g)		0	3	0.5	3	0	0.1	0.8	0.11	0	0.2	...
Apricot, medium, each		34	4	0.3	1	0.01	0.01	0.3	0.02	3	0.1	...
Apricots, dried (¹/₄ c/32 g)		59	0.3	1.4	1	0.01	0.25	0.9	0.1	3	0.2	...
Apricots, sliced (1 c/165 g)		158	16	1.5	5	0.05	0.07	1.4	0.09	15	0.4	...
Banana, dried (¹/₄ c/25 g)		3	2	0.1	0.5	0.05	0.06	0.7	0.11	3.5	0.1	1
Banana, medium, each		4	10	0.1	1	0.04	0.09	1	0.43	24	0.4	3
Banana, sliced (1 c/150 g)		4.5	13	0.2	1	0.05	0.11	1.2	0.55	30	0.5	4
Blackberries (1 c/144 g)		16	30	1.7	29	0.03	0.04	0.9	0.04	36	0.4	1
Blueberries (1 c/145 g)		4	14	0.8	28	0.05	0.06	0.7	0.08	9	0.2	...
Cantaloupe, diced (1 c/156 g)		264	57	0.1	4	0.06	0.03	1.2	0.11	33	0.2	...
Cherimoya, chopped (1 c/156 g)		1	18	...	...	0.14	0.19	0.9	0.33	28	0.4	...
Coconut, dried (¹/₄ c/29 g)		0	1.5	0.1	0.1	0.02	0.03	0.5	0.09	2.5	0.2	...
Currants, Zante, dried (¹/₄ c/36 g)		1	2	0.1	1	0.06	0.05	0.6	0.11	4	0	...
Dates, chopped (¹/₄ c/45 g)		0	0	0	1	0.02	0.03	0.7	0.1	9	0	...
Fig, fresh, medium, each		4	1	0.1	2	0.03	0.02	0.2	0.06	3	0.2	...
Figs, dried (¹/₄ c/50 g)		0	1	0.2	8	0.04	0.04	0.5	0.05	5	0.2	...
Gooseberries (1 c/150 g)		22	42	0.6	...	0.06	0.04	0.7	0.12	9	0.4	1
Grapefruit, medium, each		143	77	0.3	0	0.11	0.08	0.5	0.13	32	0.6	2
Grapefruit juice, pink (1 c/247 g)		54	94	0.1	...	0.1	0.05	0.5	0.11	25	0.5	2
Grapefruit juice, white (1 c/247 g)		5	94	0.5	0	0.1	0.05	0.5	0.11	25	0.5	2

FOOD	VITAMIN (unit)	A (mcg)	C (mg)	E (mg)	K (mcg)	THIA-MIN (mg)	RIBO-FLAVIN (mg)	NIACIN (mg)	B_c (mg)	FOLATE (mcg)	PANTO-THENIC ACID (mg)	BIOTIN (mcg)
Recommended intake for a woman*		700	75	15	90	1.1	1.1	14	1.3–1.5	400	5	30
Recommended intake for a man*		900	90	15	120	1.2	1.3	16	1.3–1.7	400	5	30
Grapefruit sections (1 c/230 g)		106	79	0.3	0	0.08	0.05	0.7	0.1	23	0.6	2
Guava, diced (1 c/165 g)		51	303	1.2	4	0.08	0.08	2.2	0.24	23	0.2	...
Honeydew melon, diced (1 c/170 g)		5	31	0	5	0.06	0.02	0.9	0.15	32	0.3	...
Huckleberries (1 c/145 g)		4	14	0.8	28	0.05	0.06	0.7	0.08	9	0.2	...
Kiwifruit, medium, each		3	70	1.1	71	0.02	0.02	0.4	0.05	19	0.3	...
Loganberries (1 c/144 g)		16	30	1.7	29	0.03	0.04	0.9	0.04	36	0.4	1
Mango, medium, each		79	57	2.3	7	0.12	0.12	1.5	0.28	29	0.3	...
Mango, sliced (1 c/165 g)		63	46	1.8	9	0.1	0.09	1.2	0.22	23	0.3	...
Orange, medium, each		14	70	0.3	1	0.11	0.05	0.6	0.08	40	0.3	1
Orange juice (1 c/248 g)		25	124	0.1	0	0.22	0.07	1.1	0.1	74	0.5	1
Papaya, cubed (1 c/140 g)		77	87	1	4	0.04	0.04	0.7	0.03	53	0.3	...
Peach, medium, each		16	6	0.7	3	0.02	0.03	1	0.02	4	0.1	0.2
Peach, sliced (1 c/77 g)		27	11	1.2	4	0.04	0.05	1.7	0.04	7	0.2	0.3
Pear, medium, each		2	8	0.2	8	0.02	0.04	0.3	0.05	12	0.1	0.3
Pear, sliced (1 c/140 g)		2	7	0.2	7	0.02	0.04	0.3	0.05	12	0.1	0.3
Pears halves, dried (¼ c/45g)		0	3	0	9	0	0.07	0.6	0.03	0	0.1	...
Pineapple, diced (1 c/155 g)		5	56	0	1	0.12	0.05	0.9	0.17	23	0.3	0.5
Plum, each		8	6	0.2	4	0.02	0.02	0.3	0.02	3	0.1	...
Plums, sliced (1 c/165 g)		26	16	1	11	0.07	0.16	0.8	0.13	4	0.3	...
Prunes, dried (¼ c/44 g)		17	0	0.5	26	0.02	0.08	0.8	0.09	2	0.2	...
Raisins, seedless, packed (¼ c/41 g)		0	1	0.1	0	0.04	0.05	0.7	0.07	2	0.1	1
Raspberries (1 c/123 g)		2	32	1.1	10	0.04	0.05	0.7	0.07	26	0.4	2
Strawberries (1 c/144 g)		1	85	0.4	3	0.03	0.03	0.7	0.07	35	0.2	2
Watermelon, diced (1 c/152 g)		43	12	0.1	0.2	0.05	0.03	0.4	0.07	5	0.3	2
VEGETABLES (RAW UNLESS STATED)												
Arugula, chopped (1 c/20 g)		24	3	0.1	22	0.01	0.02	0.1	0.02	19	...	...
Asparagus, sliced (1 c/134 g)		51	8	1.5	56	0.19	0.19	1.8	0.12	70	0.4	0.5
Asparagus spear, medium, each		6	1	0.2	7	0.02	0.02	0.2	0.02	8	0.1	...
Avocado, California, medium, each		12	15	3.4	36	0.13	0.25	4	0.5	107	2.5	6
Avocado, Florida, medium, each		21	53	8.1	...	0.06	0.16	3.5	0.24	106	2.8	...
Basil, fresh, chopped (1 c/42 g)		56	8	0.1	176	0.01	0.03	0.7	0.05	27	0.1	...
Beans, snap, green (1 c/110 g)		38	18	0.5	...	0.09	0.12	1.2	0.08	41	0.1	1
Beans, snap, yellow (1 c/110 g)		6	18	0.1	16	0.09	0.11	1.2	0.08	41	0.1	1
Beet greens, chopped (1 c/38 g)		120	11	0.6	152	0.04	0.08	0.4	0.04	6	0.1	...
Beets, sliced (1 c/136 g)		3	7	0.1	0.3	0.04	0.05	0.9	0.09	148	0.2	...

FOOD	VITAMIN (unit)	A (mcg)	C (mg)	E (mg)	K (mcg)	THIA-MIN (mg)	RIBO-FLAVIN (mg)	NIACIN (mg)	B₆ (mg)	FOLATE (mcg)	PANTO-THENIC ACID (mg)	BIOTIN (mcg)
Recommended intake for a woman*		700	75	15	90	1.1	1.1	14	1.3–1.5	400	5	30
Recommended intake for a man*		900	90	15	120	1.2	1.3	16	1.3–1.7	400	5	30
Bok choy, sliced (1 c/70 g)		156	32	0.1	25	0.03	0.05	0.5	0.14	46	0.1	1
Broccoli, chopped (1 c/71 g)		55	66	1.2	146	0.05	0.08	0.8	0.11	50	0.4	0.4
Brussels sprouts (1 c/88 g)		33	75	0.8	156	0.12	0.08	1.2	0.19	54	0.3	...
Cabbage, green, chopped (1 c/89 g)		8	29	0.1	53	0.04	0.03	0.5	0.09	38	0.1	2
Cabbage, napa, chopped (1 c/76 g)		12	21	0.1	33	0.03	0.04	0.3	0.18	60	0.1	2
Cabbage, red, chopped (1 c/89 g)		50	51	0.1	34	0.06	0.06	0.5	0.19	16	0.1	2
Cabbage, red, shredded (1 c/70 g)		39	40	0.1	27	0.05	0.05	0.4	0.15	13	0.1	1
Carrot, chopped (1 c/128 g)		771	8	0.8	17	0.08	0.07	1.5	0.18	24	0.3	6
Carrot, medium, each		433	4	0.5	8	0.05	0.04	0.8	0.1	14	0.2	4
Carrot juice (1 c/236 g)		258	9	2.7	37	0.22	0.13	0.9	...	...	0.2	...
Cauliflower, chopped (1 c/100 g)		1	46	0.1	16	0.06	0.06	1	0.22	57	0.7	2
Celery, diced (1 c/101 g)		26	4	0.3	35	0.03	0.07	0.6	0.09	43	0.3	0.1
Celery, stalk, each		14	2	0.2	19	0.01	0.04	0.3	0.05	23	0.2	0.1
Celery root, diced (1 c/156 g)		0	12	0.6	64	0.08	0.09	1.4	0.26	12	0.5	...
Chiles, hot green (1 c/150 g)		88	364	1	21	0.14	0.14	2.1	0.42	34	0.1	...
Chiles, hot red (1 c/150 g)		72	216	1	21	0.11	0.13	2.5	0.76	34	0.3	...
Cilantro (1 c/46 g)		141	16	0.9	...	0.03	0.08	0.6	0.06	29	0.3	...
Collard greens, chopped (1 c/36 g)		120	13	0.8	184	0.02	0.05	0.5	0.06	60	0.1	...
Corn, white, kernels (1 c/154 g)		0	10	0.1	0.5	0.31	0.09	3.2	0.08	71	1.2	...
Corn, yellow, kernels (1 c/154 g)		15	10	0.1	0.5	0.31	0.09	3.2	0.08	71	1.2	...
Cucumber, peeled, sliced (1 c/119 g)		5	4	0	9	0.04	0.03	0	0.06	17	0.3	...
Cucumber, unpeeled, sliced (1 c/104 g)		11	6	0.1	...	0.02	0.03	0.3	0.04	14	0.2	0.9
Dandelion greens, chopped (1 c/55 g)		136	19	2.6	151	0.1	0.14	0.4	0.14	15	0	0.2
Eggplant, cubed (1 c/82 g)		1	2	0.3	3	0.03	0.03	0.7	0.07	18	0.2	...
Garlic clove, medium, each		0	1	0	0	0.01	0	0.1	0.04	0	0	...
Jerusalem artichokes, sliced (1 c/150 g)		2	6	0.3	0	0.3	0.09	2	0.12	20	0.6	...
Kale, chopped (1 c/67 g)		515	80	0.6	547	0.07	0.09	1.1	0.18	19	0	0.3
Kelp, Japanese, chopped (1 c/80 g)		5	2	0.7	53	0.04	0.12	1	0	144	0.5	...
Leeks, chopped (1 c/89 g)		74	11	0.8	42	0.05	0.03	0.5	0.2	57	0.1	1
Lettuce, Bibb/Boston/butterhead, chopped (1 c/55 g)		91	2	0.1	56	0.03	0.03	0.3	0.05	40	0.1	1
Lettuce, iceberg, chopped (1 c/55 g)		9	2	0	13	0.02	0.01	0.1	0.03	31	0.1	1
Lettuce, leaf, chopped (1 c/36 g)		207	10	0.2	97	0.04	0.05	0.3	0.05	21	0.1	1
Lettuce, red leaf, chopped (1 c/28 g)		105	1	0	39	0.02	0.02	0.1	0.03	10	0	...
Lettuce, romaine, chopped (1 c/47 g)		162	13	0.1	57	0.04	0.04	0.3	0.04	76	0.1	1
Mushrooms, shiitake, dried (1 c/145 g)		1	4	0.2	1	0.44	1.84	21.2	1.4	236	31.7	...

FOOD	VITAMIN (unit)	A (mcg)	C (mg)	E (mg)	K (mcg)	THIA-MIN (mg)	RIBO-FLAVIN (mg)	NIACIN (mg)	B₆ (mg)	FOLATE (mcg)	PANTO-THENIC ACID (mg)	BIOTIN (mcg)
Recommended intake for a woman*		700	75	15	90	1.1	1.1	14	1.3–1.5	400	5	30
Recommended intake for a man*		900	90	15	120	1.2	1.3	16	1.3–1.7	400	5	30
Mustard greens, chopped (1 c/56 g)		294	39	1.1	278	0.04	0.06	0.7	0.1	105	0.1	...
Okra, sliced (1 c/100 g)		19	21	0.4	53	0.2	0.06	1.3	0.21	88	0.2	...
Olives, green (1 c/160 g)		24	0	4.8	...	0	0	0	0.02	1	0	...
Onion, green, each		8	3	0.1	4	0.01	0.01	0.1	0.01	10	0	0.5
Onions, green, chopped (1 c/100 g)		50	19	0.6	28	0.06	0.08	0.9	0.06	64	0	4
Onions, red/white/yellow, chopped (1 c/160 g)		0	10	0	1	0.08	0.04	0.6	0.23	30	0.2	6
Parsley (1 c/60 g)		253	80	0.4	984	0.05	0.06	1.2	0.05	91	0.2	...
Parsnips, sliced (1 c/133 g)		0	23	2	30	0.12	0.07	1.2	0.12	89	0.8	0.1
Pea pods, snow/edible (1 c/63 g)		34	38	0.2	16	0.09	0.05	0.7	0.1	26	0.5	...
Peas, fresh (1 c/145 g)		55	58	0.2	36	0.39	0.19	3.9	0.25	94	0.2	0.7
Pepper, bell, green, chopped (1 c/149 g)		27	120	0.6	11	0.09	0.04	1	0.33	16	0.2	...
Pepper, bell, green, medium, each		21	96	0.4	9	0.07	0.03	0.8	0.27	13	0.1	...
Pepper, bell, red, chopped (1 c/149 g)		234	283	2.4	7	0.08	0.13	1.8	0.43	27	0.5	...
Pepper, bell, red, medium, each		187	226	1.9	6	0.06	0.1	1.4	0.35	21	0.4	...
Pepper, bell, yellow, chopped (1 c/149 g)		15	273	1	...	0.04	0.04	1.7	0.25	39	0.2	...
Potato, baked, each (6 oz/170 g)		2	17	0	3.5	0.11	0.08	2.4	0.54	48	0.7	...
Potato, cubed, cooked (½ c/75 g)		0	6	0	1.6	0.08	0.02	1	0.21	7	0.4	...
Radish, daikon, chopped (1 c/88 g)		0	19	0	...	0.02	0.02	0.2	0.04	25	0.1	...
Radish, daikon, medium, each		0	74	0	...	0.07	0.07	0.8	0.16	95	0.5	...
Radish, medium, each		0	1	0	0.1	0	0	0	0	1	0	...
Radishes, sliced (1 c/116 g)		0	17	0	2	0.01	0.05	0.4	0.08	29	0.2	...
Radish sprouts (1 c/38 g)		8	11	...	...	0.04	0.04	1.1	0.11	36	0.3	...
Rutabaga, chopped (1 c/140 g)		0	35	0.4	0.4	0.13	0.06	1.3	0.14	29	0.2	0.1
Spinach, chopped (1 c/30 g)		141	8	0.6	145	0.02	0.06	0.4	0.06	58	0	0
Squash, acorn, cubed (1 c/140 g)		25	15	0.2	...	0.2	0.01	1.2	0.22	24	0.6	...
Squash, butternut, cubed (1 c/140 g)		1,277	50	3.5	3	0.24	0.05	3.4	0.37	65	1	...
Squash, crookneck, cubed (1 c/130 g)		10	11	0.1	...	0.07	0.06	0.8	0.14	30	0.1	...
Squash, Hubbard, cubed (1 c/116 g)		79	13	0.1	...	0.08	0.05	1.1	0.18	19	0.5	...
Squash, winter, all types, cubed (1 c/116 g)		79	14	0.1	1	0.03	0.07	0.9	0.18	28	0.2	...
Sweet potato, cubed (1 c/133 g)		967	30	0.3	2	0.1	0.08	1.2	0.28	19	1.1	...
Tomato, cherry, each		7	2	0.1	1	0.01	0	0.1	0.01	3	0	0.7
Tomato, green, chopped (1 c/180 g)		58	42	0.7	18	0.11	0.07	1.2	0.15	16	0.9	...
Tomato, medium, each		63	19	0.8	12	0.06	0.03	1	0.12	22	0.1	6
Tomato, red, chopped (1 c/180 g)		76	23	1	14	0.07	0.03	1.2	0.14	27	0.2	7

FOOD	VITAMIN (unit)	A (mcg)	C (mg)	E (mg)	K (mcg)	THIA-MIN (mg)	RIBO-FLAVIN (mg)	NIACIN (mg)	B₆ (mg)	FOLATE (mcg)	PANTO-THENIC ACID (mg)	BIOTIN (mcg)
Recommended intake for a woman*		700	75	15	90	1.1	1.1	14	1.3–1.5	400	5	30
Recommended intake for a man*		900	90	15	120	1.2	1.3	16	1.3–1.7	400	5	30
Tomato, Roma, each		26	8	0.3	5	0.03	0.01	0.4	0.05	9	0.1	2
Tomato, yellow, chopped (1 c/139 g)		0	13	...	...	0.06	0.07	1.8	0.08	42	0.2	...
Tomatoes, sun-dried (1 c/54 g)		24	21	0	23	0.28	0.26	5.8	0.18	37	1.1	...
Turnip, cubed (1 c/130 g)		0	27	0	0.1	0.05	0.04	0.7	0.12	20	0.3	0.1
Turnip greens (1 c/55 g)		0	33	1.6	138	0.04	0.06	0.6	0.14	107	0.2	...
Water chestnuts, sliced (1 c/124 g)		0	5	1.5	0.4	0.17	0.25	1.2	0.41	20	0.6	...
Yam, cubed (1 c/150 g)		10.5	26	0.6	4	0.17	0.05	1.1	0.44	34	0.5	...
Zucchini, baby, each		0	4	0	...	0	0	0.1	0.02	2	0	...
Zucchini, cubed (1 c/124 g)		12.4	21	0.1	5	0.06	0.18	0.8	0.27	36	0.2	...
NUTS AND SEEDS												
Almond butter (2 tbsp/32 g)		0	0	6.5	...	0.04	0.2	2.2	0.02	21	0.1	...
Almonds (¼ c/36 g)		0	...	9	...	0.1	0.3	2.5	0.1	16	0.1	24
Brazil nut, large, each		0	0	0.3	0	0.03	0	0.1	0	1	0	...
Brazil nuts (¼ c/35 g)		1	0	2	0	0.21	0.01	0.9	0.03	8	0.1	...
Cashew butter (2 tbsp/32 g)		0	0	0.5	...	0.1	0.06	1.9	0.09	22	0.4	...
Cashews (¼ c/33 g)		0	0	0.3	11	0.14	0.02	2	0.14	8	0.3	4
Chia seeds (2 tbsp c/20 g)		...	3	...	...	0.17	0.04	3.3	0.14	23	0.2	...
Flaxseeds, ground (2 tbsp/14 g)		0	0	0	1	0.23	0.02	0.4	0.06	12	0.1	...
Hazelnuts (¼ c/34 g)		0	2	5.1	5	0.22	0.04	1.7	0.19	38	0.3	26
Pecans (¼ c/27 g)		2	0	0.9	...	0.21	0.03	0	0.06	11	0.5	...
Pine nuts (¼ c/34 g)		0	0	3.2	18	0.1	0.08	2.1	0.03	23	0.1	...
Pistachio nuts (¼ c/32 g)		9	1	0.7	23	0.28	0.05	1.9	0.55	16	0.2	...
Poppy seeds (2 tbsp/17 g)		0	0	0.3	0	0.15	0.03	0	0.05	10	0	...
Pumpkin seeds (¼ c/35 g)		7	1	0	18	0.07	0.11	2.8	0.08	20	0.1	...
Sesame seeds, whole (2 tbsp/18 g)		0	0	0	0	0.1	0.03	0.6	0.1	12	0	2
Sesame tahini (2 tbsp/30 g)		1	0	0.7	...	0.39	0.15	1.8	0.05	29	0.2	...
Sunflower seed butter (2 tbsp/32 g)		1	1	15	...	0.1	0.09	3.2	0.26	76	2.3	...
Sunflower seed kernels (¼ c/36 g)		1	1	12.4	1	0.83	0.09	3.5	0.28	82	2.4	...
Walnuts, black, chopped (¼ c/31 g)		5	1	0.8	...	0.07	0.04	1.8	0.17	21	0.2	6
Walnuts, English, chopped (¼ c/30 g)		0	1	0.2	0.8	0.1	0.05	1.2	0.16	29	0.2	6
LEGUMES												
Adzuki beans, cooked (1 c/230 g)		1	0	...	...	0.26	0.15	1.6	0.22	278	1	...
Black beans, cooked (1 c/172 g)		0.5	...	0	...	0.42	0.1	0.9	0.12	256	0.4	...
Black-eyed peas, cooked (1 c/171 g)		1	...	0.4	2.9	0.35	0.09	0.9	0.17	...	...	...
Chickpeas, cooked (1 c/164 g)		2	2	0.6	6.6	0.19	0.1	0.9	0.2	282	0.7	...

FOOD	VITAMIN (unit)	A (mcg)	C (mg)	E (mg)	K (mcg)	THIA-MIN (mg)	RIBO-FLAVIN (mg)	NIACIN (mg)	B₆ (mg)	FOLATE (mcg)	PANTO-THENIC ACID (mg)	BIOTIN (mcg)
Recommended intake for a woman*		700	75	15	90	1.1	1.1	14	1.3–1.5	400	5	30
Recommended intake for a man*		900	90	15	120	1.2	1.3	16	1.3–1.7	400	5	30
Cranberry beans, cooked (1 c/177 g)		0	0	...	...	0.37	0.12	0.9	0.14	366	...	...
Edamame, cooked (1 c/155 g)		...	10	1	41	0.31	0.24	1.4	0.16	482	0.2	...
Great Northern beans, cooked (1 c/177 g)		0	2	...	...	0.28	0.1	1.2	0.21	181	0.5	...
Kidney beans, cooked (1 c/177 g)		0	2	1.5	5.8	0.28	0.1	1	0.21	230	0.4	...
Lentils, brown/green, cooked (1 c/198 g)		0	3	0.2	3.4	0.33	0.14	2.1	0.35	358	1.3	...
Lentil sprouts, raw (1 c/77 g)		2	13	0.1	...	0.18	0.1	0.9	0.15	77	0.4	...
Lima beans, cooked (1 c/188 g)		0	0	0.3	3.8	0.3	0.1	0.8	0.3	156	0.8	...
Mung bean sprouts, raw (1 c/104 g)		1	14	0.1	34	0.09	0.13	1.4	0.09	63	0.4	...
Navy beans, cooked (1 c/182 g)		0	2	0	1.1	0.43	0.12	1.2	0.25	255	0.5	...
Peanuts, raw (1 c/146 g)		0	0	12.2	0	0.93	0.2	17.6	0.51	350	0.4	105
Pea sprouts, raw (1 c/120 g)		10	12	0	...	0.27	0.19	3.7	0.32	173	1.2	...
Peas, raw (1 c/145 g)		55	58	0.2	36	0.39	0.19	3	0.24	94	...	...
Peas, split, cooked (1 c/196 g)		0	1	0.1	9.8	0.37	0.11	1.7	0.09	127	1.2	...
Pinto beans, cooked (1 c/171 g)		0	1	1.6	6	0.33	0.11	0.5	0.39	294	0.4	...
Soybeans, cooked (1 c/172 g)		0	3	0.6	33	0.27	0.49	0.7	0.4	93	0.3	...
Soy milk, fortified (1 c/243 g)**		134	0	0.3	7.3	0.07	0.45	1	0.08	22	0.9	9
Tempeh, raw, cubed (1 c/166 g)		0	0	...	...	0.13	0.59	4.4	0.36	40	...	...
Tofu, calcium-set, firm, raw, cubed (1 c/252 g)**		...	0	0	6	0.4	0.26	1	0.23	73	0.1	...
White beans, cooked (1 c/179 g)		0	0	1.7	6.3	0.21	0.08	0.25	0.17	145	0.5	...
GRAINS												
Amaranth, cooked (1 c/246 g)		0	...	0.5	...	0.04	0.05	0.6	0.28	...	...	...
Barley, pearl, cooked (1 c/157 g)		0	0	0	1.3	0.13	0.1	3.2	0.18	25	0.2	1
Bread, sprouted wheat (1 oz/30 g)		0	0	0.1	...	0.11	0.07	1.1	0.03	11	0	1
Bread, whole wheat (1 oz/30 g)		0	0	0.2	2.2	0.1	0.06	1.3	0.06	14	0.2	1.7
Buckwheat groats, kasha, cooked (1 c/168 g)		0	0	0.2	3.2	0.07	0.07	1.6	0.13	24	0.6	...
Buckwheat sprouts, raw (1 c/33 g)		0	1	0	...	0.07	0.05	1	0.09	13	...	...
Kamut, cooked (1 c/172 g)		7	...	...	...	0.21	0.05	4.7	0.14	21	...	...
Millet, cooked (1 c/174 g)		0	0	0	0.5	0.18	0.14	2.3	0.19	33	...	...
Oatmeal, cooked (1 c/234 g)		0	0	0.2	0.7	0.18	0.04	0.5	0.01	14	...	...
Quinoa, cooked (1 c/185 g)		0	0	1.2	...	0.2	0.2	0.8	0.23	78	...	...
Rice, brown, cooked (1 c/195 g)		0	0	0.1	1.2	0.2	0.02	2.6	0.29	8	0.6	...
Rice, white, enriched, cooked (1 c/158 g)		0	0	0.1	0	0.26	0.02	2.3	0.14	153	0.6	...

FOOD	VITAMIN (unit)	A (mcg)	C (mg)	E (mg)	K (mcg)	THIA-MIN (mg)	RIBO-FLAVIN (mg)	NIACIN (mg)	B₆ (mg)	FOLATE (mcg)	PANTO-THENIC ACID (mg)	BIOTIN (mcg)
Recommended intake for a woman*		700	75	15	90	1.1	1.1	14	1.3–1.5	400	5	30
Recommended intake for a man*		900	90	15	120	1.2	1.3	16	1.3–1.7	400	5	30
Spaghetti, white, enriched, cooked (1 c/140 g)		0	0	...	...	0.38	0.19	2.4	0.07	167	0.2	...
Spaghetti, whole wheat, cooked (1 c/140 g)		0	0	0.4	1	0.15	0.06	1	0.11	7	0.6	...
Wheat sprouts, raw (1 c/108 g)		0	3	0.1	...	0.24	0.17	5.4	0.29	41	1	...
Wild rice, cooked (1 c/164 g)		0	0	0.4	0.8	0.08	0.14	2.1	0.22	43	0.3	...
OTHER												
Maple syrup (1 tbsp/20 g)		0	0	0	0	0	0	0	0	0	0	...
Oil, flaxseed (1 tbsp/13 g)		0	0	2	0	0	0	0	0	0	...	...
Oil, olive (1 tbsp/13 g)		0	0	2	8	0	0	0	0	0	0	...
Red Star Vegetarian Support Formula nutritional yeast (3 to 4 tablespoons/16 g)		0	0	0	0	9.6	9.6	56	9.6	240	1	21
Spirulina, dried (1 tbsp/7 g)		2	1	0.4	1.8	0.17	0.26	0.9	0.02	7	...	...

Sources of data: US Department of Agriculture, Agricultural Research Service, *USDA National Nutrient Database for Standard Reference*, Release 25 (2012), ndb.nal.usda.gov. ESHA Research, The Food Processor software, version 10.12.0.

Key: c = cup; g = gram; mcg = microgram; mg = milligram; oz = ounce; tbsp = tablespoon; ... indicates that no data is available.
*For other ages, see the appendix (page 274).
**Check labels for product-specific information.

Calcium, zinc, iodine ... all the minerals you need are abundant in plant-based foods. Discover how to create a magnificent vegan diet, rich in minerals, in chapter 7.

CHAPTER 7

Minding Your Minerals

In Western cultures, there tends to be a strong, social and industry-based bias in favor of diets that rely heavily on animal products, and this has had a big impact on how most people view dietary requirements for certain minerals. Federal departments of agriculture support and protect meat and dairy producers through a variety of financial and educational programs. In addition, the meat, dairy, and egg industries are major sponsors of conferences for dietitians, physicians, educators, and other health professionals, and the nutrition research funded by these industries is biased in favor of their products. This influences many health professionals who develop nutrition education programs for consumers. On top of all of this is a massive amount of industry-funded advertising. Therefore, it isn't surprising that our minds are imprinted with messages that link calcium and strong bones with dairy consumption or iron with meat consumption. Yet plant-based diets can provide optimal amounts of these

minerals and all of the others that we need.

Minerals, Vegetables, and Animals

Carbohydrates and fat consist of three mineral elements—carbon, hydrogen, and oxygen. Protein provides these three plus nitrogen and sulfur. Many other minerals are also required for the structure and operation of our bodies, including calcium, chromium, copper, iodine, iron, magnesium, manganese, phosphorus, potassium, selenium, sodium, and zinc.

Minerals are released from decaying matter into the soil with the help of bacteria and fungi. When dissolved in water, they are then absorbed by plants. From there, minerals are picked up by plant-eating animals and move further up the food chain into the flesh of carnivorous animals. The decomposition of plant and animal matter returns minerals to the soil.

Minerals can perform a variety of roles. In the human body, minerals are part of dynamic systems in bones, fluids, and nerves. Around the clock, the body remodels bones, builds thyroid hormones and enzymes, creates new red blood cells, and maintains a precise balance between acid and alkali in body fluids. For these purposes, you need a steady supply of building materials, including specific minerals.

In this chapter, you'll learn about those minerals and how they function. We'll also provide tips for meeting recommended intakes and increasing absorption, and discuss the wide range of tasty plant foods that can provide the minerals you need. We'll take a close look at four minerals that are of particular importance to vegans: calcium, iron, zinc, and iodine. Then we'll briefly discuss several other minerals.

For details about minerals for all stages of life, see the appendix. For recommended intakes and food sources of calcium, iron, and zinc, see table 7.2. For food sources of iodine, see table 7.1.

Mineral Absorption

Several factors influence the ease with which our bodies absorb minerals, or their bioavailability. These include cooking, the presence of certain chemical compounds, and an individual's overall mineral status.

COOKING

Minerals are soluble in water and can be lost if the cooking liquid is discarded, particularly if the food has been boiled. Steaming foods, however, results in good mineral retention.

PHYTATE

In legumes, whole grains, nuts, and seeds, the phosphorus-containing compound known as phytate, or phytic acid, binds calcium, iron, magnesium, and zinc. These phytate-mineral complexes aren't completely broken down during digestion, so some of the minerals in these foods can't be absorbed. Enzymes in these foods help release the minerals when they get wet, so soaking, sprouting, juicing, and blending plant foods all help release the minerals from the phytate so the body can absorb them.

Fermentation also helps to release minerals from phytate compounds. When plant foods are fermented, as when soy is made into tempeh or miso, more than half of the phytate complexes are broken down. Leavening bread with yeast has a similar effect on the phytate in wheat.

While too much phytate can interfere with getting an adequate supply of calcium, iron, magnesium, and zinc, phytate compounds aren't all bad. Some have antioxidant powers that appear to offer protection against cancer, cardiovascular disease, and diabetes.

OXALATES

A naturally occurring plant compound called oxalic acid can combine with certain minerals and reduce their absorption during digestion. As a result, the body can't absorb most of the calcium and some of the iron and magnesium from foods such as amaranth, beet greens, cassava, chives, parsley, purslane, spinach, and Swiss chard. However, these foods still contribute a bit of calcium to the diet. For example, your body can still absorb much of the iron and about 5 percent of the calcium in spinach. And, of course, these foods still provide many other nutrients; for example, spinach provides abundant folate, vitamin K, beta-carotene, and numerous other nutrients, along with protective phytochemicals, all of which are unaffected by oxalic acid. The bottom line is, don't dismiss the nutritional value of foods just because they contain oxalic acid.

NEED AND DOSE SIZE

Mineral absorption also can be influenced by your need at that particular moment. If your body is well stocked with iron, for example, you'll absorb iron less efficiently than someone who has very little stored iron. Also, you're likely to absorb less of a mineral consumed in a large quantity at one time, such as a 1,000mg single-dose calcium supplement, than from two doses of 500mg each.

Calcium

As discussed in chapter 2, bone health involves a complex interplay of many lifestyle factors, but a well-designed vegan diet will include vegetables and fruits associated with greater bone density and less bone loss. But even so, some vegan diets are low in calcium or otherwise fail to support lifelong bone health.

From advertising, we get the impression that calcium is the primary player in promoting bone health, but relying on that one mineral to prevent osteoporosis is like trying to win at baseball with only a pitcher on your team. You need other team members—seventeen in fact—on the bases, behind the plate, and in key spots in the outfield. The team has to include a mix of protein; essential fatty acids; the minerals boron, calcium, copper, fluoride, magnesium, manganese, phosphorus, and zinc; and the vitamins B_{12}, B_6, C, D, K, and folate. (For a discussion of many of the vitamins and other nutrients you need for healthy bones, see the section "Osteoporosis,".)

CALCIUM IN PERSPECTIVE

Calcium is the most common mineral in the body. It's also the fifth-most-common mineral in the earth's crust, present in marble, limestone, and chalk. You can get calcium directly from plant foods and from dairy milk. It is also abundant in breast milk. It is believed that prior to the advent of agriculture, humans in many parts of the world had dairy-free diets that were very high in calcium, providing from 1,500 to 3,000mg per day. However, the modern versions of many fruits and other plant foods have been bred for qualities such as sweetness, rather than nutritional excellence, and therefore are far lower in calcium than the versions available to our ancestors. In nature's calcium cycle, animal bones, the shells of marine organisms, and antlers disintegrated, returning calcium to the earth that was absorbed into plants; plus, many populations cooked bones in their soup stocks.

CALCIUM'S FUNCTIONS

Calcium is best known for its structural role in hardening bones and teeth. In addition, it helps blood to clot, allows muscles to relax, helps nerves transmit messages, and regulates cell metabolism. In addition, consuming recommended levels of calcium may help prevent high blood pressure.

Calcium levels in the blood and in the fluids between cells must be kept within a specific and narrow range. If these levels drop too low, the parathyroid gland produces a hormone that activates vitamin D, which raises blood calcium levels by increasing its absorption in the intestine, decreasing urinary calcium losses, and, if necessary, breaking down some bone.

Nutrition education campaigns and dairy advertisements may tell us that we need cow's milk to meet our nutritional needs for calcium, but for most of human history, we've gotten most of the calcium we needed from plants. Dairying appears to be a relatively recent phenomenon, occurring in the last ten thousand years and only in specific areas of the world.

Where dairy products contributed significantly to people's diets, a genetic adaptation occurred that allowed people to continue drinking milk after weaning from breast milk. Normally, after weaning the body produces much less of the enzyme lactase, which digests lactose, or milk sugar. In fact, as much as 70 percent of the world's population experiences diminished lactase production after weaning. In South America, Africa, and Asia, more than 50 percent of people over four years old are lactose intolerant and experience abdominal pain, bloating, flatulence, and diarrhea when they drink cow's milk. In some Asian countries, almost everyone is lactose intolerant.

RECOMMENDED INTAKES OF CALCIUM

The recommended calcium intake is 1,000mg per day for adults younger than fifty and 1,200mg for those fifty and older. For recommended intakes at other stages of life, see the appendix. Most people in the United States, including vegans, fall short of the recommended intake. This is particularly true of women and people older than fifty. It's important to get the recommended intake, as this reduces the risk of bone fractures, which are directly linked to low calcium levels.

CALCIUM SUPPLEMENTS

If you don't get enough calcium from your diet, you should probably take a supplement. Most calcium supplements should be taken with meals because they are absorbed better when stomach acid is present, although calcium citrate and calcium citrate malate can be taken anytime. You also can increase absorption by dividing your daily supplemental calcium into two or more doses. Vitamin D is essential for optimum calcium absorption, so be sure you also get enough vitamin D.

DIETARY SOURCES OF CALCIUM

Calcium is abundant in a wide assortment of vegetables, particularly the low-oxalate green vegetables, broccoli, bok choy, kale, napa cabbage, watercress, and collard, dandelion, mustard, and turnip greens. Other good sources are fresh and dried fruit, calcium-fortified juices, almonds, and tahini. Calcium is added to fortified nondairy milks and tofu, and in both cases, calcium absorption compares favorably with that of cow's milk. Some mineral waters are good sources; check product labels to determine which are.

SOLID SOLUTIONS FOR BETTER BONES

The following sections provide tips on how to ensure strong, healthy bones. In addition, following the recommendations in chapter 14, The Vegan Food Guide, will help ensure you get the entire team of bone-building nutrients.

Put dark green vegetables on your daily menu. Include broccoli, bok choy, collard greens, kale, and napa cabbage in your diet regularly. Some minerals (and vitamins) are lost in cooking water, so steam these vegetables or use the mineralrich cooking water in soups or when cooking grains.

Eat calcium-set tofu. Tofu is made by coagulating soy milk in either nigari (magnesium chloride) or calcium sulfate. Obviously, the type made with a calcium salt such as sulfate is what you want if you're looking to increase your intake of calcium. Check the label; the calcium content can range from 120mg to 600mg per serving. Tofu is an unusually versatile food. It can be added to everything from soup to dessert, so use it often. The isoflavones in soy foods, such as tofu, tempeh, and soy milk, also are associated with reduced risk of bone fracture.

Drink calcium-fortified beverages. Fortified nondairy milks and juices can help boost your total calcium intake.

Include almonds, almond butter, blackstrap molasses, figs, and tahini in your meals and snacks. Every time you replace 2 tablespoons (30ml) of peanut butter with an equal amount of almond butter, you increase your calcium intake by 73mg. By replacing 1 tablespoon (15ml) of jam with 1 tablespoon (15ml) of molasses, you boost your intake by a surprising 168mg of calcium. These flavorful options boost your calcium and also provide iron and zinc.

Don't keep company with the calcium thieves. Avoid alcohol, limit caffeine, and, of course, don't smoke. Keep your sodium intake below 2,300mg per day. If you are salt sensitive, have high blood pressure, or are middle-aged or older, keep your sodium intake below 1,500mg per day.

Get some sunshine (or vitamin D). Take the opportunity to stretch your legs and walk around the block on your lunch break. In addition to benefiting from the exercise, under the right conditions your body can manufacture your day's supply of vitamin D. (For more on vitamin D section entitled "Vitamin D (Calciferol)".) Take a vitamin D supplement when sunshine isn't an option.

Exercise. Some form of weight-bearing exercise, such as walking, jogging, dancing, hiking, or step classes, is essential for lifelong bone health. With bones, it's a case of use 'em or lose 'em.

Top off with a supplement. If you think you aren't getting enough calcium and other bone-building nutrients in your diet, take them in supplement form.

Iron

Iron is a precious metal when it comes to human health. As a part of red blood cells, it plays a central role in transporting oxygen throughout the body and carrying away carbon dioxide, a metabolic waste product. As part of many enzyme systems, iron also plays key roles in the production of energy, immune system functioning, and mental processes involved in learning and behavior.

Every day we lose tiny amounts of iron in cells that are sloughed from skin and the inner lining of the intestine. Naturally, people experiencing blood loss for any reason (such as ulcers or blood donation) have increased needs. Women have iron losses during menstruation and generally need an extra 30 to 45mg of iron each month, making their requirements significantly higher than those of men. Growth and the building of new cells put demands on stored and dietary iron and can deplete the small reserves of infants and children. With teens, there can be the double challenges of growth and notoriously poor eating habits. Athletes have somewhat higher requirements due to increased oxygen demands. (For more on meeting the iron needs of athletes, see chapter 13). The body is efficient at recycling iron, but once lost, iron must be replaced in the diet, perhaps augmented by supplements.

IRON IN PERSPECTIVE

Many vegetarians have lower levels of stored iron—called serum ferritin—than nonvegetarians. This common situation doesn't affect how we feel and isn't an issue as long as you regularly eat foods containing iron so you can replace any iron you lose. In fact, a lower level of serum ferritin might be an advantage, since it may help improved insulin sensitivity and reduce risk of type 2 diabetes. In addition, high serum ferritin may be linked to coronary heart disease and colon cancer.

Even with lower iron stores, vegetarians and vegans don't experience irondeficiency anemia more often than nonvegetarians. However, iron deficiency is the most common nutritional deficiency worldwide, especially among women of childbearing age, infants, and teens, so vegans in those categories need to be careful. When hemoglobin levels go below the normal range, problems begin. The body's capacity to deliver oxygen to the cells will diminish, and the person may look pale, have headaches, and feel exhausted, irritable, and lethargic. Iron deficiency is easily diagnosed, so if you have any doubts, have a lab test done.

RECOMMENDED INTAKES OF IRON

Because the iron from plant foods isn't absorbed as readily as the iron from meat, vegans and vegetarians should aim for 1.8 times as much iron as the recommended intake for nonvegetarians. Vegetarian women of childbearing age are advised to get 32.4mg of iron per day, and other vegetarian adults need 14.4mg of iron; for other ages, see the appendix and multiply the recommended intake by 1.8. However, these recommendations are based on skimpy evidence and lessthan-ideal diets. Vegans who eat plenty of foods rich in vitamin C and who don't routinely use tea, coffee, or calcium supplements are likely to need somewhat less than these high levels.

An iron supplement or iron as part of a multivitamin-mineral supplement can be a valuable addition to any diet that may be somewhat low in iron, and can be helpful for people with low or marginal iron status.

DIETARY SOURCES OF IRON

Because the iron from plant foods isn't absorbed as readily as the iron from meat, the Institute of Medicine has set the recommended intake for vegetarians at 1.8 times higher than for nonvegetarians. This decision has been a point of controversy because it was based on a diet in a single study that minimized iron absorption.

Vegetarian women of childbearing age are advised to get 32.4mg iron per day and other vegetarian adults 14.4mg (see Table 2 in APPENDIX for complete recommendations). Vegans who eat plenty of foods rich in vitamin C and who don't routinely use tea, coffee, or calcium supplements are likely to need somewhat less than these high levels.

IRON ABSORPTION

Even though the body is continually breaking down red blood cells and building new ones, it efficiently recycles the iron in old red blood cells. The body absorbs more iron when needed and less when not needed, but calcium and compounds such as phytate compounds, tannins, and polyphenols (in tea, coffee, and cocoa) decrease the amount of iron the body can absorb. If you're iron deficient or need to maximize your iron intake, avoid consuming these at the same time as your iron sources.

On the other hand, foods rich in vitamin C, such as red peppers and strawberries, or foods high in citric acid, such as citrus fruits, increase the absorption of iron. These acidic foods change the iron in plant foods into a soluble form that is readily absorbed. For example, 5 fluid ounces (150ml) of orange juice, containing 75mg of vitamin C, has been shown to increase the absorption of iron from foods eaten at the same time by a factor of four. Vegans typically eat plenty of fruits and vegetables and get over 150 percent more vitamin C than nonvegetarians. This is a definite advantage when it comes to iron absorption.

As previously mentioned, soaking, fermenting, leavening with yeast, and sprouting break down the phytate compounds in grains, beans, peas, and lentils, releasing iron and other minerals and making them easier to absorb. Compounds in onions and garlic also help increase the availability of iron (and zinc) from grains and legumes, so consider adding them to bean and grain dishes.

Zinc

Zinc is essential to cell division and plays significant roles in growth during pregnancy and from infancy through adolescence. Zinc is important to the functioning of the immune system and is necessary for wound healing and nerve development. In addition, it is crucial for the functioning of a whopping three hundred enzyme systems. Our ability to taste is highly dependent on zinc. The iris and retina of the eye and the prostate, sperm, and seminal fluid contain high concentrations of zinc, and zinc may also play an important role in regulating men's serum testosterone levels.

Adequate zinc intake is particularly important during periods of growth, from gestation and birth through adolescence. Severe zinc deficiency shows up in stunted growth, reduced immune function, diarrhea, poor appetite, and an impaired ability to taste. Marginal zinc deficiency can be difficult to detect, but it's more likely than severe zinc deficiency in North America, particularly among low-income children and pregnant women, sometimes resulting in babies being born prematurely.

RECOMMENDED INTAKES OF ZINC

The recommended daily intake for zinc is 8mg for women and 11mg for men. However, vegan diets often include more substances that inhibit zinc absorption, so needs may actually be 50 percent higher. Vegans with low caloric intakes or who rely on refined foods may have poor zinc intakes.

In most studies to date, vegans met or exceeded the recommended intake for zinc, but in two studies, vegans' average zinc intake was about 10 percent short of the recommended amount. To be on the safe side, include foods rich in zinc every day. As with iron, soaking, fermentation, leavening with yeast, and sprouting can greatly improve the bioavailability of zinc. Garlic also promotes absorption, so consider adding garlic to hummus, cooked rice, and other legumes and grains.

DIETARY SOURCES OF ZINC

Zinc is generally present in the same vegan foods as iron: seeds, nuts (especially cashews), legumes, tofu, and whole grains, including oats and brown rice. Seeds and seed butters can be zinc superstars in a vegan diet. Therefore, hummus on whole-grain bread or crackers is a particularly zinc-rich combination. Note that diets that rely heavily on refined foods are usually low in zinc, since refining strips the zinc from food.

Iodine

Iodine is a mineral required in only miniscule amounts, but it is absolutely critical to life and health. It is an essential part of thyroid hormones (both T_3, or triiodothyronine, and T_4, or thyroxine), and most of the organ systems in the body are influenced by these hormones. Iodine is essential for energy metabolism, and iodine deficiency can result in either depressed or accelerated metabolic function, known as hypothyroidism or hyperthyroidism, respectively.

Hypothyroidism can result in a growth called a goiter, in which the thyroid gland becomes greatly enlarged in its efforts to trap iodine. Other symptoms of iodine deficiency are skin problems, weight gain, and increased cholesterol levels—all of which can be reversed with sufficient iodine in the diet. Fibrocystic breast disease can also result from iodine deficiency.

Iodine deficiency during pregnancy has tragic consequences. Adequate levels of thyroid hormones are crucial while an infant's brain is developing during gestation. Insufficient iodine causes an irreversible condition known as cretinism, a completely preventable developmental disability.

RECOMMENDED INTAKES OF IODINE

Adults require 150mcg of iodine per day. For recommended intakes at other stages of life, see the appendix. It's preferable to consume the recommended intake of iodine in small but frequent amounts several times a week, rather than to consume a large dose less frequently. Vegans may not get enough iodine unless they use iodized salt, eat sea vegetables, or take a multivitamin-mineral supplement that contains iodine; otherwise a vegan diet is likely to provide only about 10 percent of recommended levels. That said, it's still important to monitor overall iodine intake, as excessive amounts can cause goiter, burning in the throat, and other problems.

DIETARY SOURCES OF IODINE

Much of the planet's iodine is found in ocean water. The amount of iodine in soil varies greatly from one region to another, so some crops are rich in iodine whereas others lack this mineral. Since 1924, US salt processors have voluntarily added iodine to table salt as a way to provide this essential nutrient to the general population and prevent the tragedies of iodine deficiency that used to be common in some areas. Adding iodine has proven to be powerfully effective, but it isn't mandatory everywhere. Plus, sea salt typically doesn't contain significant amounts of iodine. Be sure to check the label of the salt you buy; not all varieties contain iodine.

In the United States and Canada, about 1/2 teaspoon (2ml or 2g) of iodized salt is supposed to deliver the day's recommended intake of 150mcg of iodine. In practice, amounts may vary from one sample of iodized salt to another. Popular salty vegan ingredients, such as tamari, soy sauce, Bragg's Liquid Aminos, and miso, aren't iodized.

Plants that are grown in iodine-rich soil can be good sources of this mineral, however iodine levels of produce generally aren't known, so it's hard to determine your intake from foods. Sea vegetables (sometimes called seaweeds), can be excellent sources of iodine; however, amounts can vary as much as eightfold from one batch to another, so it's hard to be sure how much iodine you're getting. It can also be challenging to find a supplier who provides accurate information about iodine content of their products. Although hijiki (a type of sea vegetable) is rich in minerals, it isn't a suitable choice because it commonly contains excessive amounts of arsenic, which is both toxic and carcinogenic.

Amounts of iodine also can vary depending upon how sea vegetables are dried and stored. To confirm the amounts in salts and sea vegetables, check product labels, and consider contacting manufacturers who provide iodine levels of their products. Note that levels of iodine in these products can sometimes be quite high, in which case eating large amounts of them or eating them frequently can cause you to exceed the tolerable upper limit. Supplements are carefully standardized, so the quantities of iodine in those tend to be reliable. Table 7.1 provides some guidance on iodine levels, though as we said before, actual amounts can vary significantly.

SPECIAL ISSUES WITH IODINE

Several nutritious foods, such as soy foods, flaxseeds, cruciferous vegetables (broccoli and cabbage), peanuts, pine nuts, peaches, pears, strawberries, spinach, and sweet potatoes, contain goitrogens. These are substances that can interfere with thyroid metabolism *if and only if* a person is iodine deficient. The solution is not to avoid these foods; instead, ensure a reliable source of iodine in the daily diet. Cooking can reduce help to reduce goitrogens in foods.

Water pollutants known as perchlorates, which are by-products of solid fuels, and various minerals from fertilizers and pesticides can also amplify thyroid problems in people who are iodine deficient or whose intakes are low. Finally, selenium deficiency can worsen a marginal iodine deficiency.

TABLE 7.1. Iodine in salt and dried sea vegetables

SOURCE	AMOUNT SUPPLYING 150 mcg OF IODINE	AMOUNT SUPPLYING TOLERABLE UPPER LIMIT OF IODINE (1,100 mcg)
Iodized sea salt or table salt	½ tsp (2 ml)	4 tsp (20 ml)
Noniodized sea salt or table salt	Not a source of iodine	Not a source of iodine
Arame	½ tsp (2 ml)	3½ tsp (18 ml)
Dulse granules	½ tsp (2 ml)	3¼ tsp (16 ml)
Kelp	Less than ⅟₁₆ tsp (0.3 ml)	Scant ½ tsp (1.5 ml)
Nori	1½ sheets	10½ sheets
Wakame	1⅛ tsp (5.5 ml)	2 tbsp plus 2 tsp (40 ml)

Sources of data: ESHA Research, The Food Processor software, version 10.12.0. Eden Foods edenfoods.com. Crohn, D. M., "Perchlorate Controversy Calls for Improving Iodine Nutrition," *Vegetarian Journal* no. 2 (2006).

Key: mcg = micrograms, ml = milliliters, tsp = teaspoons, tbsp = tablespoon

Other Important Minerals

Here's a quick rundown of other minerals vegans may want to consider when planning a healthful diet: chromium, copper, magnesium, manganese, phosphorus, potassium, selenium, and sodium. Fortunately, most vegan diets easily meet or exceed the requirements for these.

CHROMIUM

Adult daily recommended intake: Women: 25mcg to age fifty, then 20mcg. Men: 35mcg to age fifty, then 30mcg.

Functions: Supports the action of insulin. Helps metabolize carbohydrates.

Key plant sources: Apple, broccoli, dark chocolate, grapefruit juice, grape juice, kiwifruit, leek, orange, and whole grains.

Special issues: Measurement of chromium content of food is challenging; limited data is available.

COPPER

Adult daily recommended intake: 900mcg.

Functions: Helps form enzymes that play key roles in energy metabolism, helps protect against free radical damage, and is essential to brain and nervous system function.

Key plant sources: Lentils, mushrooms, nuts, seeds, and whole grains.

Special issues: Vegan intakes are typically more than adequate.

MAGNESIUM

Adult daily recommended intake: Women: 310mg to age thirty, then 320mg. Men: 400mg to age thirty, then 420mg.

Functions: An essential component of bones, teeth, muscles, and cell membranes. Supports transmission of nerve impulses and affects muscle contraction. Plays a role in energy production and DNA building. Good magnesium status is associated with lower blood pressure and lowered risk for diabetes, heart disease, and stroke.

Key plant sources: Leafy green vegetables, other vegetables, fruits, whole grains, and nuts.

Special issues: Vegan intakes are typically adequate.

MANGANESE

Adult daily recommended intake: Women: 1.8mg. Men: 2.3mg.

Functions: Supports enzyme activity. Required for bone and cartilage formation and wound healing.

Key plant sources: Coconut, leafy vegetables, legumes, pineapple, raspberries, tea, nuts, and whole grains.

Special issues: Vegan diets easily meet and exceed recommended intakes.

PHOSPHORUS

Adult daily recommended intake: 700mg.

Functions: A structural component of bone. Involved in the production and storage of energy from food.

Key plant sources: Dried fruit, garlic, legumes, nuts, tomato, and whole grains.

Special issues: Vegan diets typically provide intakes above recommended levels. Diets high in sodas can be too high in phosphorus. Using antacids that contain aluminum can lead to phosphorus deficiency.

POTASSIUM

Adult daily recommended intake: 4,700mg.

Functions: Essential for transmission of nerve impulses, including beating of the heart. May reduce risk of osteoporosis, strokes, high blood pressure, and kidney stones when levels are adequate.

Key plant sources: Banana, barley, dark leafy greens, dried fruit, legumes, papaya, parsnip, potato, pumpkin, and tomato. It is a myth that bananas are the most concentrated source; Brussels sprouts, cantaloupe, green beans, grapefruit, strawberries, and tomato all provide more potassium per calorie.

Special issues: Vegan diets provide far more potassium than nonvegetarian diets, yet some may not reach recommended levels. It takes plenty of fruit and vegetables to reach the recommended intake, so get your 9 servings!

SELENIUM

Adult daily recommended intake: 55mcg.

Functions: An antioxidant that protects cells from damage by free radicals. Reduces risk of cancer and heart disease. Helps regulate thyroid function.

Key plant sources: Beans, Brazil nuts and other nuts, seeds, and whole grains.

Special issues: American and British vegans tend to meet or exceed recommended intakes.

SODIUM

Adult daily recommended intake: To age fifty, sodium intakes ranging from 1,500mg to an upper limit of 2,300mg are suggested. Intakes should range from 1,300-1,500mg from age fifty to seventy and 1,200 to 1,500mg after age seventy.

Functions: Maintains the proper amount of fluid between cells. Allows transmission of nerve impulses. Plays a role in pancreas functions. Replenishes sodium lost through perspiration, urine, and tears.

Key plant sources: Among North Americans, most sodium comes from processed foods; only 6 percent comes from table salt, and 5 percent is added during cooking. Whole foods provide much safer, smaller amounts than processed foods.

Special issues: Higher intakes can be problematic for older people, African-Americans, and people with diabetes, high blood pressure, or chronic kidney disease. For all of these groups, sodium intake should be at the lower end of the recommended range. The average American consumes almost 3,500mg of sodium per day.

Three Rules for Getting Enough Minerals

Making sure you get enough of the minerals you need isn't difficult, particularly for vegans. Just remember these three rules:

1. Eat *whole* plant foods. Minerals are found in all the different food groups, but many are lost in the refining process. Follow the recommendations in chapter 14, The Vegan Food Guide.

2. Get enough calories. If you're on a weight-loss diet, take a multivitaminmineral supplement.

3. Check food labels. Consider using some foods that are fortified with calcium, zinc, iron, and iodine.

TABLE 7.2. Minerals in vegan foods

FOOD	MINERAL (unit)	CAL-CIUM (mg)	COPPER (mcg)	IRON (mg)	MAGNE-SIUM (mg)	MANGA-NESE (mg)	PHOS-PHORUS (mg)	POTAS-SIUM (mg)	SELE-NIUM (mcg)	SODIUM (mg)	ZINC (mg)
Recommended intake for a woman*		1,000	900	14–32 (8–18)**	310–320	1.8	700	4,700	55	1,200–1,500	8
Recommended intake for a man*		1,000	900	(14) 8**	400–420	2.3	700	4,700	55	1,200–1,500	11
FRUITS											
Apple, medium, each		8	37	0.2	7	0	15	148	0	1	0
Apricot, medium, each		5	27	0.1	4	0	8	91	0	0	0
Apricots, dried (¼ c/33 g)		20	...	1.5	...	...	...	520	...	1	...
Apricots, sliced (1 c/165 g)		21	129	0.6	16	0.1	38	427	0	2	0
Banana, dried (¼ c/25g)		5	98	0.3	27	0.1	19	373	1	0	0.1
Banana, medium, each		6	90	0.3	32	0.3	26	422	1	1	0.2
Banana, sliced (1 c/150 g)		8	117	0.4	40	0.4	33	537	2	2	0
Blackberries (1 c/144 g)		42	238	0.9	29	0.9	32	233	1	3	0.8
Blueberries (1 c/145 g)		9	83	0.4	9	0.5	17	112	0	1	0.2

FOOD MINERAL (unit)	CAL-CIUM (mg)	COPPER (mcg)	IRON (mg)	MAGNE-SIUM (mg)	MANGA-NESE (mg)	PHOS-PHORUS (mg)	POTAS-SIUM (mg)	SELE-NIUM (mcg)	SODIUM (mg)	ZINC (mg)
Recommended intake for a woman*	1,000	900	14–32 (8–18)**	310–320	1.8	700	4,700	55	1,200–1,500	8
Recommended intake for a man*	1,000	900	(14) 8**	400–420	2.3	700	4,700	55	1,200–1,500	11
Cantaloupe, diced (1 c/156 g)	14	64	0.3	19	0	23	417	1	25	0.3
Cherimoya, chopped (1 c/156 g)	16	110	0.4	27	0.2	42	459	...	11	0.3
Coconut, dried (¹/₄ c/29 g)	7	231	1	26	0.8	60	157	5	11	0.6
Crab apples sliced (1 c/110 g)	20	74	0.4	8	0.1	16	213	...	1	...
Currants, Zante, dried (¹/₄ c/36 g)	31	169	1.2	15	0.2	45	321	0	3	0
Dates, chopped (¹/₄ c/37 g)	69	367	1.8	77	0.5	110	1,168	5	4	0.5
Durian, chopped (1 c/243 g)	15	503	1	73	0.8	95	1,059	...	5	0.7
Fig, fresh, medium, each	18	35	0.2	8	0	7	116	0	0.5	0.1
Figs, dried (¹/₄ c/50 g)	81	143	1	34	0	33	338	0	5	0.3
Gooseberries (1 c/150 g)	38	105	0.5	15	0.2	40	297	1	2	0.2
Grapefruit, medium, each	54	79	0.2	22	0	44	332	0	0	0.2
Grapefruit juice, pink (1 c/247 g)	22	80	0.5	30	0	37	400	0	2	0.1
Grapefruit sections (1 c/230 g)	28	108	0.2	18	0	18	320	3	0	0.2
Grapes (1 c/160 g)	16	0	0.6	11	0.1	32	306	0	3	0.1
Guava, diced (1 c/165 g)	33	170	0.5	16	0.2	41	469	1	5	0.4
Honeydew melon, diced (1 c/170 g)	10	41	0.3	17	0	19	388	1	31	0.2
Huckleberries (1 c/145 g)	8.7	82	0.4	9	0.5	17	112	0	1	0.2
Kiwifruit, medium, each	26	99	0.2	13	0	26	237	0	2	0.1
Loganberries (1 c/144 g)	42	238	0.9	29	0.9	32	233	1	1	0.8
Mango, medium, each	21	228	0.3	19	0	23	323	1	4	0.1
Mango, sliced (1 c/165 g)	17	181	0.2	15	0	18	257	1	3	0.1
Orange, medium, each	52	59	0.1	13	0	18	237	1	0	0.1
Orange juice (1 c/248 g)	27	109	0.5	28	0	42	496	0	2	0.1
Papaya, cubed (1 c/140 g)	34	22	0.1	14	0	7	360	1	4	0.1
Peach, medium, each	6	67	0.2	9	0.1	20	186	0	0	0.2
Peach, sliced (½ c/77 g)	10	116	0.4	15	0.1	34	323	0	0	0.3
Pear, sliced (½ c/70 g)	15	135	0.3	12	0.1	18	196	0	2	0.2
Pear halves, dried (1 c/180 g)	61	668	3.8	59	0.6	106	959	0	11	0.7
Pineapple, diced (1 c/155 g)	20	153	0.4	19	1.8	12	178	0	2	0.2
Plums, dried (¹/₄ c/30 g)	15	91	0.3	12	0.1	15	220	1	4	0.2
Plums, sliced (1 c/165 g)	6.6	71	0.2	12	0.1	16	289	1	0	0.2
Prunes (1 c/174 g)	73	478	1.6	70	0.5	117	1,244	1	3	0.7

FOOD	MINERAL (unit)	CAL-CIUM (mg)	COPPER (mcg)	IRON (mg)	MAGNE-SIUM (mg)	MANGA-NESE (mg)	PHOS-PHORUS (mg)	POTAS-SIUM (mg)	SELE-NIUM (mcg)	SODIUM (mg)	ZINC (mg)
Recommended intake for a woman*		1,000	900	14–32 (8–18)**	310–320	1.8	700	4,700	55	1,200–1,500	8
Recommended intake for a man*		1,000	900	(14) 8**	400–420	2.3	700	4,700	55	1,200–1,500	11
Raisins, seedless, packed (¼ c/41 g)		21	131	0.8	13	0.1	42	309	0	5	0.1
Raspberries (1 c/123 g)		31	111	0.9	27	0.8	36	186	0	1	0.5
Strawberries (1 c/144 g)		23	69	0.6	19	0.5	35	220	0	1	0.2
Watermelon, diced (1 c/152 g)		11	064	0.4	15	0.1	17	170	1	2	0.2
VEGETABLES (RAW UNLESS STATED)											
Arugula, chopped (1 c/20 g)		32	0	0.3	9	0.1	10	73	0	5	0.1
Asparagus, sliced (1 c/134 g)		32	253	2.9	19	0.2	70	271	39	3	0.7
Asparagus spear, medium, each		4	...	0.1	...	...	...	46	...	0	...
Avocado, California, medium, each		22	294	1.1	50	0.3	93	877	1	14	1.2
Avocado, Florida, medium, each		30	945	0.5	73	0.3	122	1,067	0	6	1.2
Basil, fresh, chopped (1 c/42 g)		65	122	1.3	34	0.6	30	196	0	2	0.4
Beans, snap, green/yellow (1 c/110 g)		41	76	1.1	28	0.2	42	230	1	7	0.2
Beet greens, chopped (1 c/38 g)		44	73	1	27	0.1	16	290	0	86	0.1
Beets, sliced (1 c/136 g)		22	102	1.1	31	0.4	54	442	1	106	0.5
Bok choy, sliced (1 c/70 g)		74	15	0.6	13	0.1	26	176	0	46	0.1
Broccoli, chopped (1 c/71 g)		34	32	0.6	18	0.2	47	231	2	19	0.3
Brussels sprouts (1 c/88 g)		37	62	1.2	20	0.3	61	342	1	22	0.4
Cabbage, green, chopped (1 c/89 g)		42	20	0.5	13	0.1	20	219	1	16	0.2
Cabbage, napa, chopped (1 c/85 g)		59	27	0.2	10	0.1	22	181	0.5	7	0.2
Cabbage, red, shredded (1 c/70 g)		32	12	0.6	11	0.2	21	170	0	19	0.2
Carrot, chopped (1 c/128 g)		42	58	0.4	15	0.2	45	410	0	88	0.3
Carrot, medium, each		24	32	0.2	9	0.1	25	230	0	50	0.2
Carrot juice (1 c/236 g)		57	109	1.1	33	.3	99	689	1	156	0.4
Cauliflower, chopped (1 c/100 g)		22	42	0.4	15	0.1	44	303	1	30	0.3
Celery, diced (1 c/101 g)		48	42	0.2	13	0.1	29	312	0	96	0.2
Celery, stalk, each		26	22	0.1	7	0.1	15	166	0	64	0.1
Celery root, diced (1 c/156 g)		67	109	1.1	31	0.3	179	468	1	156	0.5
Chiles, hot green (1 c/150 g)		27	261	1.8	38	0.4	69	510	1	10	0.4
Chiles, hot red (1 c/150 g)		21	194	1.5	34	0.3	64	483	1	14	0.4
Cilantro (1 c/46 g)		31	103	0.8	12	0.2	25	235	0	25	0
Collard greens, chopped (1 c/36 g)		52	14	0.1	3	0.1	4	61	0	7	0
Corn, white/yellow, kernels (1 c/154 g)		3	83	0.8	57	0.2	137	416	1	23	0.7

FOOD / MINERAL (unit)	CALCIUM (mg)	COPPER (mcg)	IRON (mg)	MAGNESIUM (mg)	MANGANESE (mg)	PHOSPHORUS (mg)	POTASSIUM (mg)	SELENIUM (mcg)	SODIUM (mg)	ZINC (mg)
Recommended intake for a woman*	1,000	900	14–32 (8–18)**	310–320	1.8	700	4,700	55	1,200–1,500	8
Recommended intake for a man*	1,000	900	(14) 8**	400–420	2.3	700	4,700	55	1,200–1,500	11
Cucumber, peeled, sliced (1 c/119 g)	17	84	0.3	14	0.1	25	162	0	2	0.2
Cucumber, unpeeled, sliced (1 c/104 g)	15	34	0.3	11	0.1	21	150	0	2	0.2
Dandelion greens, chopped (1 c/55 g)	103	94	1.7	20	0.2	36	218	0	42	0.2
Eggplant, cubed (1 c/82 g)	7	67	0.2	11	0.2	20	189	0	2	0.1
Endive, chopped (1 c/50 g)	26	0	0.4	8	0.2	14	157	0	11	0.4
Garlic clove, medium, each	5	9	0.1	0.8	0	5	12	0	1	0
Jerusalem artichokes, sliced (1 c/150 g)	21	210	5	25	0.1	117	644	1	6	0.2
Kale, chopped (1 c/67 g)	90	194	1.1	23	0.5	38	299	1	29	0.3
Kelp, fresh, chopped (1 c/80 g)	134	104	2.3	97	0.2	34	71	1	186	1
Leeks, chopped (1 c/89 g)	53	107	1.9	25	0.4	31	160	1	18	0.1
Lettuce, Bibb/Boston/butterhead, chopped (1 c/55 g)	19	9	0.7	7	0.1	18	131	0	3	0.1
Lettuce, iceberg, chopped (1 c/55 g)	11	14	0.2	4	0.1	12	84	0	5	0.1
Lettuce, leaf, chopped (1 c/36 g)	20	16	0.5	7	0	16	109	0	16	0.1
Lettuce, red leaf, chopped (1 c/28 g)	9	8	0.3	3	0.1	8	52	0	7	0.1
Lettuce, romaine, chopped (1 c/47 g)	18	27	0.5	8	0.1	17	138	0	4	0.1
Mushrooms, shiitake, dried (1 c/145 g)	16	7,490	2.5	191	1.7	426	2,224	197	19	11
Mustard greens, chopped (1 c/56 g)	58	82	0.8	18	0.3	24	198	1	14	0.1
Okra, sliced (1 c/100 g)	81	94	0.8	57	1	63	303	1	8	0.6
Olives, green (1 c/160 g)	98	545	2.6	35	...	27	88	2	3,840	0.1
Onion, green, each	11	12	0.2	3	0	6	41	0	2	0.1
Onions, green, chopped (1 c/100 g)	72	83	1.5	20	0.2	37	276	1	16	0.4
Onions, red/white/yellow, chopped (1 c/160 g)	35	61	0.3	16	0.2	43	230	1	5	0.3
Parsley (1 c/60 g)	83	89	3.7	30	0.1	35	332	0	34	0.6
Parsnips, sliced (1 c/133 g)	48	160	0.8	39	0.7	94	499	2	13	0.8
Pea pods, snow/edible (1 c/63 g)	27	50	1.3	15	0.2	33	126	0	3	0.1
Peas, fresh (1 c/145 g)	36	255	2.1	48	0.6	157	354	3	7	1.8

FOOD MINERAL (unit)	CAL-CIUM (mg)	COPPER (mcg)	IRON (mg)	MAGNE-SIUM (mg)	MANGA-NESE (mg)	PHOS-PHORUS (mg)	POTAS-SIUM (mg)	SELE-NIUM (mcg)	SODIUM (mg)	ZINC (mg)
Recommended intake for a woman*	1,000	900	14–32 (8–18)**	310–320	1.8	700	4,700	55	1,200–1,500	8
Recommended intake for a man*	1,000	900	(14) 8**	400–420	2.3	700	4,700	55	1,200–1,500	11
Pepper, bell, green, chopped (1 c/149 g)	15	98	0.5	15	0.2	30	261	0	4	0.2
Pepper, bell, green, medium, each	12	79	0.4	12	0.1	24	208	0	4	0.2
Pepper, bell, red, chopped (1 c/149 g)	10	25	0.6	18	0.2	39	314	0	3	0.4
Pepper, bell, red, medium, each	8	20	0.5	14	0.1	31	251	0	2	0.3
Pepper, bell, yellow, chopped (1 c/149 g)	16	160	0.7	18	0.2	36	316	0	3	0.2
Potato, baked, each (6 oz/170 g)	26	0.2	1.87	48	0.4	121	926	0.7	17	0.6
Potato, cubed, cooked (½ c/75 g)	6	0.1	0.2	16	0.1	31	256	0.2	4	0.2
Radish, daikon, chopped (1 c/88 g)	24	101	0.4	14	0	20	200	1	...	0.1
Radish, daikon, medium, each	91	389	1.4	54	0.1	78	767	2	71	1
Radish, medium, each	1	2	0	0	0	1	10	0	2	0
Radishes, sliced (1 c/116 g)	29	58	0.4	12	0.1	23	270	1	45	0
Radish sprouts (1 c/38 g)	19	46	0.3	17	0.1	43	33	0	2	0
Rutabaga, chopped (1 c/140 g)	66	56	0.7	32	0.2	81	472	1	28	0.5
Spinach, chopped (1 c/30 g)	30	39	0.8	24	0.3	15	167	0	24	0.2
Squash, crookneck, cubed (1 c/130 g)	27	133	0.6	27	0.2	42	276	0	3	0.4
Squash, winter, all types, cubed (1 c/116 g)	32	82	0.7	16	0.2	27	406	0	5	0.2
Sweet potato, cubed (1 c/133 g)	40	201	0.8	33	0.3	63	448	1	17	0.4
Tomato, cherry, each	2	10	0	2	0	4	40	0	1	0
Tomato, green, chopped (1 c/180 g)	23	162	1	18	0.2	50	367	1	23	0
Tomato, medium, each	15	88	0.4	16	0.2	36	353	0	7	0.3
Tomato, red, chopped (1 c/180 g)	18	106	0.5	20	0.2	43	427	0	9	0.3
Tomato, Roma, each	6	37	0.2	7	0.1	15	147	0	3	0
Tomato, yellow, chopped (1 c/139 g)	15	140	0.7	17	0.2	50	359	1	32	0
Tomatoes, sun-dried (1 c/54 g)	59	768	4.9	105	1	192	1,851	3	1,131	1.1
Turnip, cubed (1 c/130 g)	39	110	0.4	14	0.2	35	248	1	87	0.4
Turnip greens, chopped (1 c/55 g)	104	192	0.6	17	0.3	23	163	1	22	0.1
Watercress, chopped (1 c/34 g)	41	0	0.1	7	0.1	20	112	0	14	0
Water chestnuts, sliced (1 c/124 g)	14	404	0.1	27	0.4	78	724	1	...	0.6
Yam, cubed (1 c/150 g)	26	267	0.8	32	0.6	82	1,224	1	14	0.4
Zucchini, baby, each	2	11	0.1	4	0	10	51	0	0	0.1

FOOD / MINERAL (unit)	CAL-CIUM (mg)	COPPER (mcg)	IRON (mg)	MAGNE-SIUM (mg)	MANGA-NESE (mg)	PHOS-PHORUS (mg)	POTAS-SIUM (mg)	SELE-NIUM (mcg)	SODIUM (mg)	ZINC (mg)
Recommended intake for a woman*	1,000	900	14–32 (8–18)**	310–320	1.8	700	4,700	55	1,200–1,500	8
Recommended intake for a man*	1,000	900	(14) 8**	400–420	2.3	700	4,700	55	1,200–1,500	11
Zucchini, cubed (1 c/124 g)	19	63	0.4	21	0.2	47	325	0	12	0.4
NUTS AND SEEDS										
Almond butter (2 tbsp/32 g)	86	288	1.2	97	0.7	168	243	1	3	1.0
Almonds (¼ c/35 g)	88	394	1.5	97	0.9	168	259	3	0	1.2
Brazil nut, large, each	8	82	0.1	18	0.1	34	31	91	0	0.2
Brazil nuts (¼ c/35g)	56	610	1.5	131	0.4	254	231	671	2	1.4
Cashew butter (2 tbsp/32 g)	14	701	1.6	83	0.3	293	175	4	5	1.7
Cashews (¼ c/33 g)	12	713	2.2	95	0.5	193	215	7	4	1.9
Chia seeds (2 tbsp/20 g)	126	185	3.1	67	0.5	172	81	11	3	0.9
Flaxseeds, ground (2 tbsp/14 g)	41	195	0.9	63	0.4	103	130	4	5	0.7
Hazelnuts (¼ c/34 g)	39	582	1.6	55	2.1	98	229	1	0	0.8
Pecans (¼ c/27 g)	19	327	0.7	33	1.2	75	112	1	0	1.2
Pine nuts (¼ c/34 g)	5	450	1.9	85	3	195	203	0	1	2.2
Pistachio nuts (¼ c/32 g)	34	416	1.3	39	0.4	157	33	2	0	0.7
Poppy seeds (2 tbsp-c/17 g)	241	275	1.6	56	1.1	143	117	0	3	1.7
Psyllium seeds (2 tbsp/19 g)	65	...	3.9	10	0.3	12	158	273	3	0.4
Pumpkin seeds (¼ c/35 g)	15	479	5.2	185	1.1	405	279	2	21	2.6
Sesame seeds, whole (2 tbsp/18 g)	176	735	2.6	63	0.4	113	84	1	2	1.4
Sesame tahini (2 tbsp/30 g)	42	483	1.3	29	...	237	138	1	11	1.4
Sunflower seed butter (2 tbsp/32 g)	39	586	1.5	118	0.7	235	23	25	1	1.7
Sunflower seed kernels (¼ c/36 g)	42	631	2.4	64	0.4	254	248	21	1	1.8
Walnuts, black, chopped (¼ c/31 g)	18	319	0.9	63	1.3	145	164	5	0	1.1
Walnuts, English, chopped (¼ c/30 g)	29	476	0.9	47	1	104	132	1	1	0.9
LEGUMES										
Adzuki beans, cooked (1 c/230 g)	64	690	4.6	120	1.3	386	1,224	3	18	4.1
Black beans, cooked (1 c/172 g)	46	360	361	120	0.8	241	611	2	2	1.9
Black-eyed peas, cooked (1 c/171 g)	41	460	4.3	91	0.8	267	475	4	7	2
Chickpeas, cooked (1 c/164 g)	80	580	4.7	79	1.7	276	477	6	11	2.5
Cranberry beans, cooked (1 c/177 g)	88	410	3.7	88	0.6	239	685	2	2	2
Edamame, cooked (1 c/155 g)	103	566	3.7	105	1.7	277	715	...	140	2.2
Falafel patties (1.7 oz/51 g)	28	130	1.7	42	0.4	98	298	0.5	150	0.8

FOOD (MINERAL unit)	CAL-CIUM (mg)	COPPER (mcg)	IRON (mg)	MAGNE-SIUM (mg)	MANGA-NESE (mg)	PHOS-PHORUS (mg)	POTAS-SIUM (mg)	SELE-NIUM (mcg)	SODIUM (mg)	ZINC (mg)
Recommended intake for a woman*	1,000	900	14–32 (8–18)**	310–320	1.8	700	4,700	55	1,200–1,500	8
Recommended intake for a man*	1,000	900	(14) 8**	400–420	2.3	700	4,700	55	1,200–1,500	11
Great Northern beans, cooked (1 c/177 g)	120	440	3.8	88	0.9	292	692	2	2	1.6
Kidney beans, cooked (1 c/177 g)	62	380	3.9	74	0.8	244	716	6	4	1.8
Lentils, brown/green, cooked (1 c/198 g)	38	500	6.6	71	1	356	730	6	4	2.5
Lentil sprouts, raw (1 c/77 g)	19	271	2.5	28	0.4	133	248	0	8	1.2
Lima beans, baby, cooked (1 c/182 g)	53	390	4.4	96	1.1	231	730	9	5	1.9
Mung bean sprouts, raw (1 c/104 g)	14	171	1	22	0.2	56	155	1	6	0.4
Navy beans, cooked (1 c/182 g)	125	380	4.3	96	1	262	708	5	0	1.9
Peanuts (1 c/146 g)	134	1,670	6.7	245	2.8	549	1,029	10	26	4.8
Pea sprouts, raw (1 c/120 g)	43	326	2.7	67	0.5	198	457	1	24	1.3
Peas, raw (1 c/145 g)	36	255	2.1	48	0.6	157	354	3	7	1.8
Peas, split, cooked (1 c/196 g)	27	350	2.5	71	0.8	194	710	1	4	2
Pinto beans, cooked (1 c/171 g)	79	370	3.6	86	0.8	251	746	11	2	1.7
Soybeans, cooked (1 c/172 g)	175	700	8.8	148	1.4	421	886	13	2	2
Soy milk, fortified (1 c/243 g)†	299	209	1	36	...	211	284	6	117	0.6
Tempeh, raw (1 c/166 g)	184	930	4.5	134	2.2	442	684	0	15	1.9
Tofu, calcium-set, firm, raw, cubed (1 c/252 g)†	315–1,721	953	3–6.7	93–146	3	305–479	373–597	25–44	10–35	2.1–4
White beans, cooked (1 c/179 g)	131	270	5.1	122	0.9	303	829	2	4	2
GRAINS										
Amaranth, cooked (1 c/246 g)	116	367	5.2	160	2.1	364	332	13	15	2.1
Barley, pearl, cooked (1 c/157 g)	17	165	2.1	35	0.4	85	146	14	5	1.3
Buckwheat groats, kasha, cooked (1 c/168 g)	12	245	1.3	86	0.7	118	148	4	7	10
Buckwheat sprouts, raw (1 c/33 g)	9	86	0.7	27	...	66	56	...	5	0.5
Kamut, cooked (1 c/172 g)	17	430	5.7	96	2	304	347	...	10	3
Millet, cooked (1 c/174 g)	5	280	1.1	77	0.5	174	108	2	3	1.6
Oatmeal, cooked (1 c/234 g)	21	170	2.1	63	1.4	180	164	13	9	2.3
Quinoa, cooked (1 c/185 g)	31	355	2.8	118	1.2	281	318	5	13	2
Spaghetti, white, enriched, cooked (1 c/140 g)	10	140	1.8	25	0.5	81	62	37	1	0.7
Spaghetti, whole wheat, cooked (1 c/140 g)	21	234	1.5	42	1.9	125	62	36	4	1.1

FOOD / MINERAL (unit)	CALCIUM (mg)	COPPER (mcg)	IRON (mg)	MAGNESIUM (mg)	MANGANESE (mg)	PHOSPHORUS (mg)	POTASSIUM (mg)	SELENIUM (mcg)	SODIUM (mg)	ZINC (mg)
Recommended intake for a woman*	1,000	900	14–32 (8–18)**	310–320	1.8	700	4,700	55	1,200–1,500	8
Recommended intake for a man*	1,000	900	(14) 8**	400–420	2.3	700	4,700	55	1,200–1,500	11
Wheat sprouts, raw (1 c/108 g)	30	282	2.3	89	2	216	183	46	17	1.8
Wild rice, cooked (1 c/164 g)	5	200	1	52	0.5	134	166	1	5	2.2
OTHER										
Dark chocolate (2 oz/60 g)	17	10	1.2	18	0	29	285	0	3	0
Molasses (1 tbsp/20 g)	41	97	1–3	48	0.3	6	293	3.6	7	0.1
Oil, olive (1 tbsp14 g)	0	0	0.1	0	0	0	0	0	0	0
Spirulina, dried (1 tbsp/7 g)	8	427	2	14	0.1	8	95	0	73	0.1

Sources of data: US Department of Agriculture, Agricultural Research Service, *USDA National Nutrient Database for Standard Reference*, Release 25 (2012), ndb.nal.usda.gov. ESHA Research, The Food Processor software, version 10.12.0.

Key: c = cup; g = gram; mcg = microgram; mg = milligram; ml = milliliter; oz = ounce; tbsp = tablespoon; ... indicates that no data is available.

*For other ages, see the appendix.

**Recommended intakes for vegetarians and vegans are set at 1.8 times greater than the recommended intakes for nonvegetarians (see page 133 for further information).¹ Check labels for product-specific information.

What is "clean eating?" It's a well-planned vegan diet, high in vitamins and minerals and bursting with phytochemicals. Read all about it, in chapter 8.

CHAPTER 8

Clean Vegan Eating

Sometimes it is said that food is to the human body what fuel is to cars. Healthy foods are considered premium fuel, and, like our vehicles, our bodies run best on clean fuel. Although the analogy is useful, it isn't entirely accurate. Food does serve as fuel for our bodies, but that's just one of its many roles. Food also provides the structural materials used to build, rebuild, and repair our tissues, along with the resources needed to manufacture brain cells, muscles, bones, hormones, and enzymes. You literally are what you eat or, perhaps more accurately, what you absorb.

The Power of the Plate

As mentioned in previous chapters, plant foods are concentrated sources of antioxidants, phytochemicals, phytosterols, fiber, vitamins, and minerals. These compounds and many others work together to support all of the body's systems, turning off disease-promoting genes, reducing inflammation, maintaining insulin sensitivity, boosting immune function, balancing hormones, protecting gastrointestinal function, reducing cholesterol levels, and controlling blood sugar levels. Although you can get many of these protective substances from supplements, research continues to show that nutrients work synergistically and are best obtained from food.

In contrast to whole plant foods, highly processed foods and animal products are generally the sources of dietary components that have been linked with disease, such as sodium, refined carbohydrates, saturated fat, cholesterol, trans-fatty acids, toxins, and chemical contaminants, such as hormones, antibiotics, and persistent organic pollutants. When eaten in excess, these compounds work together to disrupt health and promote disease.

Disease Preventers

We've covered a lot about essential nutrients: protein, fats, carbohydrates, vitamins, and minerals. Impressive as these are, plant foods continue to dazzle us with additional protective compounds, such as enzymes, phytochemicals, phytosterols, and prebiotics.

ENZYMES

The enzymes in raw plant foods help to convert specific phytochemicals into their active forms and may aid digestion. However, cooking reduces or destroys these enzymes.

To date, two plant families are known to contain enzymes that convert phytochemicals into their highly beneficial active forms. One is cruciferous vegetables, such as broccoli, broccoli sprouts, radish sprouts, Brussels sprouts, cabbage, cauliflower, kale, and turnips, and the other is allium vegetables, such as onions, garlic, and chives. By the way, sprouts are much higher in phytochemicals than the mature plants. The active phytochemicals produced in the cruciferous vegetables have remarkable detoxification effects. Most notably, they help process and eliminate carcinogens. The active phytochemicals in allium vegetables are antimicrobial and help fight bacteria, parasites, viruses, fungi, arthritis, and cancer. They can also lower cholesterol levels.

The enzymes in food may also aid digestion, though the overall contribution to digestion is very small. Enzymes start working to break down food as soon as the food is chopped, mashed, pureed, or blended—before we even begin eating it. The enzymes continue working while we chew and up until the food reaches the lower part of the stomach, where acidic conditions deactivate most of them. Food enzymes with the greatest chance of surviving stomach acid and arriving intact in the small intestine, where most digestion takes place, are those that are packaged within microorganisms, as in fermented and cultured foods.

Take-Home Message: Include many cruciferous and allium vegetables in your diet, along with a variety of sprouts. Also add cultured and fermented foods to your diet. To maximize the enzymes in vegetables and fruits, eat at least some of them raw.

PHYTOCHEMICALS

Phytochemicals are chemicals found in plants. (*Phyto* is Greek for "plant.") Plants produce phytochemicals for their own survival and protection. Some play a critical role in attracting pollinators and seed dispersers, and others act as an internal defense system, protecting plants from pests, pathogens, and potentially hostile environments. Phytochemicals play a big role in the colors, flavors, textures, and odors of plant foods.

When you eat plants, these phytochemicals go to work on your body's behalf. They support optimal health by reducing the risk of chronic disease and fighting existing diseases in multiple ways, such as by reducing inflammation and eradicating carcinogens.

All whole plant foods contain hundreds of thousands of phytochemicals. Choosing a wide variety of colorful vegetables, fruits, herbs, spices, legumes, nuts, seeds, and whole grains is the key to a diet rich in a broad range of phytochemicals. Of course, there are superstars that can help transform a good eating pattern into a phytochemical feast. Among the most noteworthy are dark leafy greens (kale, collard greens, spinach), cruciferous vegetables, sprouts, purple and blue fruits (blueberries, blackberries), herbs and spices, tomatoes, citrus fruits, legumes, nuts, seeds (flaxseeds, hempseeds), and cocoa beans.

Many factors can affect the quantity of phytochemicals in food and their bioavailability. Soil, water, climate, and the use of chemicals can all affect the phytochemical content as plants grow. Organic produce has an edge over conventional produce when it comes to phytochemical content, which makes sense, given that organic foods need more robust defenses. Refining can dramatically reduce the phytochemical content of food, especially when the most phytochemical-rich parts of the plants are removed—for instance, the germ and bran from wheat flour—or when the processing involves exposure to harsh chemicals, heat, or pressure. Some postharvest storage methods can also diminish phytochemical concentrations.

Most phytochemicals are more efficiently absorbed from raw foods. Chopping, pureeing, processing, milling, mashing, grating, and juicing all break down or remove fiber and other compounds that reduce the bioavailability of phytochemicals and other nutrients. Therefore, drinking vegetable juice can be a practical way to boost antioxidant and phytochemical intake without adding bulk to the diet. Sprouting and fermenting can also significantly enhance phytochemical content or bioavailability. For example, compared to broccoli, broccoli sprouts contain ten to one hundred times the amount of a phytochemical that has detoxifying, anticancer, and antibacterial properties and may improve insulin resistance in people with type 2 diabetes.

Cooking tends to decrease the amount of phytochemicals, and the higher the heat and the longer the food is cooked, the more significant the loss. Cooking method can also be a factor. For example, the loss of water-soluble phytochemicals is higher with boiling than steaming.

On the other hand, cooking softens plant cell walls, making it easier for the body to extract and absorb some types of phytochemicals, particularly carotenoids. For example, we absorb more of the carotenoid lycopene from cooked tomatoes than raw tomatoes, and more beta-carotene from cooked carrots than raw. In addition, including even a small amount of fat, from oil or from high-fat whole foods, improves absorption of carotenoids, whether the foods containing them are raw or cooked.

Take-Home Message: To boost phytochemical intake, eat foods with a wide range of colors within every food group. The more colorful your plate, the richer the variety and concentration of phytochemicals in your diet. Opt for organic. Eat sprouts and fermented foods, and include legumes, nuts, seeds, and whole grains in addition to vegetables and fruits.

PHYTOSTEROLS

Phytosterols, also called plant sterols or stanols, are an essential part of plant cell membranes. They are structurally similar to cholesterol, and because of this, they can inhibit our absorption of dietary cholesterol, lower total and LDL cholesterol levels, and suppress inflammation.

The diets of early humans probably provided about 1,000mg of phytosterols a day, but the average intake these days is only about 150 to 450mg. Vegetarian diets are generally higher in phytosterols, with vegan diets being highest. Raw vegan diets provide between 500 and 1,200mg of phytosterols per day, and sometimes more. Consuming about 2,000mg of phytosterols per day reduces LDL by approximately 9 to 15 percent in those with elevated cholesterol levels, but to get 2,000mg, you'd have to take supplements or eat phytosterol-fortified foods.

Although all whole plant foods contain phytosterols, the most concentrated natural sources are seeds, nuts, wheat germ, avocados, legumes, sprouts, and vegetable oils. The food industry now fortifies a variety of food products, such as margarine, cereal, and fruit juice, with phytosterols because of their cholesterol-lowering properties. While such fortified products may provide some benefit for people with elevated cholesterol levels, it makes little sense to add an otherwise unhealthful food to your diet just to boost phytosterol intake. It would make better sense to eat more plant foods. Vegans with healthful diets needn't give these products a second thought. They eat far more sterols than people on other diets, consume no cholesterol, and usually have lower cholesterol levels.

For those who do take phytosterol supplements or use phytosterol-fortified foods, intakes exceeding 2,000mg per day haven't been shown to provide added benefit, and for some people, it may cause more harm than good.

Take-Home Message: The safest and most effective way to boost phytosterol intake is to eat a whole-foods vegan diet, including higher-fat plant foods such as seeds, nuts, wheat germ, and avocados. Vegans don't need to eat phytosterolfortified processed foods.

PREBIOTICS AND PROBIOTICS

Your intestinal tract is buzzing with trillions of bacteria collectively known as gut flora or microbiota. Although thirty to forty species account for 99 percent of these microorganisms, as many as four hundred different species are known residents. These intestinal inhabitants account for a surprising 50 percent of fecal mass.

Although the body's relationship with microbiota is largely beneficial, some of these guests are more welcome than others. Benefits of preferred strains include the following:

- Boosting nutritional status by enhancing the absorption of several nutrients, maintaining amino acids, and synthesizing certain vitamins
- Breaking down fiber that the human body can't digest, resulting in the release of more than 10 percent of our daily calorie needs, improving carbohydrate and fat metabolism, and protecting against colon cancer
- Supporting immune system function, protecting against food allergies, and maintaining healthy intestinal tissues

If friendly flora aren't adequately supported, less welcome guests—more pathogenic bad bacteria—can multiply, with several ill effects:

- Toxins that injure the gut lining, making it more permeable, or leaky
- Reduced immune function
- Chronic, low-grade inflammation
- Infections
- Impaired metabolism
- Contributions to overweight and obesity

Your food choices influence whether the balance of flora is friendly or hostile. A plant-based, high-fiber diet supports good bacteria, whereas a high-fat, lowfiber diet encourages bad bacteria. The goal is not to wipe out bad bugs—you actually need some of them—but to shift the balance from bad bugs to good bugs.

Consuming probiotics can help. Probiotics are foods or supplements that contain friendly microorganisms. They arrive in the intestinal tract in an active form and exert beneficial health effects. Another option is prebiotics: indigestible, fermentable food components that stimulate the growth or activity of beneficial bacteria, usually serving as their food supply.

Fermented or cultured vegan foods that offer probiotics include nondairy yogurt and kefir, miso (if not boiled), sauerkraut, and rejuvelac (a fermented grain beverage). Consuming these foods or taking probiotic supplements can prevent or diminish complaints associated with lactose intolerance, irritable bowel syndrome, and certain types of diarrhea. Probiotics decrease cancer-promoting enzymes and toxic by-products of bad bacteria. They also appear to protect the health of the gastrointestinal tract and reduce complications associated with inflammatory bowel diseases and infection with *Helicobacter pylori,* the bacteria associated with ulcers. They can aid in the prevention of flu, the common cold, urogenital infections, and, among infants, allergies and skin disorders. Probiotics may also help reduce cholesterol levels, prevent cancer, protect against autoimmune diseases, and promote dental health.

Prebiotics are nondigestible sugars such as inulin and oligosaccharides that stimulate the growth and activity of beneficial bacteria in the digestive system. Prebiotics are found in asparagus, bananas, raw chicory, garlic, Jerusalem artichokes, leeks, onions, and sweet potatoes and are also available in foods fortified with prebiotics.

When purchasing a probiotic supplement, you'll notice that the label includes the genus and species of bacteria supplied. A probiotic containing a variety of Lactobacillus and Bifidobacteria strains is generally more effective than a singlestrain acidophilus supplement. Also, each strain of bacteria has distinct health effects. If you're using probiotics to treat a specific condition, do some research to find out what strains are most effective for your condition.

No matter what strains you use, if the microorganisms are dead, they aren't probiotics. Check the label for the expiration date. Most probiotics need to be refrigerated. To test whether a supplement is viable, you can add a spoonful to a small bowl of soymilk; leave it at room temperature and, after a day or so, check to see whether there's any bubbling or other activity indicating a living culture. Typical dosages vary with the product, but generally higher dosages (from five to ten billion colony-forming units, or CFU, per day for children, and ten to twenty billion CFU per day for adults) are associated with better outcomes.

Be aware that heat kills beneficial bacteria. If using cultured or fermented foods as a source of probiotics, don't cook them over high heat. For example, miso should be mixed with warm water and stirred into cooked dishes, rather than being boiled in a soup.

Take-Home Message: High-fiber vegan diets help promote and maintain healthy gut flora. To help restore gut flora, eat plenty of raw vegetables and fruits and add some fermented or cultured foods to your diet. Consider periodic use of a multistrain probiotic.

Disease Promoters

While focusing on whole plant foods can go a long way in promoting health and well-being, to maximize the advantages you'll also want to avoid dietary factors that can promote disease. In the sections that follow, we'll consider culprits not previously addressed.

TRIGGERS FOR FOOD ALLERGIES AND SENSITIVITIES

Although food sensitivities aren't widely recognized as playing a role in disease, adverse food reactions can contribute to disease processes. "Food sensitivity" is commonly used as an umbrella term for allergies, nonallergic food hypersensitivities, and intolerances. A true food allergy is a reaction to an allergen (usually a protein) that the immune system views as a foreign invader. The body produces antibodies against the allergen, triggering the release of histamine, which is responsible for allergy symptoms: hives, eczema, a runny nose, earaches, shortness of breath, swelling, inflammation, diarrhea, and so on. Eight foods account for 90 percent of true food allergies: milk, eggs, peanuts, tree nuts, shellfish, fish, wheat, and soy. Although allergies can begin at any age, most appear during early childhood, and in 90 percent of those cases, children outgrow them by age seven. The people most likely to remain allergic are those with severe, life-threatening anaphylactic reactions and those sensitive to peanuts or tree nuts.

Adverse food reactions that don't trigger an immune response are called nonallergic food hypersensitivities or intolerances. Though the symptoms can be similar, they may be less acute and less easily recognized than those of true food allergies. Lactose intolerance, the inability to digest lactose, the sugar in milk, is a good example of a food intolerance. Lactose intolerance commonly occurs after about age four, when production of the enzyme lactase declines in about 65 percent of people. Lactase is required by babies to digest lactose in breast milk, which is also present in cow's milk. If milk products are consumed in significant amounts after lactase levels decline, lactose in the large intestine remains undigested and causes gastrointestinal distress.

Pharmacological reactions are another type of nonallergic hypersensitivity. For example, monosodium glutamate (MSG), a flavor enhancer commonly used in Chinese food, may cause some people to have side effects similar to those of drugs, such as flushing, headaches, and abdominal symptoms. Other potentially problematic food components include sulfites in wine and dried fruit, tyramine in aged cheeses, theobromine in chocolate, and preservatives, flavorings, and coloring agents in processed foods.

Gastrointestinal reactions to food are the symptoms most strongly linked to chronic disease risk. When you're in good health, the lining of the gut serves as a highly selective barrier that facilitates the absorption of essential nutrients such as fatty acids, vitamins, minerals, antioxidants, and phytochemicals and prevents the absorption of potentially harmful substances. If the integrity of the gut wall is compromised, some of these can leak into the bloodstream, setting off immune reactions in various parts of the body and placing a significant burden on detoxification systems. This condition is often referred to as leaky gut syndrome. The lining of the gut can be breached when it's constantly in contact with the food components that cause inflammation or injury. Damage can also be caused by medications, environmental contaminants, radiation, stress, inflammatory conditions such as Crohn's disease, or an overgrowth of unfriendly gut microflora.

Once compounds leak from the gut into the bloodstream, they can wreak havoc in the system, contributing to a myriad of conditions:

- Anxiety or depression
- Asthma

- Autism
- Autoimmune diseases
- Cancer
- Cardiovascular diseases
- Celiac disease or gluten hypersensitivity
- Chronic fatigue
- Chronic low-grade inflammation
- Diabetes (type 1 and type 2)
- Gastrointestinal disorders such as diarrhea, bloating, irritable bowel syndrome, or ulcerative colitis
- Hormone abnormalities
- Insulin resistance or metabolic syndrome
- Joint and muscle issues such as chronic pain or rheumatoid arthritis
- Liver dysfunction
- Migraine headaches
- Overweight or obesity
- Skin problems such as itching, eczema, hives, acne, or psoriasis

In addition, if the epithelial cells lining the gut are damaged, they lose their ability to transport nutrients into circulation and malnutrition can result. While any food can be problematic, the foods most strongly associated with increased gut permeability are dairy products and those that contain gluten (a protein in wheat, barley, rye, spelt, triticale, and Kamut). (For more information on gluten.) Diets that promote an imbalance in gut flora, such as those high in sugar, can also adversely affect the integrity of the gut. Fortunately, with improvements in diet, the intestinal lining can regenerate and heal itself. For some individuals, supplementing with L-glutamine, probiotics, zinc, and omega-3 fatty acids may be helpful.

It's important to properly identify offending foods, but traditional allergy testing isn't helpful in identifying nonallergic food hypersensitivities. Plus, all types of allergy testing have limitations, even for the diagnosis of true allergies. To confirm a food culprit, eliminate all of the suspect foods for several weeks. If the sensitivity doesn't cause an anaphylactic response, reintroduce the suspect foods one at a time, at two- or three-day intervals, checking on reactions after each. For more information on food allergies, nonallergic food hypersensitivities, gut health, and elimination diets, see *The Food Allergy Survival Guide,* by V. Melina, D. Aronson, and J. Stepaniak (Book Publishing Company, 2004).

Take-Home Message: Nonallergic food hypersensitivities and allergies can be significant players in many disease processes. If you struggle with unsolved health issues, it's worth considering adverse food reactions as a potential contributor. In some cases, an elimination diet may be warranted.

CHEMICAL CONTAMINANTS

Food can be contaminated by hazardous materials that enter the food chain during the growing, harvesting, storage, processing, packaging, or preparation of food, including as a result of the use of agrochemicals. Unfortunately, the more polluted our world becomes, the greater our exposure to toxic contaminants. Many of these substances persist in the environment and work their way up the food chain. Ingesting various contaminants, such as arsenic, cadmium, lead, mercury, PCBs, DDT, pesticides, and hormones, has been associated with many health conditions, including cancer, diabetes, cardiovascular diseases, endocrine disruption, hypertension, and nervous system damage.

Common sources of chemical contaminants are processed foods, animal products, and conventionally grown produce. Meat, fish, and poultry can be high in contaminants due to their considerable presence in animal fodder. Therefore, vegans and vegetarians have lower exposure to almost all dietary contaminants except for agrochemicals used on conventionally grown produce, since they eat more produce than omnivores. But when all contaminants are taken into account, vegans eat fewer of them. Of course, vegans who eat mostly organic food have the lowest blood levels of agrochemical pesticides.

Although vegans have reduced exposure to chemical contaminants relative to others, there are several steps vegans can take to further reduce their risk:

- Eat organic food.
- Buy from local growers. Produce from farmers' markets tends to have fewer pesticides, even if it isn't organic.
- Grow your own organic produce. If you're short on yard space, use containers.
- Wash produce well before eating. Although pesticides get inside of foods and cannot be completely removed by washing, it will reduce total pesticide content. Peeling conventional produce also reduces pesticide content.
- Avoid highly processed foods. They often contain additives, preservatives, and products of oxidation, such as rancid fats.
- Moderate use of rice and rice products to reduce exposure to arsenic. Feed your baby a variety of cereals, rather than relying exclusively on rice cereals.
- Avoid hijiki. Although all sea vegetables can be contaminated by heavy metals and pollutants from the ocean, hijiki is particularly high in arsenic. If you do use it, soak it first and drain it well.
- Limit exposure to potentially dangerous packaging materials. Select glass containers

instead of plastic for storing and reheating food. If using plastic, purchase products free of BPA (bisphenol A). At the very least, avoid putting hot foods into plastic containers or heating foods in plastic. Avoid imported canned foods, since the cans may contain lead, and don't store food in lead-glazed or leaded glassware.

- Use cooking methods that are less likely to create toxic compounds. Steaming, stewing, and braising produce fewer by-products than frying, barbecuing, and broiling. Minimize consumption of deep-fried foods and foods cooked at high heat for long periods of time. If you cook with high heat, don't blacken or overcook foods.

- Eat more raw foods to reduce your exposure to harmful by-products of cooking. For more information, see *Becoming Raw*, by B. Davis and V. Melina (Book Publishing Company, 2010).

Take-Home Message: The primary sources of environmental contaminants are animal products, processed foods, and conventionally grown produce. Vegans have low blood levels of contaminants but can reduce these levels even more.

Which Vegan Diet Is Best?

People of all ages, genetic makeups, physical activity levels, and states of health all share two common dietary goals: to be adequately nourished, and to avoid or reverse diet-induced chronic disease. You might wonder what type of vegan diet best meets these goals. If you asked a dozen different authorities, you might receive a dozen different answers.

Many vegan diets have been touted as healthiest: low-fat, macrobiotic, Mediterranean, nutrient-dense, raw, starch-based, whole-foods, fruitarian, and the list goes on. While there are pros and cons to each, most can be designed to be nutritionally adequate. The greater challenge is teasing out the factors that provide an advantage in terms of disease prevention or treatment.

The following sections examine some common vegan diets, outlining their strengths and weaknesses and summarizing how to make each variation work for your health.

Diet: Conventional (combination of cooked and raw foods; about 30% fat)

Strengths: It isn't difficult to achieve nutritional adequacy on a conventional vegan diet, and key foods are easily accessible. It also allows greater flexibility socially. Foods are relatively accessible.

Weaknesses: With poor food choices, a conventional vegan diet may be low in foods rich in protein, iron, and zinc, such as legumes, or in calcium-rich foods.

Making it work: Eat a balance of cooked and raw foods, and use convenience foods in moderation.

Diet: Fast and Easy (high use of convenience and fast foods)

Strengths: This diet is practical and simple, and with its reliance on prepared foods, it typically includes fortified foods that boost intakes of iron and vitamins B_{12} and D.

Weaknesses: Convenience foods are high in added fats, sugars, and sodium and lower in protective phytochemicals, antioxidants, and fiber. These foods also may be expensive.

Making it work: Choose foods with short ingredient lists and less sodium, fat, and sugar. Use nutritious convenience foods such as hummus, lentil soup, and fortified nondairy milks, yogurts, and breakfast cereals.

Diet: Fruitarian

Strengths: A fruitarian diet is low in calories and fat and high in phytochemicals and antioxidants. It also avoids common allergens.

Weaknesses: Fruit may not provide enough protein, essential fatty acids, or important vitamins and minerals. It's also unsuitable for children.

Making it work: Include organic greens, nuts, seeds, and sprouted or cooked legumes.

Ensure that you're getting enough iodine and vitamins B_{12} and D.

Diet: Low-Fat (15% fat or less)

Strengths: A low-fat vegan diet minimizes harmful fats and is effective for weight loss and for treating cardiovascular diseases and type 2 diabetes.

Weaknesses: Such diets may be low in essential fatty acids and vitamin E, and absorption of minerals. They may also increase triglycerides if refined carbohydrates are emphasized. Absorption of some vitamins and phytochemicals may be impaired. In addition, a low-fat diet may not provide enough calories for children or those who are underweight.

Making it work: Eat vegetables, fruits, legumes, and whole grains and at least 1 ounce (30g) of nuts and seeds per day, including a source of omega-3 fatty acids.

Diet: Macrobiotic

Strengths: A macrobiotic diet is focused on whole foods and low in processed foods, including flour products.

Weaknesses: Such diets may not provide enough iron, zinc, lysine, essential fatty acids, or vitamins B_{12} and D. They also have a lower nutrient density due to their heavy reliance on grains.

Making it work: Include generous amounts of vegetables, fruits, legumes, nuts, and seeds. Ensure that you're getting enough iodine and vitamins B_{12} and D.

Diet: Mediterranean

Strengths: A Mediterranean diet includes generous amounts of legumes, vegetables, fruits, whole grains, nuts and seeds and limits processed foods.

Weaknesses: Such diets may be too high in fat for those who are overweight or have high cholesterol. If wine is emphasized, it may increase cancer risk.

Making it work: Rely on nuts, seeds, avocados, and olives for fat rather than oil. Ensure that you're getting enough iodine and vitamins B_{12} and D.

Diet: Nutrient-Dense

Strengths: A nutrient-dense diet emphasizes vegetables and other whole foods and provides abundant vitamins and minerals while minimizing processed foods and oil.

Weaknesses: This diet doesn't necessarily take into account harmful factors such as environmental contaminants and free radicals.

Making it work: Ensure that you're getting enough iodine and vitamins B_{12} and D. Factor in all protective dietary components as well as the potentially harmful ones (see table 8.1).

Diet: Raw

Strengths: A raw diet minimizes processed foods and avoids common allergens. It's also low in damaging dietary components, high in protective components, and avoids problems related to cooking, such as loss of nutrients and phytochemicals and formation of carcinogens.

Weaknesses: If not well planned, a raw diet may fall short of recommended intakes for protein, iron, zinc, calcium, iodine, and vitamins B_{12} and D. Food prep can be labor-intensive, and this diet can be expensive if you rely on specialty products. Raw diets aren't recommended for infants and children.

Making it work: Ensure that all of your nutritional and calorie needs are met. Eat sprouted or cooked legumes to boost protein, iron, and zinc. ("Rawfood" diets may include up to 25 percent cooked foods). Soak, sprout, juice, blend, dehydrate, and ferment foods to increase the concentration and availability of nutrients.

Diet: Starch-Based

Strengths: Starch-based diets are typically affordable and low in fat and include only moderate amounts of processed foods.

Weaknesses: Because grains provide fewer minerals and vitamins and less protein than vegetables or legumes, such diets have lower nutrient density. They may also be low in essential fatty acids and lysine and can be unsuitable for smaller people or those with small appetites.

Making it work: Eat nine servings of vegetables and fruits and at least I ounce (30g) of nuts and seeds each day. Include legumes for more concentrated protein, and select nutrient-dense starches such as quinoa and yams. Ensure that you're getting enough iodine and vitamins B_{12} and D.

Diet: Whole-Foods

Strengths: When well planned, whole-foods diets are high in antioxidants, phytochemicals, fiber, vitamins, and minerals. Such diets are also affordable and low in sodium and added fat and sugar.

Weaknesses: A diet focused on whole foods may lack iodine and vitamins B_{12} and D. Food prep can be labor-intensive.

Making it work: Include some lightly processed foods (tofu, fortified nondairy milks, and nondairy yogurt) to boost nutrient intake and make prep easier. Ensure that you're getting enough iodine and vitamins B_{12} and D.

TRANSITIONING TO A HEALTHFUL VEGAN DIET

The transition to a healthful vegan diet can be a delightful culinary adventure. When you eliminate animal products from the menu, you open up a whole new world of delights: fresh flavors, appealing textures and colors, and intriguing international influences. As you turn your focus to healthful whole plant foods—vegetables, fruits, legumes, whole grains, nuts, and seeds—opt for the cleanest choices within each of these categories, as outlined table 8.1. Also, follow the Vegan Food Guide to ensure all your nutrient needs are met!

TABLE 8.1. Clean, green food choices

FOOD CATEGORY	BEST CHOICES	CONSIDERATIONS
Vegetables	All vegetables and vegetable juices, but especially dark leafy greens	Choose organic when possible. Eat greens low in oxalates (bok choy, collard, kale, napa cabbage, watercress, and collard, dandelion, mustard, and turnip greens) for calcium. Eat at least half of your veggies raw. Focus on moist cooking methods and don't overcook. Include a fat source in salad dressings. Choose orange or yellow starchy vegetables (yams, squash). Use vegetable juices as a concentrated source of antioxidants and phytochemicals.
Fruits	All fruits, fresh, frozen, and dried	Eat mainly fresh, organic fruits and juices; cooking depletes vitamin C. Use fresh or dried fruits as sweeteners. Fruit smoothies are an almost-instant meal and very nutritious, especially if you add greens.
Legumes	Beans, lentils, peas, and their sprouts, as well as soy foods, and peanuts	Aim for 3 servings each day. Soak or sprout dried legumes before cooking. Choose organic soy products. Select fortified soymilk made with whole soybeans rather than isolates. Limit veggie meats, which are highly processed.
Whole grains	Sprouted, intact, cut or rolled whole grains and "pseudograins" (amaranth, buckwheat, quinoa, wild rice)	Sprouting dramatically increases phytochemical and lysine content and reduces compounds that inhibit nutrient absorption. Pseudograins are more nutrient dense than other grains and gluten-free. Use intact grains when possible. Moderate use of flour products even if whole-grain. Limit processed products such as flaked whole grain cereals. Minimize refined grains.
Nuts	Nuts, nut butters, and nut cheeses	Soak nuts to improve digestibility, boost phytochemical content, and decrease compounds that inhibit nutrient absorption. Walnuts provide omega-3 fatty acids. Select natural nut butters. Limit intake of roasted nuts, especially when roasted in oil and salt or coated in sugar.
Seeds	Seeds and seed butters	Sprout seeds for added nutrition. Soak them to improve digestibility, increase phytochemical content, and decrease compounds that inhibit nutrient absorption. Select natural seed butters. Use omega-3-rich seeds (chia seeds, hempseeds, and ground flaxseeds).
Sea vegetables	All except hijiki	Sea vegetables provide essential fats and iodine, but they may be contaminated if from polluted waters. Avoid hijiki due to arsenic contamination.
Concentrated fats and oils	Mechanically pressed oils rich in omega-3s or with a good balance of omega-3s and omega-6s	Limit use of added oils. Select organic oils to minimize toxins, which are concentrated when oil is extracted, and store refrigerated. For cooking, use small amounts of organic olive, canola, coconut, or high-oleic oils. Minimize use of hard fats other than coconut oil, such as margarine.
Concentrated sweeteners	Dried fruit sugars, blackstrap molasses	Minimize use of concentrated sugars. Sugars made from whole foods such as dates are more nutritious options. Blackstrap molasses is the most nutrient-rich sweetener. Choose organic.

Sources of data are listed in *Becoming Vegan: Comprehensive Edition*, by Brenda Davis and Vesanto Melina (Book Publishing Company, 2014).

The Paleo Diet: Facing the Facts

High-protein, low-carbohydrate diets often attract athletes, dieters, and health seekers of all stripes, and the "paleo" diet is an example. Its basic premise is simple—the diet humans ate in preagricultural, Paleolithic times is best suited for human health. While we can't blindly assume that what our relatively short-lived ancestors ate was necessarily optimal for human health, nutritional anthropologists have studied true Paleolithic diets extensively.

That diet essentially consisted of wild plants and wild animals, which varied with location, season, hunting and gathering skills, available tools, and so on. We know that preagricultural peoples didn't consume oil, sugar, salt, anything from a box or bag, or the milk of other mammals. Today's new paleo devotees attempt to copy the diet of our ancestors by eating meat, poultry, fish, vegetables, fruits, nuts, and seeds and, in most cases, avoiding processed foods, grains, legumes, and dairy products.

Followers apparently imagine that the nutrient intake of the new paleo diet approximates that of our Paleolithic ancestors, but they're wrong. As it turns out, vegan diets have more in common with true Paleolithic diets than the new paleo diets. This may sound like a bit of a stretch, so we did the math for you: We compared three days of recommended paleo menus from a popular paleo website with three days of recommended vegan menus from chapter 14 in this book. We also compared the average daily intakes offered by the diet true Paleolithic people ate. The results are summarized in table 8.2, which also provides dietary reference intakes (DRIs, the nutrient intake recommendations from the US National Academy of Sciences). The DRI values are for adult males and adult women who aren't pregnant or lactating. Nutrients and other dietary factors in the new paleo or vegan diet that are more similar to the true Paleolithic diet are highlighted in gray.

As you can see, new paleo intakes of protein, vitamin A, and zinc are closer to amounts in a true Paleolithic diet than in the vegan diet, but cholesterol intake is almost triple that of a true Paleolithic diet. However, vegan intakes of carbohydrate, fat, saturated fat, fiber, riboflavin, thiamin, vitamin C, vitamin E, iron, calcium, sodium, and potassium are all closer to levels in a true Paleolithic diet than in a new paleo diet.

More than 50 percent of calories in the new paleo diet come from fat, and 20 percent of calories come from saturated fat. In other words, today's paleo wannabes may be consuming twice the fat and more than three times the saturated fat of true Paleolithic people. Fiber intakes of the new paleo diet are about 30 grams per day in a 3,000-calorie diet, whereas the vegan menu provides about 80 grams of fiber. However, even the 100 percent plant-based vegan diet falls short when compared to the 104 grams of fiber consumed by our Paleolithic ancestors, who clearly ate plenty of plant foods.

Why does the new paleo diet fall flat on its face when compared to the true Paleolithic diet? The reason is that the meat and vegetables consumed today are very different from those eaten by true Paleolithic people. The wild animals eaten in Paleolithic times were far leaner than even the leanest domestic animals, and the wild plants were more concentrated in fiber and other nutrients than most of the crops commercially raised today. In addition, new paleo eaters tend to rely far more heavily on meat than did most of their ancestors.

TABLE 8.2. New paleo, true Paleolithic, and vegan diets compared

	DRI	NEW PALEO DIET	TRUE PALEOLITHIC DIET	VEGAN DIET
ENERGY (CAL/D)	2,200–2,900	3,000	3,000	3,000
MACRONUTRIENTS				
Protein (%)	10–35	32	30	15
Carbohydrate (%)	45–65	15	45–50	60
Fat (%)	15–30	53	20–25	25
Saturated fat (%)	<10	19	6	5
Cholesterol (mg)		1,308	480	0
Ratio of omega-6: omega-3		11:1	4:1–1:1	3:1
Fiber (g/d)	25–38	31	104	81
VITAMINS				
Riboflavin (mg)	1.3–1.7	2.6	6.5	4
Thiamin (mg)	1.1–1.2	2.7	3.9	3.9
Vitamin C (mg)	75–90	226	604	491
Vitamin A (mcg RAE)	700–900	2,436	3,797	1,966
Vitamin E (mg)	15	24	32.8	27
MINERALS				
Iron (mg)	8–18	25	87.4	37
Zinc (mg)	8–11	33	43.4	25
Calcium (mg)	1,000–1,200	643	1,956	2,633
Sodium (mg)	<2,300	4,193	768	1,958
Potassium (mg)	4,700	4,762	10,500	8,153

Sources of data: New paleo data is based on the average of three days (Wednesday, Thursday, and Friday) of recommended menus from the Paleo Plan website (paleoplan.com/resources/sampler-menu-meal-plan/), adjusted to 3,000 calories. True Paleolithic data is from Eaton, S. B., et al., "Paleolithic Nutrition Revisited: A Twelve-Year Retrospective on Its Nature and Implications," *European Journal of Clinical Nutrition* 51, no. 4 (1997): 207–216. Vegan data is based on the average of three days of menus from chapter 14, adjusted to 3,000 calories.

Bottom Line: The new paleo diet is a very pale imitation of the diet of early humans. The focus tends to be on consuming large quantities of meat. Plus, this dietary pattern ignores the environmental crisis that makes eating lower on the food chain an ecological imperative, the ethical issues associated with an increased demand for food animals, and the numerous health risks associated with the consumption of meat. If people want to move closer to a true Paleolithic diet, they might turn their attention to becoming vegan—it's as close to a true Paleolithic diet as most modern-day people can achieve.

THE OCCASIONAL INDULGENCE

There are few foods that haven't been "veganized." Vegan peanut butter cups, chicken nuggets, croissants, pizza, cream cheese, marshmallows, ice cream bars, mayonnaise, spare ribs, and even calamari are all readily available, and their accessibility can make the transition to a vegan diet less daunting. Still, you may wonder if these convenience foods have a place in a healthful vegan diet.

For most people, the occasional treat isn't a problem. Ultimately, the answer depends on your health and energy needs. People who are healthy and active have more dietary leeway than those who are unhealthy or inactive. If you are fighting a serious disease, we recommend that your diet be as clean as possible. Remember, all body systems are interconnected, and when one system is compromised, other systems falter. Even for vegans, too many calories or too much highly processed food can compromise health and healing.

As you progress along the vegan culinary path, you'll discover that the taste of processed, prepared foods doesn't compare to the flavors of whole, fresh foods. For example, vegan ice cream is yummy, but desserts made solely from frozen fruits, such as banana and mango, are stupendous. Over time, you're likely to find that commercial products taste too sweet, too rich, and too salty and simply lose their appeal.

Next, we tackle one of the most pervasive health problems of our century: overweight and obesity.

CHAPTER 9

Triumph over Weight

One of the great attractions of a vegan diet is the promise of slimness. It's an established part of the vegan stereotype. If you're an overweight vegan, mentioning your dietary preferences may elicit looks of surprise. Reactions, even if unspoken, often clearly say, "You don't look like a vegan." If you're overweight and adopt a vegan diet, not losing weight can be frustrating. And if you *gain* weight after becoming vegan, it can be downright exasperating. But the truth is, vegans come in all shapes and sizes, and although becoming vegan can be an effective ally in an effort to shed pounds, it doesn't guarantee weight loss.

The Costs of Overweight

Avegan diet provides remarkable protection against overweight and obesity. Vegans are leaner, having lower body mass indexes (BMI) and percentage of body fat than any other dietary group. The average vegan has a BMI of about 22, compared to a BMI of about 28 for the average American. The United States is one of the most overweight nations, with almost 70 percent of the adult population being overweight or obese. In a large study in the United Kingdom, only 2 percent of vegans were obese, compared to more than 5 percent of healthconscious meat eaters. Still, although these statistics are reassuring, they provide little consolation for overweight and obese vegans.

Overweight and obesity come with a hefty price tag. In 2008, medical costs associated with obesity in the United States were estimated at $147 billion. Excess body fat causes harmful changes to the body's basic physiology, adversely affecting blood pressure, cholesterol, triglycerides, respiration, fertility, skin and joint health, hormones, and insulin activity. More specifically, it significantly increases risk for the following debilitating and often fatal health conditions:

- **Type 2 diabetes.** The risk of type 2 diabetes is directly linked to the amount of excess body fat, particularly when fat is carried in the abdomen. As body fat increases, insulin sensitivity declines and insulin resistance increases.

- **Heart disease and stroke.** Being overweight contributes to high blood pressure, high cholesterol and triglyceride levels, and angina and can markedly increase the chance of a heart attack, stroke, or congestive heart failure.

- **Cancer.** Overweight women suffer more breast, uterine, cervical, ovarian, gallbladder, and colon cancers, while overweight men are at elevated risk for cancers of the colon, rectum, and prostate.
- **Osteoarthritis.** Excess body weight increases the risk of osteoarthritis, probably because it puts extra pressure on the joints, which erodes the cartilage that cushions and protects joints.
- **Sleep apnea.** Sleep apnea, which involves pauses in breathing during sleep, is often marked by heavy snoring and snorting breaths following sometimes fairly prolonged lapses in breathing. Risk for sleep apnea is significantly higher among overweight people.
- **Gout.** The product of high levels of uric acid in the blood, gout causes painful swelling in the joints, usually affecting one joint at a time, most commonly the big toe. Risk for gout rises progressively with increased body weight.
- **Gallbladder disease.** Being significantly overweight increases the risk of gallbladder disease and gallstones, but rapid, significant weight loss can also increase the chance of developing gallstones. Gradual weight loss of about 1 to 2 pounds (0.4 to 0.9kg) per week is less likely to trigger gallbladder attacks.

- **Polycystic ovarian syndrome.** A painful disorder marked by small cysts on the ovaries, menstrual irregularities, facial hair, acne, patches of dark skin on the neck, and weight gain, polycystic ovarian syndrome affects women of reproductive age. It's associated with insulin resistance and abdominal obesity and strongly increases the risk of type 2 diabetes, heart disease, and stroke.

You may wonder how problematic some excess weight is if you're eating a healthy vegan diet. While published research hasn't yet answered this question, there is evidence that healthful lifestyle habits are associated with a significant reduction in mortality for all people, whether of healthy weight, overweight, or obese, with the greatest benefits being observed in obese individuals. Because vegan diets are generally associated with reduced risk of chronic disease, it's understandable that overweight and obese vegans would enjoy some health advantages compared to overweight and obese omnivores. However, vegans who eat a lot of refined grains and processed foods with added fat, sugar, and salt will assuredly fare worse than health-conscious meat eaters.

Healthy Body Weight

Not all people of the same height will have the same ideal weight, despite widely held beliefs to the contrary. Healthy weight depends on bone structure, muscle mass, body fat, and build. However, the following definitions, along with body mass index (BMI; outlined in table 9.1), can be helpful in determining if a person is overweight or obese.

"Overweight" is generally defined as weighing at least 10 percent more than healthy body weight. For most people, that amounts to 10 to 30 pounds more than their healthy weight. "Obese" is generally defined as weighing at least 20 percent more than healthy body weight. For most people, that amounts to 30 or more pounds above their healthy weight.

The best way to know if your weight is within a healthy range is to determine how much of your body weight is fat. A simple tool called body mass index (BMI) is commonly suggested for estimating this. As shown in table 9.1, a BMI of 18.5 to 24.9 is in the healthy range. A BMI below 18.5 is deemed underweight, and a BMI of 25 to 29.9 is considered overweight. Obesity is generally defined as a BMI equal to or greater than 30, with a BMI of 35 or higher being severe and a BMI of 40 or more being extreme.

While BMI is a useful tool for most people, it has several significant limitations. First and foremost, it doesn't take into account differences in body composition between genders and among races, ethnic groups, or those of different ages. In addition, it's only considered to be valid for people twenty to sixty-five years old, is less precise for people less than 5 feet (1.5 meters) tall, and is of little value to bodybuilders or other people with extremely large muscles. It isn't applicable to pregnant women.

What Your Body Shape Means

Once you've figured out your BMI and have a general idea of your degree of body fat, there's one more important factor to consider: your body shape. The most common descriptors of body shape are apple and pear. If you carry the bulk of your weight above your hips (mainly in your abdomen), you have an apple shape. People who are apple shaped sometimes have a larger waist than hips. If you have an apple shape, when you gain weight, it tends to go directly to your stomach. This body shape is more prevalent in men.

If you carry excess weight in your hips, thighs, and buttocks, you have a pear shape. People who are pear shaped generally have larger hips than waist. This body shape is more common in women.

You also can easily determine whether you have an apple or pear shape by calculating your waist to hip ratio. Simply measure your waist and hips and divide your waist measurement by your hip measurement. Ratios of 0.8 or less for women and 0.9 or less for men are considered a pear shape.

Whether you have an apple or pear shape only matters if you're carrying excess weight. If you're overweight or obese, having an apple shape puts you at much higher risk for heart disease, type 2 diabetes, hypertension, and several types of cancer. For those who naturally become apple shaped with weight gain, it's critically important to maintain a healthy body weight.

TABLE 9.1. Body mass index (BMI)

Height in inches

WT(LB)	60	61	62	63	64	65	66	67	68	69	70	71	72	73	74	75	76
100	20	19	18	18	17	17	16	16	15	15	14	14	14	13	13	12	12
105	21	20	19	19	18	17	17	16	16	16	15	15	14	14	13	13	13
110	21	21	20	19	19	18	18	17	17	16	16	15	15	15	14	14	13
115	22	22	21	20	20	19	19	18	17	17	17	16	16	15	15	14	14
120	23	23	22	21	21	20	19	19	18	18	17	17	16	16	15	15	15
125	24	24	23	22	21	21	20	20	19	18	18	17	17	16	16	16	15
130	25	25	24	23	22	22	21	20	20	19	19	18	18	17	17	16	16
135	26	26	25	24	23	22	22	21	21	20	19	19	18	18	17	17	16
140	27	26	26	25	24	23	23	22	21	21	20	20	19	18	18	17	17
145	28	27	27	26	25	24	23	23	22	21	21	20	20	19	19	18	18
150	29	28	27	27	26	25	24	23	23	22	22	21	20	20	19	19	18
155	30	29	28	27	27	26	25	24	24	23	22	22	21	20	20	19	19
160	31	30	29	28	27	27	26	25	24	24	23	22	22	21	21	20	19
165	32	31	30	29	28	27	27	26	25	24	24	23	22	22	21	21	20
170	33	32	31	30	29	28	27	27	26	25	24	24	23	22	22	21	21
175	34	33	32	31	30	29	28	27	27	26	25	24	24	23	22	22	21
180	35	34	33	32	31	30	29	28	27	27	26	25	24	24	23	22	22
185	36	35	34	33	32	31	30	29	28	27	27	26	25	24	24	23	23
190	37	36	35	34	33	32	31	30	29	28	27	26	26	25	24	24	23
195	38	37	36	35	34	33	32	31	30	29	28	28	27	26	25	24	24
200	39	38	37	35	34	33	32	31	31	30	29	28	27	26	26	25	24
205	40	39	37	36	35	34	33	32	31	30	29	29	28	27	26	26	25
210	41	40	38	37	36	35	34	33	32	31	30	29	28	28	27	26	26
215	42	41	39	38	37	36	35	34	33	32	31	30	29	28	28	27	26
220	43	42	40	39	38	37	36	35	34	33	32	31	30	29	28	27	27
225	44	43	41	40	39	37	36	35	34	33	32	31	31	30	29	28	27
230	45	43	42	41	39	38	37	36	35	34	33	32	31	30	30	29	28
235	46	44	43	42	40	39	38	37	36	35	34	33	32	31	31	29	29
240	47	45	44	43	41	40	39	38	36	35	34	33	33	31	31	30	29
245	48	46	45	43	42	41	40	39	37	36	35	34	33	32	32	30	30
250	49	47	46	44	43	42	40	39	38	37	36	35	34	33	32	31	30

UNDERSTANDING YOUR BMI	
BMI less than 18.5: May indicate underweight	BMI 30–34.9: Indicates class 1 obesity
BMI 18.5–24.9: Healthy weight for most people.	BMI 35–39.9: Indicates class 2 or severe obesity
BMI 25–29.9: Indicates overweight	BMI 40 or more: Indicates class 3 or extreme obesity

There's another way to determine whether you're carrying excess weight. Simply measure your waist. A measurement greater than 32 inches (81cm) for women and 37 inches (94cm) for men suggests that you shouldn't gain any weight. A measurement of 35 inches (89cm) for women and 40 inches (102cm) for men indicates that you're overweight and weight loss could improve your health. (Note that these numbers would need to be adjusted for people with very large or very small frames.)

Being overweight or obese isn't something many people aspire to or would choose. So why are so many Americans overweight or obese? And why aren't kale-eating vegans entirely protected from this fate? Let's take a look.

The Root of the Weight Crisis

Everyone knows that overeating and insufficient activity are at the root of the obesity epidemic. It's clearly a matter of energy balance. If you eat more than you need, you gain weight. If you eat less than you need, you lose weight.

While it sounds so simple, there are a number of factors that can throw a monkey wrench into the energy-in/energy-out theory. For years, the accepted axiom regarding weight loss was that 1 pound (0.45kg) of fat contains 3,500 calories. So if you wanted to lose 1 pound (0.45kg) of fat per week, you needed to decrease food intake by 3,500 calories, increase energy output by 3,500 calories, or do some combination of the two. While this works beautifully on paper, real-life results aren't nearly as predictable.

The human body is a remarkably adaptable machine, and when survival is at stake, it hangs on to energy reserves for dear life. Therefore, the 3,500-calorie rule may overestimate weight loss for most people. For example, if you cut out 500 calories per day, you might lose 1 pound (0.45kg) per week for a few weeks, but your body would quickly adjust to the new reality and weight loss would slow or stop.

There's tremendous individual variability in this process. Two people eating the same diet and exercising the same can lose (or gain) weight at very different rates. As it turns out, for a given energy deficit (less calories consumed than used), adults with greater fat reserves can expect to lose more weight than those with fewer fat reserves. Still, even though weight loss may not be as rapid as would be expected based on the 3,500-calorie formula, small changes in energy intake can result in significant weight loss over time.

The long-held view that all calories are equal has also recently come under fire. Evidence suggests that not all calories behave the same way in the body and that some foods and food combinations promote calorie burning more effectively than others.

In addition, sleep, stress, and exposure to environmental toxins can disturb hormones that influence the storage and breakdown of fat, calorie burning, and body weight. All of these factors can weigh as heavily on vegans as nonvegans. The bottom line is, while it's true that overweight and obesity are the result of energy imbalances, the degree of imbalance is the product of a complex interplay of physical, environmental, and emotional factors.

PHYSIOLOGICAL FACTORS

Some people seem to gain weight simply by inhaling too deeply as they pass a bakery, while others can apparently devour an entire loaf of bread as an appetizer and not gain an ounce. If you fit into the former category, you might be described as metabolically efficient. Dropped on a desert island with no food, your body would preserve your fat and release its stored energy slowly to prolong your survival. The good news is that you'd probably last for weeks. The bad news is that in today's world, you're far more likely to be faced with an endless supply of energy-dense food beckoning you throughout the day. While humans are naturally drawn to this level of security, it commonly leads to weight gain and increased risk of many diseases. Those who are best able to survive famine are least able to thrive with excess. For such people, moderate food intake and vigorous physical activity are necessary.

Not surprisingly, risk of being overweight can be affected by genes, age, and gender. Men tend to burn more calories than women, and for most people, metabolism gradually declines after age forty. Very low-calorie diets and yo-yo dieting only make matters worse, as they send a strong signal to put on the metabolic brakes and conserve precious energy stores.

Less commonly, overweight and obesity can be triggered by hypothyroidism. Hypothyroidism lowers metabolic rate, triggers weight gain, and often makes people feel cold, tired, weak, and depressed. This condition can be triggered or worsened by chronic iodine deficiency, which is rare in North America due to the addition of iodine to table salt. However, those who use mostly natural, noniodized salt are at higher risk. (For more on iodine see chapter 7.)

Finally, corticosteroids, antidepressants, and antiseizure medications can slow metabolism, increase appetite, or cause water retention, all of which can lead to weight gain. (Of course, if you're taking such medications, the underlying condition may be a greater health threat than excess weight. In any event, please don't discontinue these medications without the approval and guidance of your health care provider.)

ENVIRONMENTAL FACTORS

The United States is an ideal environment for overweight and obesity. Food choices are perhaps more diverse than anywhere on the planet, and food is abundant and accessible at home, at work, and everywhere in between. Unfortunately, all too often an American meal is a heaping plate of nutritionally depleted processed or fast food, loaded with fat, salt, and sugar.

Humans are hardwired to like the flavors of fat, sugar, and salt. These flavors, which are highly diluted in nature, once gave us assurance that food was safe and nourishing. But when these flavors are concentrated in processed foods such as sodas, hot fudge sundaes, double cheeseburgers, stuffed-crust pizzas, and deep-fried doughnuts, the results are disastrous. Our innate ability to control appetite becomes unhinged because foods that contain concentrated sugar, fat, and salt are physically addictive, stimulating the same pleasure centers in the brain as heroin, nicotine, and alcohol. Essentially, they provide so much pleasure that they trigger cravings. And don't fool yourself: vegan versions of such foods can be just as problematic.

Another challenge is that portion sizes keep expanding. According to the Centers for Disease Control and Prevention, the average restaurant meal is four times larger than it was in the 1950s. A serving of soda has shot up from 7 fluid ounces (210ml) to 42 fluid ounces (1.25L). A serving of French fries, which once was 2.4 ounces (68g) is now 6.7 ounces (190g). And whereas a typical burger used to be just 3.9 ounces (111g), it is now 12 ounces (340g). No wonder the average adult is 26 pounds (11.8kg) heavier than sixty years ago! Not surprisingly, as portion sizes increase, people—vegan or not—eat more.

Vegan versions of almost every convenience food, snack food, and fast food are now yours for the taking. Today, the word *vegan* is used to provide products with a halo of health. Don't be fooled. Just because the word *vegan* is plastered on a label doesn't guarantee that a product is good for you, nor do labels of "low-calorie," "low-fat," "low-sugar," or "low" anything.

Further compounding the problem, the level of physical activity necessary in much of the world has dwindled dramatically in recent decades. Increasing numbers of people work in offices, and most drive or take public transit to and from work. Even if people want to increase their activity level, many neighborhoods lack sidewalks and safe places for outdoor exercise. People tend to devote their spare time to watching television, playing video games, surfing the Internet, and other passive activities. In addition, every possible convenience has been developed to help reduce energy expenditure: elevators, escalators, remote controls, electric mixers, bread machines, dishwashers, and even electric can openers.

Another potential trigger for weight gain—one that's less well recognized—is lack of sleep. While you might assume that less sleep means greater expenditure of calories, evidence suggests that lack of sleep promotes weight gain. This may be because people who are sleep deprived are attracted to more energy-dense foods, which can lead to overeating and weight gain. In addition, studies indicate that lack of sleep reduces insulin sensitivity, increases levels of ghrelin, a hormone that promotes hunger, and reduces levels of leptin, a hormone that curbs hunger.

A Permanent Solution

The weight-loss industry has a remarkable track record for peddling promises, marketing miracles, and delivering disappointment. Diets are generally designed to produce a calorie deficit or ensure that people take in fewer calories than they burn so they'll lose weight. Most succeed in this task.

So, if most diets succeed in producing weight loss, why do so many fail in the long run? The answer is simple: they end. If you don't have a plan for lifelong dietary and lifestyle changes, old habits return, and with them the weight. Unfortunately, in many cases, the deprivation of a diet pushes the body into conservation mode, sending metabolism into a nosedive. As a result, you may not just regain the lost weight, but also pack on a few extra pounds. This is your body's attempt to effectively prepare for the next famine.

Weight-loss diets are generally a lesson in frustration, but this doesn't mean you have to give up on weight loss. You just need to find a more effective longterm solution. Three simple steps will help you redirect your goals so weight loss becomes a by-product of bigger and better things: make health your goal, think positively, and build healthful habits.

STEP 1: MAKE HEALTH YOUR GOAL

Dump the dieter's mentality of thinness at all costs and redirect your focus to health. Make it your top priority. The ultimate test of anything that promises to peel off pounds is one simple question: Does it support and promote optimal health? If the answer is yes, it has passed the litmus test and will be a useful ally. If the answer is no, don't even give it a second thought. If it compromises health, it's worse than useless.

Every single cell of your body is a product of the food you put in your mouth; food provides the body's basic structural materials. Resist the urge to select foods on the basis of their caloric content or perceived effectiveness as diet foods. Instead, select foods on the basis of their ability to nourish and protect your body. Before you bite into a sugar-free diet cookie made with white flour, partially hydrogenated vegetable oil, and artificial sweeteners, ask yourself whether those are the best materials for rebuilding your brain cells, or any other cells for that matter. Keep your eyes squarely on the goal.

Establish an environment that will effectively reset your metabolic machinery. Do what you can to calm inflammation and minimize your exposure to toxins (more on how these factors affect weight shortly). This will help ensure that the hormones that affect hunger, metabolism, and weight aren't compromised.

STEP 2: THINK POSITIVELY

Hold on to your dreams. No matter how far away they might seem, know that every step you take in the right direction is worth celebrating. Being on the right path, even if just inching your way to your goal, is more important than where you are on that path. Listen carefully to your body. It communicates with you constantly and honestly. Let it guide you as you gradually reclaim your health.

Fear of failure is often the greatest stumbling block, breeding negative thoughts that can effectively crush your spirit. In this journey, there are no reprisals or exams. There's nothing to fear. Take on only what you're ready and able to take on. Push out any negative thoughts with positive affirmations. Remind yourself that you will achieve what you've set your sights on and that nothing anyone else does or says can extinguish your enthusiasm.

As you work to develop positive habits, be prepared for stumbling blocks and resistance. Don't beat yourself up when things don't go according to plan. Instead, use each disappointment as a valuable lesson about what works and what doesn't.

STEP 3: BUILD HEALTHFUL HABITS

One of the greatest challenges in the quest for wellness is to break old, destructive habits and replace them with habits that truly support and promote health. Many repetitions are required to transform a behavior into a habit.

Bad habits are hard to break because they arise to fill a need. Identify that need and consider the costs and benefits of using the habit to fill that need. You may find it helpful to keep a log for a couple of weeks to make you more conscious of your behavior. If a habit doesn't serve you, it's time to replace it with something that does. Fill the need with anything that will improve your well-being and make you feel better about yourself. For example, if your diet descends into the abyss of junk food while watching television after dinner, fill your evenings with television-free activities. Create a new routine and follow it faithfully for a set period of time. One month is a good goal. If you set a time frame for yourself, it makes sticking to the routine a little easier. Once you've repeated a behavior for a month, you're well on your way to turning it into a new habit. To make your plan foolproof, be sure to surround yourself with a network of supportive friends and family.

Preparing for the Journey

The following guidelines will help ensure your success in the journey to freedom from excess pounds and the related risk of chronic diseases.

Get a physical exam. Have testing done to determine your blood pressure and levels of thyroid hormones, cholesterol, triglycerides, blood sugar, vitamin B_{12}, vitamin D, iron, and CRP (measure of inflammation). If you're on prescription medications, make sure your health care provider knows about your new health plan. As you regain your health, it's important to closely monitor your condition, as you may need to reduce or eliminate certain medications (with the guidance of your health care provider).

Keep a three-day food and activity diary. Keep track of everything you eat and drink for three full days. (Excellent online sites and apps can assist you in this task.) Try to include at least one weekend day. Include the following information:

- Type and amount of food consumed
- Time of day you ate
- Where you ate
- Preparation method used
- Reason for selecting the food
- Degree of physical hunger on a scale of 0 to 5 (0 being not hungry and 5 being famished)
- How you felt before eating the food
- How you felt after eating the food

In addition, note all of your activities, from gardening to grocery shopping. Include any exercise or other fitness activities and be specific about duration. Keep track of your sleeping patterns: when and where you slept, how long, and how well. Also note anything you did to take care of yourself, such as getting a massage or pedicure, prayer time, meditation, or enjoyable social activities. Finally, record of all addictive substances you used, such as cigarettes, alcohol, or recreational drugs. Simply writing these things down provides a powerful reality check.

Set both short-term and long-term health goals. When setting goals, be specific. They should be measurable and attainable. The primary focus shouldn't be weight loss, but rather improving your fitness level, increasing your fiber intake, eating more leafy greens, reducing your cholesterol level, and so on. Tackle goals one at a time, so you don't feel overwhelmed. Even small changes can produce big health rewards.

Deliver yourself from temptation. Get rid of unhealthful foods and beverages that tempt you. You don't need that kind of pressure. Take them to a food bank or homeless shelter, give them away, or throw them out. If others in your household don't want you to give these things away, explain what you're doing and why, and respectfully request their support. Be sure to express gratitude for whatever sacrifices they are willing to make.

Restock your pantry. Eating healthfully isn't about deprivation. Highly healthful food can be more delicious than the unhealthy food it's replacing. Go shopping for items that meet your new standards. Select recipes that you'd like to try, and gather all the ingredients required. Consider investing in some high-quality food preparation equipment if you can.

Take a few steps outside your comfort zone. If you've been eating a lot of junk food or fast food, you may need to learn how to prepare healthful food. Begin by making a few simple meals. Try at least one new recipe every day or two, even if it's just a salad dressing. Experiment with dehydrating, juicing, or sprouting or soaking beans and nuts.

Reclaiming Your Health

No one else can achieve health for you. No doctor or dietitian can eat for you, exercise for you, or manage stress for you. You hold the power to transform your life and reclaim your health. Becoming vegan is an extraordinary first step. The next step is becoming a truly healthy vegan.

Before we discuss specific food choices, we think it will be helpful for you to understand why you need to make the recommended changes. Dietary choices that work against your body can compromise all body systems. While you may feel as though your body is failing you, there's a good chance that you're failing your body. Your body depends on your dietary choices for survival. Below are six health goals, each of which will help explain why food choices recommended later in this chapter are necessary.

OVERCOME FOOD ADDICTIONS AND CRAVINGS

Although it sounds a little extreme, we encourage you to think of ultraprocessed foods laden with fat, sugar, or salt as drugs. To break your addiction, you have to stop eating them. While breaking a food addiction isn't easy, replacing addictive foods with foods that are of real value to your health has amazing results. Your body can restore its balance and free you from the addiction. When you reach this point, cravings are far less likely, and your body will also be better able to handle the occasional addictive food.

To overcome a food addiction, you need to keep your blood sugar levels stable. Eat meals containing a good balance of protein, carbohydrate, and fat. For example, if you eat cereal for breakfast, top it with nuts and seeds. Use unsweetened nondairy milk. Eat legumes, tofu, or tempeh at lunch and dinner. Consider including legumes at breakfast to give you staying power through the morning. Avoid caloric beverages, sugar, and artificial sweeteners.

Eliminate deep-fried foods. Steer clear of ultraprocessed foods. Also be aware of any food allergies, which are one of the less well-recognized causes of cravings. Ironically, people often crave the very foods they're allergic to, and for growing numbers of people, wheat or gluten seems to be an issue.

CONTROL INFLAMMATION

Inflammation is one of the key forces behind overweight, obesity, insulin resistance, diabetes, heart disease, dementia, and just about every other chronic disease. Dietary factors can generate inflammation in many ways. Overweight can trigger inflammation. Healthy fat cells produce a balance of proinflammatory and anti-inflammatory hormones. When fat cells become overfilled with fat, production of proinflammatory hormones increases, while production of antiinflammatory hormones decreases. This imbalance promotes insulin resistance.

Other common contributors to inflammation are food sensitivities and allergies. Once again, gluten can be especially problematic. Environmental contaminants, chronic stress, and deficiencies of certain nutrients, particularly vitamin D and omega-3 fatty acids, can also promote inflammation. Fortunately, the abundant vegetables, fruits, legumes, whole grains, nuts, seeds, herbs, and spices in a whole-foods, high-fiber, plant-based diet don't just help prevent overweight and obesity; they also provide an array of anti-inflammatory compounds.

IMPROVE DIGESTION

An unhealthy gut can contribute to obesity and disease. There are two key issues here: leaky gut syndrome and bacterial imbalance in the intestinal tract. We'll address this issue briefly here; for more information, see "Food Sensitivities" in section entitled "TRIGGERS FOR FOOD ALLERGIES AND SENSITIVITIES".

The foods most commonly associated with leaky gut syndrome are gluten-containing grains (wheat, spelt, Kamut, rye, barley, and triticale), dairy products, and ultraprocessed, packaged convenience foods such as sugar and highly refined flour.

There's no question that good food feeds good bacteria and bad food feeds bad bacteria. Low-fat, high-fiber diets with plenty of vegetables help keep guthealthy bacteria flourishing. High-quality probiotic products can help reestablish a healthy gut flora.

AVOID TOXINS

There is increasing awareness of a connection between accumulation of body fat and environmental contaminants such as BPA, heavy metals, persistent organic pollutants, and pesticides. While you can't completely eliminate your exposure to these compounds, you can minimize it. You can also reinforce the body systems that help neutralize and excrete these compounds.

Fortunately, vegans may be at an advantage on both counts. Animal products, including fish, are high on the food chain, so they contain higher concentrations of environmental toxins. These are, of course, not included in vegan diets. Eating organic foods whenever possible will further reduce exposure. Vegans also tend to eat a lot of cruciferous vegetables (broccoli, cabbage, cauliflower, and the like), which are rich in phytochemicals that support detoxification. Numerous vitamins, minerals, amino acids, phytochemicals, and antioxidants play a role in this process, so good nutritional status is important.

ENHANCE YOUR NUTRITIONAL STATUS

Although vegans tend to eat more nutrient-rich vegetables and fruits and have higher intakes of fiber and many phytochemicals, antioxidants, and other nutrients, shortfalls are not uncommon. Even if you think you're doing everything right, when you limit calories in an effort to lose weight, you can easily miss out on nutrients, particularly vitamin B_{12}, vitamin D, and iodine. In addition, it's important to make sure you're getting enough protein, iron, zinc, calcium, magnesium, and selenium. Follow the vegan food guide, and if your diet still falls short, take supplements to meet your needs. (See chapters 3, 6, and 7 for details.)

When cutting back on calories, focus on eating foods with a lot of nutrients per calorie. The best choices are vegetables (especially leafy greens), legumes, fruits, nuts, seeds, and intact whole grains (rather than grains that have been processed or ground into flour). When you fuel your body with high-quality, organic, whole plant foods, it shifts gene expression, reducing your risk for overweight, obesity, and chronic disease.

BALANCE HORMONES AND BOOST METABOLISM

Boosting metabolism is the holy grail of seekers of slimness everywhere, but how fast your body burns calories depends on numerous factors. Optimal health and metabolism are highly dependent on the functioning of the many systems that produce and release hormones, including thyroid and stress hormones.

Thyroid hormones control metabolism and can have a significant impact on body weight. Vegans, especially those who avoid iodized salt, sea vegetables, and supplements can be low in iodine, which is needed in the production of thyroid hormones. Insufficient selenium and vitamin D can also adversely affect thyroid function.

Cortisol is a hormone that helps deliver the appropriate type and quantity of carbohydrate, fat, and protein to body tissues. Under chronic stress or calorie deprivation, cortisol levels rise and fat is shuttled into fat deposits in the abdomen. Called visceral fat, these deposits are associated with insulin resistance. Elevated cortisol is also associated with increased appetite and cravings for fat and sugar.

The keys to balancing all of these hormones and boosting metabolism is to consume a whole-foods, nutrient-dense, plant-based diet that emphasizes foods with a low glycemic load, take supplements if needed, manage stress, and get enough physical activity.

Getting Healthy

So far in this chapter, you've learned about the roots of the overweight and obesity crisis and about the essential steps required to achieve and maintain a healthy body weight for life. Now, let's turn our attention to designing a delicious vegan diet that supports you in this process.

EAT AT LEAST SIX SERVINGS OF NONSTARCHY VEGETABLES DAILY

One serving is 1 cup (250ml) of raw vegetables or 1/2 cup (125ml) cooked. In their natural state, vegetables are the most nutrient-dense foods on the planet. Aim for every color of the rainbow: at least three servings of green vegetables, including dark leafy greens, and at least one each of red, orange-yellow, purpleblue, and white-beige each day. Eat a variety of raw vegetables daily. Cooked vegetables are most nutritious when lightly steamed rather than boiled. Limit serving sizes of starchy vegetables, such as sweet potatoes and corn, to no more than 1/2 cup (125ml) once or twice a day.

LEARN TO LOVE LEGUMES

Beans, lentils, and peas are the powerhouses of the plant kingdom when it comes to protein, iron, and zinc. They are also among the richest sources of fiber, which contribute to satiety and provide staying power between meals. Lentils, split peas, or fresh peas (in or out of the pod) are great choices for people trying to slim down because they are extremely low in fat but high in nutrients and fiber. Lentils, mung beans, and dried peas are the best legumes for sprouting.

Tofu and tempeh, which are made from soybeans, are also nutrient-rich choices.

Eat at least three 1/2-cup (125ml) servings of legumes per day. In addition to beans, peas and lentils, options include tofu, tempeh, unsweetened soy milk, some protein powders, and some vegan meats. If need be, begin with smaller servings and gradually increase portion sizes over a couple of weeks to give your body time to adjust to the increased fiber intake. Add beans to stews, soups, and salads or use them to make patties, loaves, and spreads.

GO EASY ON GRAINS

Once you've met the recommended number of servings for vegetables, fruits, legumes, and nuts and seeds (see chapter 14 for details), add grains to meet your energy needs. As your calorie needs decrease (for example, as a result of aging, menopause, reduced physical activity, and so on), decrease your consumption of grains. Most people trying to lose weight should limit grains to not more than 1/2 cup (125ml) per meal, but people with higher energy needs can afford to include more grains in their diets.

Focus on intact whole grains, such as quinoa, wild rice, buckwheat, oat groats, and barley. One of the most healthful ways to prepare grains is to sprout them. Add sprouted grains to salads or use them as breakfast cereal. (Add them to a bowl of fruit and nondairy yogurt and top with seeds.) Cut and rolled grains are also options, although they are less desirable than intact whole grains because processing them damages or destroys some of their nutrients. Because each stage of processing further diminishes nutrients and increases impact on blood sugar, it's best to minimize consumption of all types of ground grains and flour, even if they are whole-grain. This includes most whole-grain breads, crackers, pretzels, cookies, and other baked goods. Completely avoid highly refined grains, such as white rice and products made with white flour. Also avoid processed cereals with added sugar and salt.

If you're avoiding foods that contain gluten, don't substitute packaged glutenfree foods made with processed, refined ingredients. Instead, use gluten-free whole foods, such as cooked quinoa, millet, brown rice, wild rice, or buckwheat.

SATISFY YOUR SWEET TOOTH WITH FRESH FRUIT

Fruit is nature's candy—with the added bonus of vitamins, antioxidants, and fiber. Eat all of the edible parts of fruit, including skins and seeds, which often contain the highest amounts of fiber and phytochemicals.

While it may take time to get used to thinking of a piece of fruit as dessert, there are ways to make it more appealing. Simply slicing fruit and arranging it creatively on a plate makes it seem special. Make a fruit salad and top it with a bit of plain nondairy yogurt. For a delectable frozen dessert, process frozen berries, peeled bananas, and cubed pineapple and mango in a blender, food processor, or juicer until smooth. Alternatively, put frozen fruit in a blender with a little nondairy milk or yogurt and process until very smooth.

If you have high blood sugar, limit fruit to three or four servings per day. One serving is 1 cup (250ml) of fresh fruit, 1 medium fruit, or 1/2 cup (125ml) of fruit juice or cooked fruit. Limit dried fruit to 1/4 cup (60ml) per day since it's very high in natural sugars.

GET FATS FROM NUTS, SEEDS, AND AVOCADOS

Although nuts, seeds, and avocados are high in fat and packed with calories, they are unexpected weight-loss allies. They are loaded with phytochemicals, plant sterols, and healthy fats, and because they contain a lot of fiber, they're also highly satisfying. Still, portion sizes are important. Reasonable daily intakes for weight loss are half of a small avocado and 1 to 2 ounces (30 to 60g) of nuts and seeds. Consuming a mixture of chia seeds, flaxseeds, hempseeds, and walnuts will ensure a good balance of essential fatty acids. Include one or two Brazil nuts to boost selenium. Soaking nuts and seeds reduces compounds that interfere with absorption of nutrients, increasing their nutritional value.

MAKE THE MOST OF HERBS AND SPICES

Herbs and spices are health heroes. Not only do they make foods taste better, they do so without adding sodium or fat. Several herbs and spices have shown promise as weight-loss allies due to their ability to boost metabolism, calm inflammation, or balance blood sugar levels. Among these spicy superstars are black pepper, cardamom, cayenne, cinnamon, cloves, cumin, ginger, mustard seeds, oregano, rosemary, and turmeric. Grow your own herbs on a windowsill. Most are hardy plants that may produce year-round. Herbs can also be frozen or dehydrated for later use.

LIMIT PROCESSED AND CONVENIENCE FOODS

Throughout this book, we've talked about how processed, convenience foods are at the bottom of the barrel when it comes to supporting health. Not all processed foods are bad news, however. Good choices include frozen herbs, low-sodium canned beans in BPA-free cans, frozen shelled edamame, some sprouted breads, organic fruit and nut bars, and some jarred tomato sauces. Read the ingredient list; if you can't pronounce the ingredients, it quite possibly isn't real food.

MINIMIZE CONCENTRATED SWEETENERS AND AVOID ARTIFICIAL SWEETENERS

Whether sugar comes from high-fructose corn syrup or organic dehydrated cane juice is less important than the *amount* of sugar you eat. Regardless of the source, sugar is sugar, and it's full of empty calories.

Avoid artificial sweeteners. They won't assist you in your quest for health, and they may negatively affect metabolism and appetite control. If you must sweeten your coffee or tea, using stevia would be a reasonable option. (For more information, see box entitled "Are Sugar Substitutes Safe?".)

LIMIT FATS AND AVOID PARTIALLY HYDROGENATED OILS

Although fats and oils are extracted from whole foods, processing strips them of fiber, minerals, phytochemicals, and even fat-soluble vitamins. It's best to use them sparingly. Fats and oils contain about 120 calories per tablespoon

(15ml), and per weight, they contain about 2.5 times more calories than protein or carbohydrates. Avoid margarines and other foods containing partially hydrogenated fats and oils, as they contain trans fats, which are strongly linked to many health conditions, including insulin resistance.

Mechanically pressed oils (preferably organic) are the best choices, being rich in essential fatty acids. However, they shouldn't be used for cooking because they are damaged by heat. If you use other oils, 1 tablespoon (15ml) is the upper limit if you're trying to lose weight, and less is better.

AVOID SNACKING

Cut out snacks unless you're genuinely hungry. If you do snack, stick to raw vegetables, raw fruits, legumes, nuts, or seeds. Other acceptable snacks include plain popcorn and seasoned sea vegetable snacks.

RELY ON WATER

Water is the best thirst quencher, and it's calorie-free. If possible, use a filter that eliminates chlorine, lead, nitrates, microorganisms, and other environmental contaminants without removing minerals such as calcium and magnesium.

Herbal teas can also be healthful choices, and green tea has been shown to slightly boost metabolism and may aid in weight loss. For added nutrition with minimal calories, vegetable juice (especially green juices or tomato juice) or wheat grass juice are good options. If you want something sweet to drink, try sparkling water with a splash of pure fruit juice or have a sweet herbal tea, such as apple cinnamon.

While some beverages are good sources of nutrients, you're generally better off getting those nutrients from whole foods because they provide greater satiety, which is so helpful in weight management. If you consume nutritious highercalorie beverages such as fresh fruit juices, fruit smoothies, and nondairy milks, think of them as food rather than drinks. They often contain 100 to 150 calories per cup (250ml). Smoothies made from a combination of fruit, greens, and seeds, with 400 to 500 calories per 3-cup (750ml) serving, can be healthful meal replacements, but if you use them in this way, limit it to one per day.

Beware of most other beverages. It's easy to underestimate their contribution to calories. For example, 12 fluid ounces (375ml) of lemonade, fruit punch, or soda contains 120 to 150 calories and has little or no nutritional value; 12 fluid ounces (375ml) of beer contains 110 to 170 calories; 1 1/2 fluid ounces (45ml) of distilled spirits has about 110 calories; 1 1/2 fluid ounces (45ml) of liqueur has 150 to 190 calories; and 4 fluid ounces (125ml) of wine has about 80 calories. Of course, these numbers don't include any added cocktail mixes.

Are Weight-Loss Aids Helpful?

Weight-loss aids are designed to block the absorption of fat or carbohydrate, stimulate thermogenesis (fuel burning), increase metabolism, or suppress appetite. Research hasn't shown them to be particularly effective. Those containing stimulants, such as caffeine, ephedrine, and synephrine, can cause insomnia, irritability, restlessness, anxiety, and, in the long term, dependency and exhaustion. It's best to avoid them. Some food-based supplements, such as green tea or green tea extract and certain types of food fiber may help prevent weight gain over time and are relatively safe. Weight-loss aids are unnecessary, but if you want to use one, stick with food-based products that support health.

Also avoid calorie-free beverages containing artificial sweeteners. They can confuse your appetite control center and metabolic hormones and are of no value to health.

Making the Most of Your Menu

Simple menus to get you started can be found in chapter 14, including a basic 1,600-calorie menu and a 2,000-calorie menu. These menus can be adjusted to suit your energy needs and food preferences. Most people should eat at least 1,600 calories per day (or 1,400 calories for those who are very small) because it can be difficult to meet all of your nutritional requirements on fewer calories.

Very low-calorie diets can also trigger the body to slam on the brakes on metabolism, making it even more difficult to shed unwanted pounds. The 1,600-calorie diet menu in chapter 14 provides a reasonable blueprint for most people with weight-loss goals. The 2,000-calorie diet in chapter 14 may be more appropriate for active individuals or larger men.

To enhance the nutritional, hormonal, and metabolic advantages of these basic diets, here are a few practical tips:

- Add extra greens or other nonstarchy vegetables, including sprouts.
- Be generous with herbs and spices such as turmeric, ginger, and garlic.
- Substitute green tea for coffee.
- Choose higher-fiber fruits, such as berries, apples, pears, and figs.

- Use unsweetened fortified nondairy milks, such as plain soy or rice milks, instead of sweetened or flavored varieties.
- When using tofu, pick a brand that's high in calcium.
- Select breads made with sprouted grains or higher-fiber breads. Better yet, substitute whole grains for bread.
- Eat fruit instead of drinking fruit juice.
- Drink plenty of water.
- Consider nutritional supplements. For most people, reasonable additions include 1,000mcg of vitamin B_{12} twice a week, daily supplementation with 25mcg (1,000 IU) of vitamin D and 150mcg of iodine, and a high-potency probiotic taken daily for two weeks and twice weekly thereafter.

Beyond Food

Losing weight involves more than simply restricting food intake. Certain lifestyle changes go hand in hand with a good diet to improve your health and support your efforts to achieve and maintain a healthful weight:

LET THE SUN SHINE IN

Strive for thirty to sixty minutes of fresh air and sunshine a day. Sunshine helps the body manufacture vitamin D and may benefit the body in other ways that haven't yet been identified. There's no doubt that the sun's rays have healing powers for both the body and soul. (For more on vitamin D, see section entitled "Vitamin D (Calciferol)".)

MAKE EXERCISE A PRIORITY

Plan to exercise daily or at least five days a week, for forty-five to sixty minutes per day. The best exercise for you depends on your age, current fitness level, state of health, and personal preferences. (For more details on types of exercise and designing an exercise program, see chapter 13).

If you haven't exercised in a long time, begin with walking or an activity that you're comfortable with. Start with ten to fifteen minutes of walking two or three times a day and increase the duration gradually. As you get stronger, incorporate a balance of cardio, strength, and flexibility exercises in your program. The best choice for burning calories and for overall health is moderate aerobic activity, such as brisk walking, combined with resistance training, such as working out with light weights. Be sure to stretch well after working out. Consider adding focused stretching routines, such as yoga or Pilates, into the mix.

Ultimately, it's best to include a wide variety of activities in your exercise program: walking, jogging, biking, swimming, hiking, yoga, racket sports, aerobics classes, and so on. The more you vary the intensity, duration, and type of activity, the more fit you'll become. Also be sure to choose activities you enjoy, as you'll be far more likely to stick with them.

Try to do something physical after eating. This is one of the most effective changes you can make, because muscles at work quickly use up circulating sugar, avoiding an insulin surge. This prevents excess blood sugar from being stored as fat and keeps sugars from damaging body tissues. There's some wisdom in the old Chinese saying "Walk one hundred steps after dinner, and you'll live to be ninety-nine years old."

Also increase your activity level in general, not just through exercise. Every physical movement you make helps increase your energy expenditure. For example, gardening, walking while shopping or at work, grating carrots, cleaning the house, making your bed, bathing your dog, and so on. In fact, this type of activity can make a bigger difference in your energy expenditure than exercise. Take full advantage of every opportunity you have to move your body, especially if you have to sit much of the day.

GET ADEQUATE SLEEP

Insufficient sleep can result in weight gain, compromise physical and mental performance, and contribute to death and disease.

Requirements for sleep vary with age, gender, lifestyle, stress, and even genetics. If you wake up spontaneously and feel refreshed and alert for the whole day, you've had a good sleep. For most adults, this requires seven to eight hours of sleep, but some people require as little as six hours, while others need nine hours. Listen to your body.

Sleeping well requires adequate preparation. Doing activities that calm and soothe you just before bedtime, such as taking a warm bath or reading, can help. (Watching the late news while sipping on an espresso probably doesn't fall into this category!) Set a regular bedtime and stick to it as much as possible. It's important that your bedroom be free of light and noise. If your neighborhood is noisy or brightly lit at night, consider investing in an eye mask, light-blocking window shades, or earplugs. Do whatever you can to make your sleeping environment peaceful and inviting.

MANAGE STRESS

While stress is normal and even potentially beneficial, ongoing severe stress can wreak havoc with your immune system, trigger mindless or binge eating, and increase the risk of death and disease. Incorporating stress management techniques into your daily routine will increase your ability to handle excess stress when it arises. A healthful vegan diet, exercise, adequate sleep, and getting fresh air and sunshine are all important, but attitude is the trump card when it comes to dealing with stress. For many people, a practice such as prayer, meditation, or yoga can be helpful. Building healthy relationships with friends, family, and colleagues can also help you cope with stress.

AVOID ADDICTIVE SUBSTANCES

Alcohol contains about 7 calories per gram—almost twice the amount in carbohydrate or protein—so, not surprisingly, it can be an important contributor to overweight and obesity. Worse, consuming any alcohol at all increases the risk of cancer, and excessive drinking can contribute to high blood pressure, liver disease, impaired immunity, and heart failure.

Of all personal choices, smoking tobacco is thought to be the greatest threat to health. Although smoking slightly increases metabolic rate, that isn't worth dying for. Surprisingly, nicotine also can significantly increase risk of overweight and obesity in infants of mothers who smoked during pregnancy.

Next, we'll discuss the flip side of the weight coin: underweight. In chapter 10, those who need to gain weight will learn how to do so healthfully on a whole-foods vegan diet.

CHAPTER 10

Overcoming Underweight

In a world with a burgeoning epidemic of overweight and obesity, being underweight is an anomaly. Yet for those who struggle with being too thin, it can be more challenging to gain a pound than it is for someone who's overweight to lose a pound.

Although underweight affects people of both genders, it's less often considered a problem for women, in whom thinness is prized. Men feel a different sort of pressure around body shape. While low body fat is desirable, being skinny isn't. The goal for men is a buff body, so their quest is to accumulate sufficient muscle.

If you see yourself as underweight, regardless of the reason, rest assured that a vegan diet can help you achieve a healthy body weight. Our goal in this chapter is to help you do that.

The Downside

About 1.6 percent of Americans are underweight as defined by the World Health Organization and the Centers for Disease

Control, having a body mass index (BMI) less than 18.5. (For more on the BMI, see the section "Healthy Body Weight,", and table 9.1.) A BMI of 17 to 18.4 is considered mildly underweight, a BMI of 16 to 16.9 is considered moderate, and a BMI below 16 is considered severe. These values aren't necessarily accurate for everyone. For example, a small-boned person may not be underweight with a BMI of 18, while a large-framed person could be underweight with a BMI of 20.

The number of underweight Americans has steadily declined from about 4 percent in the early 1960s. While comparable statistics for American vegans aren't available, most vegans do have healthy body weights and BMIs in the normal range. In a culture plagued by overweight, they are generally lucky to have lower BMIs and less body fat than lacto-ovo vegetarians or the general population. However, vegans, and particularly raw-food vegans, do seem to experience higher rates of underweight compared to the general population.

While most people would rather be underweight than overweight, being underweight is also associated with several negative health issues. The most significant is increased mortality. People who are underweight experience higher death rates than normal or overweight individuals but lower rates than obese individuals. Studies suggest a direct relationship between BMI and mortality: as BMI decreases, mortality decreases, right up to the point of being clinically underweight, at which point mortality increases as weight decreases. However, this finding is controversial because there is also evidence suggesting that people with good lifestyle habits who restrict calories live longer. While research is limited, the critical factor appears to be lifestyle and nutritional status. Being underweight is riskiest for people who smoke, are inactive, or eat few fruits and vegetables. On the other hand, the Oxford Vegetarian Study reported increased death rates from all causes except cancer in people with BMIs less than 18. Since it isn't easy to meet needs for all nutrients on low-calorie diets, it makes sense to strive to meet your body's energy needs and avoid being underweight, if possible.

Here are a few other health problems associated with being underweight:

- **Nutritional imbalances.** If you're underweight because you don't get enough calories, you may not be getting all the nutrients you need. This can lead to a weakened immune system and less protection against infection. Deficiency in just one nutrient can impair the immune response, even when the deficiency is mild. In addition, underweight people, particularly women of childbearing age, have a higher risk for iron deficiency, which results in weakness, fatigue, and irritability.

- **Hormonal imbalances.** Being underweight can influence the production and action of hormones in both men and women. In women, low body fat can prevent ovulation and menstruation, reducing fertility. If conception does occur and weight gain is insufficient, the baby is at risk and is more likely to be small for its gestational age. In underweight men, sperm count and semen quality can be significantly reduced.

- **Weakness, fatigue, and reduced muscle mass.** If you don't eat sufficient calories, the body first mobilizes energy from glycogen (the stored form of carbohydrate). When it exhausts its glycogen, it then uses body fat. When those reserves are depleted, it will try to get energy from protein, which decreases muscle mass, leading to weakness and fatigue.

- **Osteoporosis.** Underweight individuals—both men and women—are at risk for bone breakdown and decreased bone density, elevating the risk of osteoporosis.

Determining Your State of Health

Careful consideration of the following factors will help you determine whether your low body weight poses a health risk and weight gain is warranted. In general, if you lack energy and are weak, often sick, and take a long time to recover, chances are your weight is too low. Of course, it's important to rule out any underlying disease that could be causing these symptoms. On the other hand, if you're generally in good health, energetic, seldom sick, and quick to recover from illness, you may be at a healthy body weight even though your BMI is low.

Body frame. If you have a small frame, your BMI may indicate that you're underweight when you actually aren't. For example, a healthy, small-boned woman who is 5 feet 4 inches (1.63m) tall and weighs 107 pounds (52kg) has a BMI of 18.4, which is technically underweight. However, considering her bone structure and health status, she's likely at a healthy weight. On the other hand, a largeframed woman may appear to have a healthy weight according to her BMI but actually be underweight. For example, a woman with a large bone structure who's 5 feet 4 inches (1.63m) tall and weighs 116 pounds (56.4kg) may be underweight even though her BMI of 20 is well within the healthy range.

Gender. Men tend to have larger bones and muscles than women, so at any given height, men generally weigh more than women, even when their body fat is lower. While the BMI ranges are the same for men and women, it's relatively common for men to be underweight when their BMI is between 18.5 and 20—above what is technically classified as underweight.

Lifestyle. If you're underweight as a result of unhealthy lifestyle practices such as substance abuse or a poor diet, you could be at risk for disease. However, if you eat a healthy plant-based diet, avoid addictive substances, and engage in regular physical activity, your weight-related health risks would be lower.

Causes of Underweight

Underweight is relatively rare in populations with abundant food supplies. Technically, underweight is the result of not consuming enough calories for the energy expended, just as overweight is the result of too many calories for the energy expended. However, just as with overweight and obesity, the causes are far more complex than energy-in, energy-out. People become underweight for a variety of reasons, including genetics, illness, medications and other drugs, and psychological factors.

Genetics. Just as someone can be genetically predisposed to overweight, it's also possible to be predisposed to underweight. We all know entire families who exhibit "lean genes." If you're underweight and have a high metabolism, you require more food than other people of similar height and weight but still don't seem to gain a pound. Becoming vegan and eliminating high-calorie meat and dairy products may cause weight loss, since you'll replace those foods with others that are generally lower in fat, lower in calories, and higher in fiber. Fortunately, there are simple steps you can take to ensure a healthy weight without consuming animal products (discussed later in this chapter).

Illness. Many diseases can cause weight loss or result in being underweight. Gastrointestinal diseases can prevent the absorption and metabolism of foods or trigger chronic diarrhea. Metabolic and hormonal disorders can alter appetite control, metabolic rate, or energy needs, resulting in less hunger, reduced food intake, or rapid burning of calories consumed.

Medications and chemical dependencies. Certain medications can cause underweight, so in a sense, this is another way in which illness can be involved. In addition, drugs, alcohol, and tobacco can reduce appetite, speed metabolism, and compromise energy intake.

Psychological factors. Here are some of the more common psychological factors that can contribute to underweight:

- **Depression.** Those who are overwhelmed by depression commonly lose interest in eating and sharing meals with others.
- **Eating disorders.** Anorexia nervosa results in significant, sustained, and often severe weight loss. (For an in-depth look at eating disorders, see *Becoming Vegan: Comprehensive Edition*, by B. Davis and V. Melina, Book Publishing Company, 2014.)

- **Stress.** While some people respond to stress, anxiety, and other forms of psychological pain by eating, others have a diminished appetite and avoid food.

- **Cultural pressure.** Our society promotes thinness, especially in women. This reinforces eating behaviors that promote restrictive eating, such as skipping meals or curbing appetite by smoking, gum chewing, or other means.

- **Abuse.** One consequence of physical or emotional abuse can be withdrawal and a subconscious effort to occupy as little space as possible—to become invisible. One way to achieve that is to become as thin as possible.

OTHER FACTORS

- **Habits.** Skipping meals, avoiding between-meal snacks, avoiding higherfat foods, and restricting portion sizes can all lead to insufficient intake of calories, especially in those with a high metabolic rate.

- **Hunger.** Worldwide, the most common cause of underweight is inadequate access to food or hunger. While this is less common in more affluent areas of the world, such as North America, it may be more prevalent in the West than is recognized.

- **Overactivity.** Underweight may be the product of an overactive lifestyle: too much exercise, work, volunteering, and so on. When activities demand a lot of time and energy, there may be an energy imbalance or insufficient time to eat well.
- **Social factors.** Behaviors related to food are affected by family patterns and styles of social interaction. People who like to eat with others but are usually alone for meals may eat less than they need to. If one family member chooses to drastically change his or her diet, to treat a health condition, for example, another family member might follow suit to offer support and not eat enough as a result.

Great Gains for Vegans

Whether you decide to actively pursue weight gain may largely depend on your perception of your body. For the most part, men tend to be more highly motivated to correct underweight than women because of the way society views thinness in men versus women. However, as a vegan, you may want to broaden your goals. Your personal example is your most powerful tool to shift others toward a more compassionate and sustainable lifestyle. If you're underweight and generally unhealthy, your example probably won't create the kind of inspiration you may have hoped for.

Perhaps it's time to renew your commitment to health and take the steps necessary to achieve a healthy weight. The most effective approach to weight gain isn't so different from that for weight loss: permanent lifestyle changes that include a combination of diet and exercise. While exercise might seem counterintuitive if you're trying to gain weight, building and maintaining lean body tissue is critical to success, so make it a priority. As you plot your course forward, consider the rest of this chapter to be your blueprint for weight gain.

Eating to Gain

Many lifestyle factors come together to influence body weight. Fortunately, most of these factors are within your control. They fall into two main categories: diet and lifestyle. Let's begin by considering the multiple ways of adjusting your food intake to better support health and achieve your target body weight.

MAKE GOOD HEALTH YOUR TOP GOAL

Think of food as the raw materials with which you'll rebuild your body. The best building blocks are foods that provide not only calories but also an abundance of antioxidants, phytochemicals, and other nutrients. Even if you don't gain weight as quickly as you'd like, you'll soon notice that you have increased energy, better concentration, fewer illnesses, and improved mood.

Because you can afford to eat extra calories, it may be tempting to load up on vegan junk foods, such as chips, candy, and sweet desserts. While the occasional indulgence is fine, these foods shouldn't be dietary staples. An unhealthful diet can lead to heart attacks, strokes, cancer, and other afflictions, regardless of body weight.

INCREASE FOOD INTAKE

The typical formula for weight gain is that you need to add between 500 to 1,000 calories to your diet daily to gain 1 to 2 pounds (0.45 to 0.9kg) per week. However, this is actually an underestimate for some people. Most underweight adults require about 2,500 to 4,000 calories per day to gain weight, and athletes need even more. To accomplish this, select energy-dense vegan foods, with an emphasis on whole foods, and increase your serving sizes. In chapter 14, you'll find sample high-calorie menus, one offering 2,500 to 2,800 calories per day, and another providing 4,000 calories. Table 10.1, below, presents general guidelines on daily number of servings from each food group for 2,500- and 4,000-calorie diets. In addition to boosting your intake of calories, this strategy will ensure that you get all of the nutrients you need. (See table 14.1, in chapter 14, for information about each food group, including serving sizes.) Ideally, these foods should be consumed throughout the day, including a bedtime snack and other snacks as desired.

EAT MORE OFTEN

It's difficult to take in enough calories if you eat only one or two meals a day. Aim for three meals a day, plus at least two hearty snacks. Don't skip meals or go to bed on an empty stomach. If you're likely to forget to eat, use a timer to remind yourself. If your mornings are rushed, make your lunch and snacks the night before.

Including just one additional snack of 500 calories each day could result in a weight gain of 1 pound (0.45kg) a week. Here are a few snack options that each provide approximately 500 calories:

- 3/4 cup (185ml) trail mix (nuts, seeds, and dried fruits)
- 2/3 cup (160ml) nuts
- A smoothie (such as the Protein Power Smoothie in chapter 10)
- An almond butter and banana sandwich plus 1 cup (250ml) soy milk or hot chocolate made with soy milk

- 3/4 cup (185ml) granola, 1 banana, and 1 1/2 cups (375ml) soy milk
- 20 crackers, 2 ounces (60g) vegan cheese, 4 vegan deli slices, and 10 olives

TABLE 10.1. Suggested daily food servings* for weight gain

FOOD GROUP	AVERAGE CALORIES PER SERVING	DAILY SERVINGS IN A 2,500-CALORIE DIET	DAILY SERVINGS IN A 4,000-CALORIE DIET
Vegetables	40	5	7
Fruits	75	4	6
Legumes	120	5	9
Grains	75	8	13
Nuts and seeds	160	4	6
Fats and oils†	40	4	7

*See the Vegan Food Guide in Chapter 14 for serving sizes in each food group.
†1 serving = 1 teaspoon

- 1 vegan muffin or energy bar, 1 cup (250ml) coconut yogurt, and 1 apple
- 2 ounces (60g) baked pita chips with 1/2 cup (125ml) each of salsa, refried beans, and guacamole

SNEAK IN EXTRA CALORIES

Whole plant foods, especially fruits and vegetables, can be high in fiber, low in fat, and relatively low in calories, filling you up without providing sufficient calories for weight gain. The following tips will help you to add calories to a whole foods diet while also boosting nutrients and flavor:

- Garnish salads with beans, nuts, seeds, tofu, or avocado, and use dressings made with high-quality oils or tahini.
- Top steamed vegetables with a creamy sauce made from tofu or nuts.
- Include tofu, nuts, or seeds in stir-fries, casseroles, and pasta dishes.
- Top diced fruits with nondairy yogurt and granola.
- Cook hot cereals, such as whole grains or oats, in nondairy milk rather than water. Add chopped nuts, seeds, and dried fruits.
- Spread nut butter on English muffins or toast.
- Use full-fat nondairy milk instead of lighter varieties.
- Top vegan ice cream with nuts, dark chocolate, and berries.
- Dip cut-up fruit in a vegan avocado-chocolate mousse.
- Add cashew cream or coconut milk to soups and sauces. To make cashew cream, puree 1/2 cup (125ml) of cashews with 1 cup (250ml) water.

USE BEVERAGES TO YOUR ADVANTAGE

The beverages you choose can make a significant difference in your overall energy intake.

For example, 1 cup (250ml) of fruit juice typically provides 120 to 180 calories (freshly squeezed is best); 1 cup (250ml) of soy milk provides 100 to 120 calories; and a soy-fruit shake, 300 to 500 calories. These energy-rich beverages can be an easy way to increase calories. However, it's best to limit the liquids you consume with meals, since low-calorie soups or calorie-free beverages such as coffee and tea can fill you up. If you have difficulty eating larger portions at mealtime, try drinking beverages primarily between meals.

EAT HIGHER-FAT WHOLE FOODS

Vegan diets are generally higher in fiber and lower in fat than nonvegan diets, and that can interfere with gaining weight. The easiest way to add energy without adding too much fiber or volume is to increase the fat. About 20 to 30 percent of your calories should come from fat. Among the most energy-dense vegan foods are nuts, seeds, soy foods, coconut, nondairy alternatives (milk, cheese, yogurt, and so on), avocados, nutritious baked goods, and oils. Table 10.2 shows the approximate calorie content of some high-calorie vegan foods.

TABLE 10.2. Calorie content of higher-fat foods

FOOD	SERVING SIZE	CALORIES
Avocado	1 medium	340
Carrot cake	1 slice	400
Hearty cookie	2 cookies	300
Nuts (except peanuts)	½ c (125 ml)	360–480
Peanuts	½ c (125 ml)	415
Pumpkin muffin	1 large muffin	400
Soy milk	1 c (250 ml)	120–160
Soy nuts	½ c (125 ml)	390
Tofu (firm)	½ c (125 ml)	183
Unrefined oil	1 tbsp (15 ml)	120

Source of data: US Department of Agriculture, Agricultural Research Service, USDA National Nutrient Database for Standard Reference, Release 25 (2012), and estimates based on popular vegan recipes for baked goods.

Key: c = cup; tbsp = tablespoon.

The following sections provide tips on how to incorporate more of these higher-fat, nutritious foods into your meals and snacks.

Nuts and Seeds

Try to add 1/2 to 1 cup (125 to 250ml) of nuts and seeds to your daily diet. They're highly nutritious and conveniently portable. Although soy nuts are legumes, they have similar advantages and can be used in much the same way. Here are just a few ideas on how to boost your consumption of these nutritional powerhouses:

- Keep nuts and seeds wherever you spend most of your time so you can snack at will.
- Use nuts and seeds as a base for vegan cheeses or sauces.
- Add them to stir-fries, baked goods, pancakes, and waffles.

- Use them to make veggie roasts, burgers, and pâtés.
- Sprinkle them on salads.
- Eat power bars based on nuts or seeds.
- Spread nut and seed butters on bread, apple slices, or celery sticks.
- Mix nut and seed butters into salad dressings.

Tofu

Tofu is wonderfully versatile, low in fiber, and relatively high in fat. Here are some tips on adding tofu to your diet:

- Add soft tofu to shakes or use it in desserts, such as puddings.
- Eat scrambled tofu for breakfast.
- Use flavored tofu or tofu salads in sandwiches.
- Add cubed tofu to stir-fries, stews, curries, and soups.
- Use mashed tofu in lasagna.
- Sauté chopped, sliced, or grated tofu with a little oil, tamari, nutritional yeast, and herbs and use it as a salad topping.
- Use tofu as a base for veggie roasts, burgers, pâtés, and dips.
- Try marinated baked or barbecued tofu as a dinner entrée.
- Experiment with tofu especially in desserts. Add it to cheesecakes, cakes, muffins, and cookies.

Dairy Alternatives

Today, you can find vegan replacements for most dairy products. Some are based on soy, while others are made from almonds, rice, coconut, hempseeds, grains, or root vegetables. These products continue to be improved and are often tasty and nutritious. However, some contain partially hydrogenated oils, sugar, preservatives, and other unhealthful ingredients, so be sure to read ingredient lists.

A great option is to prepare some of your own nondairy foods. Many cookbooks and online resources offer recipes for almond or hempseed milk, fermented nut cheeses, fruit-based ice cream, and nondairy yogurts. If you use commercial soy milk, choose one that's full-fat and made with organic soybeans. Because nondairy foods can significantly increase your energy intake, they're well worth adding to your diet. Here are a few suggestions on how to do so:

- Use nondairy milk or yogurt in smoothies and on cereal.
- Replace water with soy milk when making puddings, pancakes, waffles, breads, muffins, and other baked goods.
- Enjoy a simple dessert of nondairy yogurt, berries, and granola or nuts.
- Use vegan sour cream as a base for dips or as a topping for soups. For an optimally

healthy product, you may want to make your own using cashews or tofu.

- Add vegan mayonnaise to sandwiches and salads. Again, you can make your own using cashews or tofu.
- Experiment with nut-based cheeses.

Avocados

Avocados pack a lot of calories into a small and delectable fruit. Here are some delicious ways to use them:

- Dress up a salad with wedges of avocado.
- Mash avocados with lemon juice for dips, sandwich spreads, and toppings.
- Add avocado chunks to salsa.
- Use avocado slices in sandwiches and pita pockets.
- Add diced avocado to pasta or quinoa salads.

Sweet Treats

If you start with the right ingredients, sweet treats can make a valuable contribution to your daily calorie count. Here are some tips on how to keep sweet treats healthful:

- Go raw. Raw desserts, such as vegan cheesecakes, pies, cookies, and brownies, are outrageously delicious and usually high in healthful calories, since they're based on nuts, coconut, and dried and fresh fruits.

- Replace some or all of the fat in baked goods with nuts, seeds, or coconut or their butters.
- Try ground flaxseeds, which are a great source of omega-3 fatty acids, as an egg replacer. For each egg in a recipe, whisk together 1 tablespoon (15ml) of ground flaxseeds and 3 tablespoons (45ml) of water.
- Substitute cooked and mashed dried fruits for all or part of the sugar in your treat recipes.
- Use high-quality oils instead of hydrogenated fats in baking.

BE GENEROUS WITH CARBOHYDRATES

A high-carbohydrate diet helps muscles work harder for longer periods of time and spares protein from being used as an energy source. Between 55 and 65 percent of your daily calories should come from carbohydrates. The most concentrated sources are grains and starchy vegetables. Excellent choices are pseudograins, such as quinoa, buckwheat, and amaranth, and colorful starchy vegetables, such as yams, corn, winter squash, and purple potatoes. Here are some suggestions to stoke your creativity with carbs:

- Soak or sprout grains to use in cereals, salads, breads, and raw or baked treats and desserts.

- Use cooked whole grains in salads, stews, pilafs, and cereals.
- Add cooked yams or sweet potatoes to salads.
- For a one-two punch of grains and high-carb legumes, enjoy bread with hummus or other legume-based spreads.
- Add potatoes to curries, stews, and scrambled tofu.
- Enjoy breads, muffins, pancakes, and waffles made with whole-grain flours and wheat germ.
- Add corn to salads, soups, and stews.

PUSH PLANT PROTEIN

Vegan diets can fall short on protein, particularly when they include only minimal legumes, nuts, and seeds. If your muscle mass is low, build it up by eating 1.2 to 1.7 grams of protein per kilogram (2.2lb) of body weight per day (g/kg/d). If you don't need to build muscle, 1.2g/kg/d is sufficient. Calculate your needs based on your ideal body weight rather than your actual body weight. For example, if you weigh 120 pounds (54kg), but your healthy weight is 145 pounds (66kg), aim for at least 80 grams of protein per day (66kg x 1.2g/kg = 79.2g).

Include a good source of protein in every meal. Table 10.3 provides simple suggestions for substituting protein-rich foods for lower-protein foods. For a comprehensive list of plant foods and the amounts of protein they contain, see table 3.3, also see table 11.3.

SAVOR SMOOTHIES

Smoothies are an exceptional vehicle for adding protein, calories, and nutrients to your diet. If you're having difficulty meeting your protein needs, adding vegan protein powder to a smoothie is a great option. A wide variety of products are available with protein derived from hempseeds, peas, rice, soy, and other foods. The easiest and most delicious way to use protein powder is to add it to a smoothie.

TABLE 10.3. Substitutions to boost protein

INSTEAD OF:	PROTEIN (g)	CHOOSE:	PROTEIN (g)
Brown rice, 1 c (250 ml)	5	Quinoa, 1 c (250 ml)	8
Corn nuts, 2 oz (60 g)	5	Soy nuts, 2 oz (60 g)	24
Cornflakes, 1 c (250 ml)	2	Oatmeal, 1 cup (250 ml)	6
Garden salad, 4 c (1 L), with Italian dressing, 2 tbsp (30 ml)	4	Kale salad, 4 c (1 L), with tahini dressing containing 1 tbsp (15 ml) tahini	12
Margarine, 2 tbsp (30 ml)	0	Peanut butter, 2 tbsp (30 ml)	8
Orange juice, 1 c (250 ml)	2	Protein Power Smoothie (page 194), 2½ c (625 ml)	40
Pretzels, 1 oz (30 g)	3	Pumpkin seeds, 1 oz (80 g)	9
Vegetable soup, 1 c (250 ml)	2	Lentil soup, 1 c (250 ml)	9
Rice milk, 1 c (250 ml)	1	Soy milk, 1 c (250 ml)	8
Tomato sandwich on whole-grain bread	6	Tomato sandwich on whole-grain bread with 2 oz (60 g) vegan deli slices*	21
Tomato sauce, 1 c (250 ml)	3	Tomato sauce, 1 c (250 ml) with 2 oz (60 g) vegan ground round	15
Vegan mayonnaise-based dip, ¼ c (60 ml)	0	Hummus, ¼ c (60 ml)	5
Vegetable stir-fry, 3 c (750 ml)	6	Vegetable stir-fry, 3 c (750 ml), with ½ c (125 ml) firm tofu*	26

Source of data: US Department of Agriculture, Agricultural Research Service, *USDA National Nutrient Database for Standard Reference*, Release 25 (2012).

Key: c = cup; g = gram; L = liter; ml = milliliter; oz = ounce; tbsp = tablespoon.

*Check labels for product-specific information.

Protein Power Smoothie

Makes 2 1/2 cups (625ml)
If you like your smoothies ice-cold, use frozen fruit. Alternatively, add a few ice cubes before blending. This smoothie provides about 500 calories and 40 grams of protein, depending on choice of protein powder.

1 scoop protein powder
1 banana
1 cup (250ml) berries, chopped peaches, or other fruit
1 1/2 cups (375ml) soy milk
Put all the ingredients in a blender and process until smooth. Serve immediately.

Be creative with smoothie boosters and variations. High-fat boosters, such as avocados, oils, and nuts and seeds and their butters add valuable calories. Foods rich in antioxidants and phytochemicals, such as kale, carob powder, cocoa powder, goji berries, and spices can help boost health. Nondairy yogurts or probiotic powders provide beneficial bacteria. Try one or more of the following to boost the protein in any smoothie, including the Protein Power Smoothie, above.

• For a green smoothie, add 2 cups (500ml) of chopped kale, 1/2 small avocado, or both.

- Chocolate lovers can add 1 to 1 1/2 tablespoons (15 to 22ml) of cocoa or carob powder.
- For a boost in beneficial bacteria, add 1/2 cup (125ml) of nondairy yogurt.
- To increase essential fatty acids, add 1 tablespoon (15ml) of cold-pressed oil rich in omega-3s, such as flaxseed, hempseed, or chia seed oil. For optimum nutrition, choose one with added DHA. Alternatively, add 2 tablespoons (30ml) of hempseeds, flaxseeds, or chia seeds.
- To support healthy bacteria in your intestinal tract, add 1/4 teaspoon (1ml) of powdered probiotics.
- Add healthful, flavorful herbs and spices such as cinnamon, cloves, ginger, and nutmeg to fruit smoothies, and fresh herbs, such as basil, mint, and oregano, to green smoothies.
- For added protein and healthy fat, add 1 tablespoon (15ml) of nut butter.
- Add 2 tablespoons (30ml) of goji berries. (Soak dried goji berries for at least four hours and drain before using.)

MAKE EATING A PRIORITY

If you never seem to have real food around the house and eat mainly out of boxes and bags, it's time for some lifestyle adjustments in keeping with your weight-gain goals. Making specific plans about meals will help you succeed in your quest. Here are a few things you might try:

- Make a weekly menu, prepare a shopping list, and select a weekly shopping day. (See *Cooking Vegan* by V. Melina and J. Forest, Book Publishing Co., 2012)
- If you can't cook, take lessons. Go with a friend and make it fun.
- Make eating a social event. Eat with friends and family more often. Host a potluck, invite someone to dinner, or enjoy a meal at a vegetarian restaurant.
- Invest in simple vegan cookbooks and try a few new recipes each week.
- Buy a slow cooker. In the morning, throw in a combination of ingredients, such as grains, veggies, and beans or tofu and let it cook all day.
- Plan to spend time cooking on the weekends or whenever you have time. Make one or two main dishes, a soup, and some healthy baked goods. Prepare enough to last several days. Freeze leftovers for days when you don't have time to cook.
- Keep your pantry, fridge, and freezer well stocked with healthful foods that you enjoy eating: trail mix, power bars, muffins, healthy cookies, frozen bananas dipped in melted

chocolate and rolled in nuts, vegan cheesecake ... you get the picture.

- Stash a few goodies at work, in your car, in your purse or backpack, or anywhere that you spend a lot of time.

FUEL YOUR APPETITE

You may rarely feel hungry, perhaps because you have a small appetite or a small stomach. While appetite can be affected by mood, stress, and physical activity, some simple food and nutrition tips can help kick it into high gear:

- Increase your food intake gradually, allowing your stomach to expand over time so you'll be able to comfortably eat more.
- Focus on foods that take up less space in the stomach per calorie. Examples include nuts, seeds, dried fruits, beans, avocados, and tofu. Mashing and pureeing foods can also help reduce their volume.
- Surround yourself with tempting aromas. Bake bread or buy frozen dough and bake it at home. Simmer a few cinnamon sticks and cloves in a pot of water. Walk past food stands, bakeries, and restaurants that entice you.
- Tantalize your senses with beautiful pictures of food in magazines and cookbooks. Then try the recipes!

- Make mealtimes enjoyable. Create a low-stress atmosphere with candles, a pretty table setting, soft music, and, if possible, pleasant company.
- Use big bowls, plates, cups, and cutlery. Using larger dishes, forks, and spoons has been shown to increase total food intake.
- Eat several courses. When you include a variety of different smells and tastes, it's easier to tempt your taste buds. Instead of one big plate of food, try having four sequential courses.
- Honor your hunger. Eat when you feel the least bit hungry. If you know you should be eating something, but are not hungry, drink something. Have carrot juice, freshly squeezed orange juice, hot chocolate, or a smoothie.
- Avoid foods that cause you gastrointestinal distress. This can reduce your appetite and food intake.

KEEP A FOOD DIARY

You may want to log your food intake. You can even do this online; there are free sites for this. If you have a smartphone, you can also download free apps for this purpose. Keeping track of your food intake will help you understand your eating habits, likes, dislikes, and tendencies. Adjusting what you do is easier if you know where you're starting and understand the challenges.

BE CAUTIOUS ABOUT WEIGHT-GAIN AIDS

There are dozens of weight-gain aids in the marketplace, but most are designed for bodybuilders who aren't underweight. Do your research and know the risks and benefits before trying a new supplement.

While some may prove helpful, others are a waste of money and may even be harmful. The US Food and Drug Administration provides online information about bodybuilding products that contain ingredients considered to be unsafe.

Your health care provider may suggest appetite stimulants to support your weight-gain efforts. While these can be effective, some have undesirable side effects. It's best to use other strategies to increase food intake.

CONSIDER SUPPLEMENTS

If your diet hasn't been particularly healthful in the past, consider taking a multivitamin-mineral supplement until you improve your nutritional status. Select one that provides zinc, magnesium, chromium, selenium, and possibly iron. (However, it's a good idea to have your iron level tested to see if you need additional iron, since excesses can be dangerous.) We also recommend that you include supplements of vitamin B_{12}, vitamin D (if exposure to sunshine is insufficient), and iodine (if you don't use iodized salt)—as we do for all vegans.

Building a Bigger Body

The second piece of the weight-gain puzzle is lifestyle. Let's explore the lifestyle changes you can make to put on healthy pounds.

Set realistic goals. Determine a target weight. Aim to gain 1 or 2 pounds (0.45 to 0.9kg) per week. Be realistic; if your natural body type is tall and slim, don't expect to be transformed into the Hulk overnight. While it is possible to gain muscle, your body may fight it every step of the way. You may have to work twice as hard as the average person to gain the same amount of weight. Consistency is the key to producing results, but even with regular training, most men will gain no more than 20 pounds (9kg) of lean tissue per year, and women will gain about half that much.

Do resistance training. Even if you have no desire to build big muscles, moderate resistance training is the best way to promote muscle growth and ensure that the weight you gain includes a healthful balance of muscle and fat. Resistance training is often done with free weights or weight machines, but you can also use resistance bands or your own body weight, with push-ups or pull-ups, for example. Here are some tips to optimize the effectiveness of resistance training:

- Work with a professional trainer who can tailor your program to meet your personal goals and abilities and who will follow your progress.
- Train only two or three times per week to allow your muscles sufficient time to recover and grow between workouts.
- Aim for thirty- to sixty-minute workout sessions, and keep the pace moderate to intense. Begin with light weights and increase gradually as you perfect your form.
- Change your exercise routine every six to eight weeks to keep your muscles challenged (and your interest up).
- Warm up for five to ten minutes before strength training and cool down for five to ten minutes afterward.
- Drink plenty of water.

Don't overdo aerobic exercise. It's tough to gain weight while training for a marathon. Aerobic exercise boosts metabolism and burns calories, which can work against you when you're trying to gain weight. On the other hand, aerobic exercise improves overall health, enhances cardiovascular and respiratory function, and keeps body fat low, so don't avoid it altogether. A reasonable compromise is to do a moderate amount of aerobic activity, such as thirty to sixty minutes, two or three times a week.

Get some R & R. Physical and emotional stress can affect your metabolism, appetite, and hormones and prevent weight gain. Consider doing yoga, tai chi, qigong, meditation, or other relaxation therapies. Take little relaxation breaks throughout the day, and pamper yourself from time to time. Be sure to get sufficient sleep; it restores energy and allows muscles to recuperate and grow. For most adults, seven to nine hours a night is reasonable. If your life is so busy that you often forget to eat, it's time to rethink your priorities and simplify your life.

Avoid addictive substances. In addition to damaging health, alcohol, tobacco, and recreational drugs can alter your metabolism and interfere with appetite, especially if consumed regularly or to excess. If you struggle with addiction, it's probably a contributing factor to your weight challenges. Take a step in a positive direction and seek professional help.

Listen to your body. Everyone's body is unique, and people function optimally at different sizes and shapes. If you're constantly tired, you may need more sleep or more food. If you're always sore, you may be training too much. (That said, some underweight people probably shouldn't trust their instincts where food is concerned because their hunger and satiety mechanisms may be compromised. In that case, eating specific amounts at designated times each day can be very helpful.)

Pregnancy, breast-feeding, and raising children to be healthy eaters can present special nutritional challenges. The next chapter explores the dietary issues unique to these stages of life and simple ways to adapt a vegan diet to ensure that dietary needs are met during these critical times.

CHAPTER 11

From Pregnancy On: Nourishing Strong Children

As we've seen throughout this book, a well-balanced vegan diet can be an excellent path to health. But when the conversation shifts to the best diets for pregnancy, babies, and children, emotions often set in. We become vulnerable to the opinions of well-meaning people we love, and we may begin to question our decisions. A parent may wonder whether a diet that's great for the average adult will also be good for moms-to-be, babies, and children.

We assure you that eating a healthful vegan diet during pregnancy and while breast-feeding will give your baby the best possible start and will set the stage for a lifetime of good health for your entire family. This chapter discusses how a well-balanced vegan diet can contribute to a healthy pregnancy and a healthy baby, how it can help ensure an abundance of

nutritious breast milk and superb health and well-being for growing children and teens.

The Research

If you're already vegan, don't be surprised if your doctor questions your diet or doesn't know a lot about vegan diets. A physician may get only three hours of nutrition training, and the focus of that training isn't vegan nutrition. You can point out that the Academy of Nutrition and Dietetics has voiced its support for vegan diets, including during pregnancy, lactation, childhood, and adolescence. Share a copy of their position on vegetarian diets (see Resources). If health professionals, family members, or friends don't know how to put together a nutritionally adequate vegan diet, they may not be sure it's possible and advise against it. Like all pioneers, you'll need to do some research and have some facts on hand. You might also consider sharing some tasty vegan meals with doubters.

For More on Specific Nutrients

This chapter outlines requirements for specific nutrients at many phases of life (pregnancy, lactation, infancy, and through to adolescence). For more information on specific vitamins and minerals, and for complete details on

nutritional requirements for all stages of life, see chapters 6 and 7 and the appendix.

Studies have shown few or no significant health differences between babies born to vegetarian moms versus nonvegetarians. In fact, where differences exist, vegetarian moms are at an advantage in some regards. They are less likely to give birth to infants with health problems related to excessively high birth weights, and also less likely to develop gestational diabetes, especially if they were physically active while pregnant.

Getting enough iron is a concern during any pregnancy. However, pregnant vegetarians have been shown to have higher intakes of dietary iron than meat eaters. Nonheme iron, the type in plant foods, has been linked to better birth weights. Vegetarian moms are also more likely to take iron supplements.

The largest study to date on the health of pregnant vegans and their pregnancy outcomes was completed in 1987. It examined the maternity records of 775 vegan women from The Farm, a community in Summertown, Tennessee. Their diet was centered on soy foods, grains, fruits, and vegetables, most of which were organic and grown on The Farm. The women took prenatal supplements with iron and calcium, received regular prenatal care, and had active lifestyles. They didn't smoke cigarettes or drink alcohol, and only rarely did they drink coffee.

Two important findings emerged from this research. First, the infants were all of normal weight, and second, only one, or 0.13 percent, of the vegan moms developed preeclampsia, a dangerous condition that includes high blood pressure, fluid retention, and protein loss in the urine and can result in harm and even death to mother and baby. In the general population, preeclampsia affects 5 to 10 percent of expectant moms.

Some studies have shown less favorable pregnancy outcomes among vegan women, particularly among women on restrictive macrobiotic diets who were unwilling to take vitamin and mineral supplements, and among moms whose diets were low in calories and lacked vitamin B_{12}. Also, earlier studies on pregnant vegans were carried out long before fortified vegan foods and nutritious vegan convenience foods became widely available. Now almost every supermarket stocks hummus, tofu, nondairy beverages fortified with calcium and vitamin D, and vegetarian meats fortified with vitamin B_{12}.

The message we can take from all of this is that vegan diets can support healthy pregnancies as long as moms ensure they're getting enough calories and nutrients, as is the case for anyone on any diet.

Preparing for Pregnancy

Even before you become pregnant, you need to prepare to host a new life. If you're planning to get pregnant any time in the next few years, start making the necessary changes in your diet now. By the time you're pregnant, your nutrient reserves will be in good shape and you also will have established eating patterns that are health promoting for you and your family.

One step is to get your weight where you'd like it to be *before* you become pregnant. Check table 9.1 to determine your body mass index (BMI). This will give you a good idea of whether your weight is in the optimal range. You don't want to be following a weight-loss diet during any stage of pregnancy. If your BMI is in the overweight or obese range, weight reduction can decrease your risk of gestational diabetes, high blood pressure, and preeclampsia. If you're underweight, gaining enough weight for a normal BMI can increase your chances of becoming pregnant and decrease your chances of having a preterm birth or an underweight infant. See chapters 9 and 10 for tips on losing or gaining weight.

No matter what your weight, make sure your diet is rich in folate. Folate deficiency in the mother in early pregnancy can result in spina bifida and other neural tube defects in the baby. Getting enough folate shouldn't be difficult, since beans, greens, and oranges are excellent sources of this vitamin. It is extremely important that you enter pregnancy with abundant reserves of this nutrient, because they will be drawn upon frequently for nine months. See section entitled "Folate (Vitamin B_9, Folic Acid)" and for more information on folate in chapter 11.

It may be advisable to take a prenatal multivitamin-mineral supplement or a supplement specific to pregnancy. Ask your health care provider about this. Choose a supplement that includes vitamin B_{12}, vitamin D, choline, iodine, iron, and zinc. Avoid herbal supplements and botanical remedies unless you discuss them with your health care provider.

Vegan Nutrition During Pregnancy

The nutrients your baby needs for growth come entirely from you. Although you need only in the range of 10 to 15 percent more calories during the second and third trimesters, your need for specific vitamins and minerals can increase significantly over your pre-pregnancy requirements (shown in the appendix), in some cases doubling. Your food selections really matter. Fortunately, designing a nutritionally adequate vegan diet for pregnancy is not only possible, it's also less challenging than you might think.

Recommended intakes for certain vitamins and minerals during pregnancy and lactation are shown in table 11.1. As you can see, recommendations for some nutrients, such as calcium and vitamins D and K, don't change, whereas the need for some increases during lactation, and the need for yet others decreases during lactation. For many nutrients, simply eating greater quantities of a wide variety of healthful vegan foods will easily ensure adequate intakes. Also note that adequate intake of omega-3 fatty acids is essential, as outlined in section entitled "Back to the Essentials" and section entitled "OMEGA-3 FATTY ACIDS". A daily DHA supplement of 200 to 300mg is commonly recommended during pregnancy.

TABLE 11.1. Recommended intakes for pregnant or breast-feeding women ages nineteen to fifty

NUTRIENT	RECOMMENDED INTAKE DURING PREGNANCY	RECOMMENDED INTAKE WHILE BREAST-FEEDING
Calcium	1,000 mg	1,000 mg
Iodine	220 mcg	290 mcg
Iron*	49 mg (27 mg)	16 mg (9 mg)
Magnesium**	350 or 360 mg	210 or 320 mg
Zinc	11 mg	12 mg
Vitamin A (carotenoids)	(2,450 IU) 770 mcg RAE	(4,290 IU) 1,300 mcg RAE
Vitamin C	85 mg	120 mg
Vitamin D	(600 IU) 15 mcg	(600 IU) 15 mcg
Vitamin E	(22.5 IU) 15 mg	(28.5 IU) 19 mg
Vitamin K	90 mcg	90 mcg
Vitamin B_{12}	2.6 mcg	2.8 mcg
Thiamin	1.4 mg	1.4 mg
Riboflavin	1.4 mg	1.6 mg
Niacin	18 mg	17 mg
Pantothenic acid	6 mg	7 mg
Vitamin B_6	1.9 mg	2.0 mg
Folate	600 mcg	500 mcg

Sources of data: Institute of Medicine summaries. Mangels, R., *The Everything Vegan Pregnancy Book* (Axon, MA: F+W Media, 2011). Linus Pauling Institute, Micronutrient Information Center, "Micronutrient Needs during Pregnancy and Lactation" (2012), lpi.oregonstate.edu/infocenter/lifestages/pregnancyandlactation.

*The recommended intake of iron shown here is for vegans and other vegetarians and is higher than that for nonvegetarians (shown in parentheses). However, the need for a higher intake among vegetarians and vegans is controversial, and actual need may be less.

**For magnesium, the first amount is the recommended intake for women nineteen to thirty years of age; the second is for those older than thirty.

Key: IU = International Units, mcg = microgram, mg = miligram; RAE = Retinol Activity Equivalents

FIRST TRIMESTER

You'll need few if any added calories during the first trimester. Average weight gain during the first trimester is 3.5 pounds (1.6kg). Underweight women gain about 5 pounds (2.2kg) during this time; overweight women typically gain about 2 pounds (0.9kg). For overall weight gain recommendations, see table 11.2.

Morning sickness can be the first sign of pregnancy for many women. Fortunately, it often subsides after the first trimester. Dry, low-fat carbohydrate foods, such as crackers, seem to help morning sickness because they are digested quickly, creating less opportunity for queasiness as they rapidly pass through the stomach. Eating a few crackers upon waking seems to help some women. Eating ginger cookies or sipping ginger tea may be beneficial. Sometimes the nausea is actually due to hunger, so eat often, relying on small meals and frequent snacks. Crackers with hummus is a nutritious combination, as is lentil or bean soup with toast. If you feel too queasy to eat solid food, drink juice, water, soy milk, or miso broth. If you're unable to eat or drink adequate amounts of fluids for twenty-four hours, contact your health care provider.

TABLE 11.2. Weight gain in pregnancy

FACTORS DETERMINING WEIGHT-GAIN GOALS	TOTAL WEIGHT GAIN RECOMMENDED	AVERAGE RATE OF WEIGHT GAIN PER WEEK IN SECOND AND THIRD TRIMESTERS
Normal or optimal prepregnancy weight (BMI 18.5–24.9)	25–35 lb (11.5–16 kg)	0.8–1 lb (0.35–0.45 kg)
Underweight before pregnancy (BMI < 18.5)	28–40 lb (12.5–18 kg)	1–1.3 lb (0.45–0.59 kg)
Overweight before pregnancy (BMI 25–29.9)	15–25 lb (7–11.5 kg)	0.5–0.7 lb (0.23–0.32 kg)
Obese before pregnancy (BMI ≥ 30)	11–20 lb (5–9 kg)	0.5 lb (0.23 kg)
Adolescent	30–45 lb (14–20.5 kg)	(variable)
Normal or optimal prepregnancy weight with twins	37–54 lb (17–24 kg)	(variable)

Sources of data are listed in *Becoming Vegan: Comprehensive Edition*, by Brenda Davis and Vesanto Melina (Book Publishing Company, 2014).

Though the recommended intake of protein doesn't increase during the first trimester, make sure you emphasize foods that are rich in protein and iron to help build the additional blood your body must create. In addition, focusing on high-protein legumes (beans, peas, and lentils) can reduce the risk of gestational diabetes, and their fiber will help with constipation. (See "How Much Protein Do We Need,", for information on protein needs, which are based on body weight.)

SECOND AND THIRD TRIMESTERS

By the fourth month of pregnancy, you'll need more calories. The average weight gain during this time is 1 pound (0.45kg) per week. (See table 11.2.) You'll probably gain a little more than that if you're underweight. If you're overweight, you may gain a little less. On average, you'll need to eat an additional 340 calories per day in the second trimester, and 452 additional calories daily during the third. (See chapter 14 for menus at different calorie levels, and table 3.3, for the number of calories in various foods.) At this important stage, choosing nutrient-rich foods is crucial.

Specific Nutrients

In the sections that follow, we'll take a look at some of the nutrients of greatest concern during pregnancy. We'll also discuss substances to avoid and provide some suggested menus. Then our focus will shift to nutritional requirements during lactation in similar detail.

PROTEIN

Starting in the fourth month of pregnancy, your recommended protein intake increases by 25 grams per day. If you're expecting twins, double that amount. Table 11.3 shows various foods that provide 15 grams of protein based on the serving sizes listed in the left-hand column. (Some of these are hearty servings, but you'll probably have a growing appetite.) It makes sense to include at least one protein-rich food in each meal and most snacks, especially as these foods often provide iron, zinc, folate, and choline as well.

TABLE 11.3. Foods that provide 15 grams of protein per serving

	CALORIES	IRON (mg)	ZINC (mg)	FOLATE (mcg)
LEGUMES				
Black beans, cooked (1 c/250 ml)	230	3.6	1.9	256
Chickpeas, cooked (1 c/250 ml)	270	4.7	2.5	282
Edamame, cooked (1 c/250 ml)	165	3.2	2.0	454
Lentils, cooked (scant 1 c/220 ml)	201	5.8	2.2	314
Peanut butter (¼ c/60 ml)	379	1.2	1.9	47
Peanuts, raw (½ c/125 ml)	427	1.6	2.4	106
Pea pods, snow/edible, raw (5.5 c/1.3 L)	226	11.2	1.5	226
Tempeh, crumbled (½ c/125 ml)	160	2.2	1.0	20
Tofu, firm, cubed (6 tbsp/100 g)	140	2.6	1.5	27
LEGUME (OR NUT) AND GRAIN COMBINATIONS				
Sandwich of peanut butter or almond butter (2 tbsp/30 ml) on whole wheat bread (2 slices/60 g)	330	2.0	2.0	37–52
Soy milk (1 c/250 ml) with oat cereal (2 c/500 ml)	320	4.0	2.2	77
Veggie burger with bun (check labels)	208	1.4	1.4	100
GRAINS				
Bread, whole wheat (4 slices/120 g)	277	2.7	2.0	56
Pasta, white, enriched, cooked (1¾ c/435 ml)	387	3.1	1.2	179
Pasta, whole wheat, cooked (2 c/500 ml)	347	3.0	2.3	14
Quinoa, cooked (2 c/500 ml)	444	5.5	4.0	155
Rice, brown, cooked (3 c/750 ml)	649	2.5	3.7	23
NUTS AND SEEDS				
Almonds (½ c/125 ml)	411	2.7	2.2	36
Hazelnuts (¾ c/185 ml)	636	4.8	2.5	114
Pumpkin seeds (6 tbsp/90 ml)	361	4.3	3.8	28
Sunflower seeds (½ c/125 ml)	410	3.7	3.5	159

Sources of data: US Department of Agriculture, Agricultural Research Service, *USDA National Nutrient Database for Standard Reference*, Release 25 (2012), and estimates based on popular vegan recipes for baked goods.

Key: c = cup; g = gram; L = liter; ml = milliliter; tbsp = tablespoon

Although raw vegan diets can be healthful and slimming for adults, we don't advise 100 percent raw diets for pregnant women or for children. Take a look at the amount of pea pods you need for 15 grams of protein in table 11.3! Instead, include some cooked legumes. (For a more extensive list of foods and their protein content, see table 3.3. You also can see replacements that increase your protein intake in table 10.3.)

IRON

Whether the diet is vegan, vegetarian, or omnivorous, iron deficiency can be a concern for women. Many fail to meet the recommended intakes, especially during pregnancy, when the body's blood supply increases by 40 to 50 percent in order to deliver oxygen to the baby and supporting tissues. Iron supports neurological development and is required for the fetus to build up iron stores, especially during the third trimester. Adequate iron intakes during pregnancy are linked with reduced likelihood of preterm births and with larger birth weights.

During pregnancy, when women need more iron, nature steps in and greatly increases the ability to absorb iron from plants, especially during the second trimester. Also, the monthly losses that normally occur during menstruation obviously don't occur during pregnancy, making more iron available for mother and baby.

Pregnant women are advised to consume 27mg of iron per day. Because some plant foods contain substances that limit iron absorption, such as phytate compounds, pregnant vegetarians are advised to get 1.8 times as much iron as nonvegetarians, which would make their recommended intake 49mg per day. But there is some question as to whether vegans need that much, since their diets are already high in vitamin C, which greatly increases iron absorption. In any case, vegan diets tend to be high in iron, with studies repeatedly showing that vegans consume more iron than nonvegetarians.

Supplements providing 30mg of iron are commonly prescribed for pregnant women. It's best to combine such a supplement with an iron-rich diet. Large doses of supplemental iron can be toxic, so don't exceed the amount recommended by your health care provider. Here are some suggestions for effectively meeting your requirement for iron:

- Eat iron-rich foods, such as beans, blackstrap molasses, dried fruit, leafy greens, lentils, seeds, soy foods, whole grains, and fortified grain products.
- Eat foods rich in vitamin C, such as bell peppers, citrus, and tomatoes, when you eat iron-rich foods, in order to increase absorption of the iron.
- Take a prenatal supplement that includes iron or take a daily supplement of 30mg of iron. A good strategy is to take the supplement between meals, with orange juice.
- Avoid coffee and all types of tea (including black, green, and even some herbal teas, such as chamomile and peppermint), which can decrease the absorption of iron.

ZINC

Zinc is required for cell differentiation, in which cells change to perform particular functions in the body. This mineral is also involved in cell replication, which is fundamental to growth. Insufficient intake during pregnancy has been linked with preterm deliveries, low birth weights, prolonged labor, and other problems. Recommended daily intakes increase from 8mg before pregnancy to 11mg during pregnancy or 12mg for pregnant teens. Fortunately, absorption of this mineral increases during pregnancy.

Many foods high in protein and iron, such as beans, also are rich in zinc. Other good sources include asparagus, cashews, corn, mushrooms, peanuts, peas, quinoa, seeds, tahini, tofu, and fortified cereals and veggie meats.

CALCIUM

Though a growing fetus needs calcium for bone building, a woman's recommended intake for this mineral, which is 1,000mg between the ages of nineteen and fifty, doesn't increase during pregnancy and lactation. As with iron and zinc, the body becomes more efficient at absorbing calcium during pregnancy. However, note that most vegans don't meet recommended levels, so pay attention to your calcium intake. If you don't get enough calcium, your body will take calcium from your bones to make up the difference.

Many plant foods are excellent sources of calcium, including almonds, blackstrap molasses, bok choy, broccoli, Chinese cabbage, collard greens, figs, kale, okra, and tofu (if calcium-set). You should also include calcium-fortified foods such as orange juice, nondairy beverages, and cereals to help you meet your daily requirement.

IODINE

Iodine is an essential component of thyroid hormones. Tiny amounts of this mineral are required for normal development of the infant's brain and central nervous system and to avoid the tragedy of cretinism, a preventable form of brain damage that occurs in babies when the mother is deficient in iodine during pregnancy.

Not all prenatal supplements contain iodine, so make sure yours does. The recommended daily intake is 220mcg per day. Most supplements contain only 150mcg. However, if you add 1/4 teaspoon (1ml) of iodized salt over the course of the day, you'll add 70mcg of iodine and meet the recommended intake while avoiding excessive sodium intake.

Some vegans tend to use sea vegetables as a source of iodine, but this isn't ideal, since the amount of iodine can vary so much from one batch to another. If the package has a label, check to see if it lists iodine content (many don't). Iodine drops also are a possibility and deliver a known quantity of iodine per drop. Be aware that there is an upper limit for daily iodine intake, which is 900mcg for teens and 1,100mcg for adults, pregnant or not.

VITAMIN D

The recommended daily intake for women for vitamin D is 15mcg (600 IU), whether or not she is pregnant. This vitamin plays many roles, including aiding in the absorption of calcium. During pregnancy, insufficient vitamin D may increase the risk of preeclampsia. Some experts recommend that all pregnant and lactating mothers take 50mcg (2,000 IU) of vitamin D per day through the winter months in order to maintain sufficient vitamin D levels.

VITAMIN B^12

It's essential that pregnant women get sufficient vitamin B_{12}, whether from diet or supplements. If not, the baby has an increased risk of neural tube defects, brain damage, being born prematurely, seizures, and even death. In addition, if a mother's vitamin B_{12} levels are low, levels of this vitamin will be low in her breast milk, so the infant won't get enough vitamin B_{12}.

In addition to the tragic outcomes for babies and their families, this also hurts the reputation of vegan diets, which have so much going for them. Medical associations have taken stands against vegan diets based on such tragedies. It's important to understand your B_{12} needs and how to meet them, and to spread the word to other women. In short, all pregnant women should take one of the following:

- A daily supplement that includes at least 25mcg of vitamin B_{12}.
- A supplement that contains 1,000mcg of vitamin B_{12} two or three times a week.
- Three servings of food fortified with vitamin B_{12} each day—for example, breakfast cereals, veggie meats, or Red Star Vegetarian Support Formula nutritional yeast. Make sure each serving contains at least 4mcg of vitamin B_{12}, with the label showing that each serving contains at least 60 percent of the daily requirement for this vitamin.

FOLATE

Crucial for building the baby's DNA and for other aspects of growth, folate is also needed for the development of the neural tube, which develops into the brain and spinal cord. Vegans are likely to get enough folate since they eat plenty of beans, greens, and oranges. However, the recommended intake of folate for pregnant women can be complex. A pregnant woman should get 600mcg of folate per day. The body utilizes folate from food quite readily. A pregnant vegan could get her day's supply of folate from I cup (250ml) of orange juice, 3 cups (750ml) of romaine lettuce, and I cup (250ml) each of cooked quinoa and black beans.

A synthetic version of folate, called folic acid, is used in supplements and fortified foods such as breads, pasta, rice, flour, cereals, and other enriched grain products. The body converts folic acid to folate, but there's no reliable way to tell how much folate the body obtains as a result. Although it's safe to get plenty of natural folate from food, preliminary evidence suggests a link between high intakes of folic acid and some cancers. Therefore, it may be prudent to limit your intake of folic acid supplements to 600mcg per day; the benefits of folic acid supplements in early pregnancy outweigh the possible risks. A diet that includes plenty of folate-rich plant foods can easily meet recommended intakes, but a supplement is recommended especially if your appetite is poor.

OMEGA-3 FATTY ACIDS

Essential omega-3 fatty acids are key nutrients needed before, during, and after pregnancy. The long-chain omega-3 fatty acids docosahexaenoic acid (DHA) and eicosapentaenoic acid (EPA) are critical building blocks for development of the baby's retinas, brain, and central nervous system. We all have the ability to convert ALA to EPA and DHA, but pregnant women have superpowers in this regard. Even so, vegans have lower levels of DHA and EPA, including in their breast milk, than nonvegetarians, so many experts suggest that pregnant and nursing vegans take supplemental DHA and EPA. Aim for a ratio of omega-6 to omega-3 fatty acids between 2 to 1 and 4 to 1. (For more on omega-3 and omega-6 fatty acids, see section entitled "GETTING ENOUGH OMEGA-3S".)

During pregnancy and lactation, it's essential to consume adequate alphalinolenic acid (ALA), which the body can convert into EPA and DHA. Good sources of ALA are chia seeds, hempseeds, walnuts, ground flaxseeds, and their oils.

Certain dietary habits affect the ability to convert ALA to DHA. The body makes DHA most efficiently when we limit our intake of trans-fatty acids and oils high in omega-6 fatty acids (corn, cottonseed, safflower, sesame, and sunflower oils), and when we eliminate processed and deep-fried foods made with these oils and fats. Foods containing trans-fatty acids that inhibit DHA production include some margarines, crackers, cookies, pastries, and any food that lists "partially hydrogenated vegetable oil" on the label.

There may be a health advantage to the infant if the mother includes a direct source of vegan DHA, such as a microalgae-based DHA supplement or foods and oils that are fortified with algae-derived DHA. A combination of DHA and EPA is also suitable, as the body can convert EPA to DHA.

Avoiding the Bad Guys

Alcohol is toxic to developing brain cells. Avoid it entirely throughout pregnancy. It passes from your blood directly through the placenta, and the baby's liver isn't mature enough to handle it. There's no point in getting stressed if you had a few drinks early in pregnancy, before you knew that you were embarking on this great adventure, but now that you know, don't use alcohol.

The same goes for tobacco and marijuana. The amount of caffeine that's safe isn't certain, but a small amount—a maximum of 200mg per day—is commonly considered safe. Note that 1 cup (250ml) of coffee contains 100 to 200mg, 1 cup (250ml) of tea has 40 to 75mg, 12 ounces (360ml) of cola has 40 to 60mg, and 1 ounce (30g) of dark chocolate has about 15mg.

The placenta can filter out toxins of a certain size, but it can't totally protect a fetus, so do your part by not letting in toxic substances in the first place. That includes pesticides, so be sure to choose organic foods whenever possible.

Exercise

Staying active during pregnancy has plenty of advantages. It makes you feel good, it keeps you fit and shapely (even when round), and it tones your muscles to aid in delivery. While you shouldn't ski, scuba dive, in-line skate, do gymnastics, ride horseback, or do activities where you might fall, plenty of possibilities remain. Swimming, water aerobics, prenatal yoga, and walking are all good choices. If you jogged and cycled before you were pregnant, it may be fine to continue. Aim to get at least thirty minutes of exercise daily. If you aren't accustomed to exercise, are concerned, or have a high-risk pregnancy, check with your doctor.

Meal Ideas

Let's take a look at how you can incorporate all of the nutrients discussed above into a delicious vegan diet that's ideal for you and your baby. Each day, try to eat at least three servings of grains, three servings of legumes, five servings of vegetables, four servings of fruit, and one serving of nuts or seeds. Make sure six servings of these foods are high in calcium.

The sample menu that follows incorporates those recommendations. It also features protein-rich foods at every meal and snack, and no calories are wasted on sugar or other refined foods that don't deliver nutrients to you and your baby. Potassium, choline, and folate come from vegetables, fruits, and beans. The high fiber intake helps prevent constipation, and drinking plenty of water and exercising will also help with this. The beans, hummus, soy foods, cereal, and nuts or seeds deliver zinc and iron, but not quite as much iron as recommended during pregnancy.

We recommend taking a prenatal supplement to provide vitamin B_{12} and additional vitamin D, iodine, and iron.

As indicated in the list of variations below the menu, you can substitute different foods and still be assured that you're meeting your nutritional requirements. Be aware that this plan doesn't leave a lot of room for soft drinks, sweets, chips, and oily snacks, so when you want to enjoy a treat, choose something based on whole foods, such as homemade ice creams made from frozen fruit, or cookies and bars made with whole-grain flour, nuts, and dried fruit.

Before you review the menu, we'd like to set the record straight on soy foods, which seem to be a magnet for rumors. To some extent, this can be traced back to messages put out by competing industries, rather than to authentic research. In some cases, studies that cast a negative light on soy used birds as research subjects. One was a report on two people who unwisely consumed twelve to fourteen servings of soy foods per day for many months. That said, if you have thyroid problems and your iodine status is low, you shouldn't eat soy until you get enough iodine and the thyroid problems are resolved; after that, soy shouldn't be a problem. In general, feel free to have one to three servings of soy foods per day during pregnancy and while breast-feeding.

SAMPLE PREGNANCY MENU

BREAKFAST

I cup (250ml) cereal with 1/2 cup (125ml) blueberries or other fruit and I cup (250ml) fortified soy milk

I slice whole-wheat toast with 2 tablespoons (30ml) almond butter or seed butter

I cup (250ml) freshly squeezed orange juice or fruit

SNACK

1/2 cup (125ml) carrot sticks with 1/4 cup (60ml) hummus

LUNCH

Sandwich with 1/2 cup (125ml) seasoned tofu and lettuce on 2 slices whole-grain bread

2 cups (500ml) tossed salad with 1/2 avocado and 2 tablespoons (30ml) Liquid Gold Dressing

SNACK

2 figs or I piece other fresh fruit

2 tablespoons (30ml) nuts, peanuts, or seeds

I cup (250ml) fortified soy milk

DINNER

I cup (250ml) beans and I/2 cup (125ml) brown rice

I/2 to I cup (125 to 250ml) cooked kale with lemon juice

I cup (250ml) tomato slices

Nutritional analysis: calories: 2,135; protein: 97g (18% of calories); fat: 85g (34% of calories); carbohydrate: 271g (48% of calories); dietary fiber: 60g; calcium: 1,400 to 2,109mg (depending on choice of tofu, nuts, and fruit); iron: 22mg; magnesium: 791mg; phosphorus: 1,817mg; potassium: 4,938mg; selenium: 94mcg; sodium: 1,451mg; zinc: 15mg; thiamin: 3.2mg; riboflavin: 3.4mg; niacin: 23mg; vitamin B_6: 2.8mg; folate: 754mcg; pantothenic acid: 6.1mg; vitamin B [12]: 5.1mcg; vitamin A: 1,581mcg RAE (5,271 IU); vitamin C: 234mg; vitamin D: 5.5mcg (200 IU); vitamin E: 18mg (27 IU); vitamin K: 497mcg; omega-6 fatty acids: 21g; omega-3 fatty acids: 5.9g

VARIATIONS

- Substitute similar items, such as different types of fruits, vegetables, and beans.
- For an equally high-protein menu without soy, use a different fortified nondairy milk, increase the hummus in the snack to 1/3 cup (160ml), and replace the tofu with 1 cup (250ml) of lentils.
- For an alternative source of omega-3s, replace the Liquid Gold Dressing with 2 tablespoons (30ml) of ground flaxseeds, 2 teaspoons (10ml) of flaxseed oil, or a handful of walnuts.

Fueling the Milk Machine

For a multitude of reasons, breast-feeding is the best option for both babies and moms. When it isn't possible, commercial soy-based infant formula is a safe and healthful alternative.

Nature has done a superb job of designing human breast milk. It contains the perfect balance of protein, fat, and carbohydrate. It's easy for the baby to digest. The proportions of protein and sodium are ideal for the infant's kidneys. Vitamins, minerals, and protective compounds abound, as does DHA, which builds brain and eye tissues. Breast milk also contains a number of protective substances, helps the gastrointestinal system mature, and guards against gastrointestinal illness.

Breast-fed babies are less likely to develop colds, ear infections, stomach upsets, allergies, and asthma. They are also less likely to be overweight as children or adults and more likely to do well in school. They have a reduced risk of childhood leukemia, diabetes, and heart disease. In addition, the mother's body automatically adjusts the composition of the milk as the baby grows so that it always meets the baby's changing nutritional requirements from birth to toddlerhood.

The American Academy of Pediatrics and the World Health Organization recommend breast-feeding exclusively for the first six months before introducing solid food. If possible, breast-feeding should continue for at least another six months, and longer as desired by mother and baby. The natural age of weaning is between two and four years. At the age of four, lactase, the enzyme that breaks down the milk sugar lactose, naturally declines. However, even a short period of breast-feeding is beneficial, so just do the best you can given any practical considerations you face. Vegetarian and vegan moms tend to nurse their babies longer than nonvegetarians, and this is an excellent trend.

In terms of advantages for mothers, those who breast-feed lose baby weight more quickly, especially if breast-feeding lasts at least six months. Breast-feeding also reduces mothers' risk of diabetes and breast and ovarian cancers later in life. Breast-feeding is convenient. You don't have to warm bottles and cart a lot of equipment with you whenever you and your baby venture out. It also gives you superb one-on-one time with your baby, often providing some of the sweetest moments of parenting.

Vegan and vegetarian mothers offer their babies a further advantage by breast-feeding: they have fewer toxins in their milk than nonvegetarian moms. Sadly, the levels of potentially toxic environmental pollutants commonly found in breast milk would prevent its sale as a food for infants. But breast milk from vegetarian moms typically contains only a fraction of those levels. Given that, imagine the advantages of a vegan diet of *organic* food.

Breast-feeding moms need plenty of calories, protein, and other nutrients. During the first six months of breast-feeding, you need 330 to 500 extra calories per day. (Naturally, if you have multiple infants, such as twins, you'll need even more.) If you need to lose some baby weight, stick with about 330 extra calories per day. If your weight is already back where you want it, eat about 400 extra calories per day. Of course, how much you eat depends on the baby's appetite too. If your little one is voracious, you may need more calories. After the baby begins eating solid food, you'll need fewer calories. As in pregnancy, eating small frequent meals is a good way to ensure that you're getting enough calories.

While nursing, you could continue using the same sample pregnancy menu adding a little extra avocado or nut butter or other sources of vitamin E, and be assured that you're meeting all of your basic nutrient requirements, with two exceptions. You'll need to get more pantothenic acid and vitamin A, so we'll discuss these two nutrients first.

PANTOTHENIC ACID

Pantothenic acid is needed for building essential cell components and neurotransmitters, and for energy production. You need more while you're breast-feeding, but a good vegan diet can provide enough. Whole grains are good sources of this vitamin; in refined grains it's been stripped away. You can get the additional pantothenic acid you need for the day if you eat another half avocado, add 3/4 cup (185ml) of sweet potato or mushrooms, or eat 2 cups (500ml) of cooked oatmeal with a big banana for breakfast. Other good sources of pantothenic acid include broccoli, legumes, mushrooms, nutritional yeast, nuts, and seeds, such as sunflower seeds.

VITAMIN A

Vitamin A allows cells to carry out specific tasks, and its effects are diverse. It's needed for the growth of bones and teeth, for reproduction, and to build and regulate hormones. Vegans get vitamin A from the carotenoids in orange, yellow, red, and green fruits and vegetables. The sample pregnancy menu provides enough to meet your needs from carrots, kale, lettuce, tomatoes, and fortified soy milk. Carotenoids are also found in apricots, broccoli, cantaloupe, leafy greens, mangoes, nectarines, papayas, peppers, persimmons, plantains, prunes, pumpkin, squash, sweet potatoes, turnips, and sea vegetables. For other sources, see table 6.2.

VITAMIN B₁2

Babies require vitamin B_{12} for the normal development of brain, nerve, and blood cells. Without it, the baby's brain won't develop normally, resulting in neurological problems. This can occur even if the mother shows no symptoms of vitamin B_{12} deficiency, so it is critical that nursing moms get enough vitamin B_{12}. Breast milk doesn't include vitamin B_{12} from the mother's stores, so nursing moms must eat foods fortified with vitamin B_{12} or take a B_{12} supplement daily or a larger supplement twice a week (see VITAMIN B_{12} in chapter 11. Supplements are a better choice than fortified foods because the amounts are more carefully standardized.

PROTEIN

Nursing mothers need to get as much protein as in the second and third trimesters of pregnancy. Legumes, whole grains, greens, and vegetables provide plenty of protein, along with iron, zinc, calcium, other minerals, and many B vitamins.

IRON

Women require less iron while breast-feeding than during pregnancy, since the body is no longer building its blood supply for gestation, or for menstruating. Breast milk provides adequate amounts of iron in a form that's easily absorbed by the baby. The recommended intake for nursing vegans and vegetarians is 16mg per day.

ZINC

Mothers need slightly more zinc while breast-feeding than during pregnancy—12mg instead of 11mg per day. Some of the best sources of zinc are seeds, particularly pumpkin and sunflower seeds and sesame tahini; nuts, especially cashews; every kind of bean, pea, and lentil; peanuts; soy foods; whole grains, including barley, brown rice, oats, whole wheat products, and wheat germ; plus asparagus, corn, mushrooms, spinach, and dark chocolate. Some breakfast cereals, nondairy milks, veggie meats, and energy bars are fortified with zinc.

CALCIUM

Mothers need just as much calcium—1,000mg per day—while nursing as during pregnancy. While lactating, the body goes through changes that enhance its absorption of calcium. The mother's body may also draw on calcium stores in her bones for breast milk. Consuming more calcium doesn't seem to prevent this, but fortunately, studies have shown that after weaning, the mother's bone mineral content will be restored.

VITAMIN D

Breast milk is low in vitamin D, and levels vary according to the mother's sun exposure, her dietary intake, and whether she takes a vitamin D supplement. The American Academy of Pediatrics recommends that all infants and children, including adolescents, get at least 10mcg (400 IU) of vitamin D daily beginning soon after birth.

OMEGA-3 FATTY ACIDS

The section on omega-3s earlier in this chapter discussed ways to enhance the body's stores of DHA. However, the most reliable way of increasing DHA in breast milk is to take supplemental DHA. Although these are commonly made using fish oil, vegan DHA supplements made from DHA-rich algae (the same place the fish get their DHA) are available. Supplementation isn't absolutely essential, but taking 200 to 300mg of DHA per day will help boost your DHA status. Another option is to eat DHA-fortified foods and oils. In addition, because this essential fat is so important during the third trimester, premature babies should receive supplemental DHA, as they aren't yet able to synthesize DHA. Formulas for premature infants include DHA.

FLUIDS

If your body is going to make milk, you need to drink lots of liquids. You will feel thirsty often, so keep water, juice, soy milk, or smoothies on hand all day. Be sure to keep beverages near the comfortable chair that you use for nursing so you can sip while your baby nurses.

Formula Feeding

There can be good reasons to use infant formula as your baby's primary source of nutrition or as an occasional option. The American Academy of Pediatrics recommends iron-fortified infant formula as the only acceptable substitute for breast milk during the first year because it can help prevent iron-deficiency anemia. Infants born prematurely are at highest risk for iron deficiency because their iron stores can be very low. Full-term infants are usually born with iron stores sufficient for their first six months, until solid foods are introduced. Formula contains higher levels of iron than breast milk, but the iron from breast milk is absorbed more easily. Infant formula also supplies adequate amounts of vitamins D and B_{12}, but it lacks many of the immune-protective compounds found in breast milk.

Standard formulas are based on cow's milk or soy milk and are fortified to contain roughly the same nutrients as breast milk at similar levels. If you wish to avoid animal products, use soy formula. (However, soy formula isn't suitable for preterm infants or those with congenital thyroid problems. For more information on this, see the "Infant Formula" section of "Soy: What's the Harm?" at veganhealth.org/articles/soy_wth.)

Several of the infant formulas available in North America are close to vegan. As this book goes to press, the single nonvegan component is vitamin D_3 derived from lanolin from sheep's wool. With sufficient consumer demand, more companies might choose to use vitamin D 2 or vegan vitamin D_3 from lichen.

Please be aware that most cases of malnutrition in vegan infants can be traced to homemade infant "formulas" that are grossly nutritionally inadequate. Never feed a baby homemade formula, and never substitute regular dairy or nondairy milk for formula or breast milk. Using regular dairy or nondairy milk or homemade formula can lead to poor child development or even tragic, disastrous health problems, *including death.* Babies need specific nutrients in certain amounts. Beverages other than breast milk and infant formula don't provide all of the nutrients they require. The only safe and nutritionally adequate types of milk for the first twelve months of life are breast milk and commercial infant formula.

Resources and Websites for Pregnancy and Lactation

Good nutrition during pregnancy and lactation is crucial to giving infants an healthy start in life, but space doesn't permit us to address this important topic in greater detail. Here are a few resources that provide more details:

• *The Everything Vegan Pregnancy Book,* by R. Mangels (Adams Media, 2011). The title says it all.

• *Cooking Vegan,* by V. Melina and J. Forest (Book Publishing Company, 2012). Tasty high-protein recipes, complete with nutritional analyses.

• *Raising Vegetarian Children,* by J. Stepaniak and V. Melina (McGraw-Hill, 2003). An entirely vegan book packed with practical tips, recipes, and menus.

• "Pregnancy and the Vegan Diet" at vrg.org/nutrition/veganpregnancy.htm. **An**

Internet resource offeredby the Vegetarian Resource Group.

• "Vegetarian Diets in Pregnancy" at vegetariannutrition.net/docs/Pregnancy-Vegetarian-Nutrition.pdf. An Internet resource offered by the Academy of Nutrition and Dietetics.

For a more extensive edition of this book, fully referenced and for health professionals, see *Becoming Vegan, Comprehensive Edition: The Complete Reference to Plant-Based Nutrition*, by B. Davis and V. Melina (Book Publishing Company, 2014).

Food Allergies

If anyone in the baby's family has a history of allergies, seek advice from a dietitian, nurse, doctor, or clinic regarding the introduction of foods beyond breast milk. The potential to develop an allergy is an inherited characteristic. However, the tendency to react to specific foods isn't inherited. Pediatricians and allergy specialists can provide individualized guidance. Early introduction of solid foods, especially before three months of age, has been linked with the development of food allergies, and it's a primary reason experts recommend against introducing solid foods until the baby is six months old. Your baby may have a reduced risk of developing celiac disease if you wait until after six months to introduce foods with gluten. However, giving gluten- and wheat-containing foods after the six-month mark has been found to *lessen* risk of celiac disease. Breast-feeding seems to play a protective role in reducing reactions to gluten or potential food allergens. Breast-feeding may support the immune system and the maturation of the intestinal tract so they can more effectively perform their protective functions.

For all infants, and especially those with a family history of allergies, it's wise to introduce foods one at a time and then wait at least three or four days to see if there's any reaction before introducing another new food. Mixed foods shouldn't be introduced until the individual ingredients have been consumed without reaction. Signs of food allergy can appear on the skin as red or itchy patches, which may be eczema or hives; in the respiratory tract as a stuffy nose, wheezing, or runny eyes; or in the gastrointestinal tract as colic that doesn't go away, frequent spitting up, or diarrhea. In extreme cases, the baby's lips, face, eyes, or ears may swell, and the baby may have trouble breathing. This can signal a medical emergency, so if this happens, take your baby to an emergency room immediately.

In the past, the medical community advised parents to delay the introduction of highly allergenic foods, but now that advice has come into question. Needlessly restricting the diet can be problematic and lead to nutrient shortages that are entirely unnecessary. Follow the advice of your physician.

However, we will share information on foods that are more likely to be allergenic so you can be alert to potential issues when (or if) you introduce them. These include fish, shellfish, eggs, milk, peanuts, tree nuts, soy, wheat, sesame seeds, and sulfites (for example, in dried fruit). Foods generally considered less likely to trigger allergic reactions include apple (cooked), apricot, avocado, banana, barley, beet, blueberries, broccoli, carrot, cauliflower, green beans, kale, millet, oats, parsnip, peach, pear, plum, potato, prunes, rice, quinoa, squash, sweet potato, tapioca, and yam.

Note that children who react to a particular food in raw form sometimes don't react to the same food when it's cooked.

Introducing Solid Foods

Several decades ago, The Farm in Tennessee was the focus of another study, this time looking at the growth and development of 288 vegan children who were born and raised there. The children ate nutritious vegan foods, including full-fat, fortified soy milk. Researchers found that infants born at The Farm had normal birth weights and that their growth was typical of predominantly breast-fed children. Their average weights and heights were within normal ranges and fell between the twenty-fifth and seventy-fifth percentiles. So if well-meaning friends and relatives question the safety of raising children on a vegan diet, you can say you have solid medical science on your side.

Up to about six months of age, babies typically need only breast milk or formula, but then things start to change. The baby's intestinal tract matures, decreasing the possibility of allergic responses to foods.

In addition, the baby's supply of iron, which is stored during gestation, starts to run low. In a few cases, this happens as early as four months. By six months of age, nursing babies should receive complementary foods to provide about 1mg of iron per kilogram (2.2lb) of body weight per day. If insufficient iron-rich solid foods are consumed, a supplement is recommended. In most cases, formula-fed babies don't need an iron supplement, since formula is fortified with iron. Parents are generally advised to provide supplemental iron to preterm breast-fed babies and a special iron-enriched formula to those who are formula-fed, as these babies have low iron reserves. However, inappropriate iron supplementation can lead to iron overload, so these infants should be carefully monitored by their physicians.

What about Raw Diets for Growing Children?

Scientific studies haven't established the adequacy of raw diets for growing children. In fact, extremely restrictive and high-fiber diets, such as fruitarian diets, can be too low in calories, protein, and some vitamins and minerals and have been linked to cases of severe malnutrition and even infant deaths. We don't recommend raw vegan diets for infants and children, although including some raw foods is great!.

Beginning solid foods at the right stage has many benefits, including helping children avoid weight problems later on. For example, formula-fed babies who eat solid foods before four months of age are six times more likely to be obese at age three.

Babies show that they are ready for solid foods when they can sit, hold up their head, and pick up a morsel of food and put it in their mouth. Another sign is when they show interest in the foods that family members are eating. When a baby reaches this stage, don't wait too long to introduce solid foods. If you miss this period of fascination with new tastes and textures, the child may become a picky eater. However, be sure that a major component of the baby's diet remains breast milk or formula until at least age one, and perhaps age two or older.

Parents typically begin with pureed food. As babies progress beyond that stage, it's important to make sure they get enough calories. Use full-fat soy foods, such as tofu and soy yogurt. Other sources of concentrated calories and nutrients include avocados, nut and seed butters, and bean spreads. You may wish to include some refined grain products (such as pasta) in addition to whole grains.

Rely on cooked foods such as thick soups and stews, as cooking generally makes food more digestible. Cookies, muffins, puddings, and shakes can also be highly nutritious foods if you use healthful ingredients.

BOOSTING BABY'S IRON STORES

Because babies' iron stores tend to start running low at six months, when solid foods are usually introduced, be sure to include iron-rich foods early on. Iron-fortified commercial infant cereals generally are a good first choice as you introduce solid foods; two tablespoons (30mL) dry iron-fortified oat cereal provides enough iron for the day. Vary your grains. Well-cooked, pureed whole grains such as oats, barley, or quinoa are good options, but provide less iron than fortified cereals. In the past, many people recommended against giving babies wheat early on. However, recent research shows that including wheat as a starter food for breast-fed babies may reduce their risk of celiac disease and sensitivity to wheat. Mix cereals or grains with some breast milk or formula. Iron-rich foods to try include Cream of Wheat and pureed broccoli, green beans, kale, peas, or sweet potatoes.

At around seven months, follow up with additional iron-rich foods, such as well-cooked lentils and beans, mashed tofu, soy yogurt, grated or peeled and cooked vegetables, and fruits. Prune juice is a good source of iron, and citrus fruit or a bit of citrus juice will increase absorption of dietary iron.

EXPANDING THE MENU

When babies are eight to nine months old, they begin to enjoy finger foods. Try chunks of pita bread or tortilla, teething biscuits, different shapes of pasta, unsweetened cereal, pieces of rolls or pancakes, unsalted crackers, steamed tofu cubes, and soft fruits like avocado, banana, kiwi, mango, melon, or papaya.

At nine to twelve months, most babies are ready to join family meals and can start eating what the family eats: mixed dishes, stews, grated raw carrot and apple, and veggie meats. After each new food seems well accepted, include it regularly. Soon your family can share ratatouille, stir-fries, lentil curries, chili, pasta dishes, vegan pizza, risotto, roasted veggies, and more. Just omit the salt and salty seasonings, such as Bragg

Liquid Aminos, tamari, or soy sauce, from your baby's portion.

Meals for Babies

Table 11.4 outlines sample meal plans for babies ages six to eighteen months. Babies need 3 to 4 cups (24 to 32 floz, or 750ml to 1 liter) of breast milk or infant formula over the course of the day. That amount will naturally decrease between twelve and eighteen months of age. Although fortified soymilk is an acceptable milk alternative after 12 months of age, iron-fortified infant formula is preferable until age two. After six months or as the baby begins to eat more solid food, add some sips of water, especially when the weather is warm.

SUPPLEMENTS AND FOOD SOURCES FROM BIRTH TO EIGHTEEN MONTHS

The sample menus meet the recommended intakes for all nutrients, except for vitamins B_{12} and D, which can be obtained from fortified foods and supplements. After you introduce solid foods, regularly include well-cooked broccoli and firm tofu for calcium, avocado and seed butters for vitamin E, and plenty of fruits and vegetables for potassium, along with abundant breast milk or formula.

TABLE 11.4. Sample meal plans for babies six to eighteen months old

TIME	6 TO 9 MONTHS	9 TO 12 MONTHS	12 TO 18 MONTHS
Early morning	Breast milk or formula	Breast milk or formula	Sleep in! (Or wish you could.)
Breakfast	¼ to ½ c (60 to 125 ml) infant cereal mixed with breast milk, formula, or water 1 to 4 tbsp (15 to 60 ml) soft fruit in small pieces	¼ to ½ c (60 to 125 ml) infant cereal mixed with breast milk, formula, or water Small pieces of whole-grain toast Soft fruit in small pieces Breast milk or formula in a cup	1 small pancake; toast with tahini; or ½ c (125 ml) oatmeal ½ banana or ½ c (125 ml) applesauce Breast milk or ¾ c (185 ml) formula in a cup
Morning snack	Breast milk or formula	Breast milk or formula Soft fruit in small pieces	Small whole wheat bun or 2 or 3 crackers, spread with 2 tbsp (30 ml) hummus Breast milk or ½ c (125 ml) formula
Lunch	1 to 4 tbsp (15 to 60 ml) mashed or soft vegetables 1 to 6 tbsp (15 to 90 ml) pureed well-cooked beans, lentils, or peas; steamed tofu or tempeh; or soy yogurt Soft fruit in small pieces Breast milk or formula	2 to 4 tbsp (30 to 60 ml) mashed or soft vegetables or fruit 2 to 6 tbsp (30 to 90 ml) soft cooked beans, peas, or lentils; steamed tofu or tempeh; veggie burger; or soy yogurt Breast milk or formula in a cup	½ to ¾ c (125 to 185 ml) lentil soup ½ veggie burger or sandwich ½ cup (125 ml) berries or fruit, such as cooked peeled pear Breast milk or ½ c (125 ml) formula in a cup
Afternoon snack	Breast milk or formula	Breast milk or formula Soft vegetables or fruit in small pieces	½ c (125 ml) soy yogurt with fruit Water in a cup
Supper	1 to 4 tbsp (15 to 60 ml) mashed or soft vegetables 1 to 6 tbsp (15 to 90 ml) pureed cooked beans, peas, or lentils 1 to 4 tbsp (15 to 60 ml) soft fruit in small pieces Breast milk or formula	2 to 6 tbsp (30 to 90 ml) cooked potato or pasta 2 to 6 tbsp (30 to 90 ml) pureed cooked beans, peas, or lentils; steamed tofu or tempeh; or soy yogurt Soft vegetables or fruit in small pieces Breast milk or formula in a cup	¼ cup (60 ml) cooked beans, peas, or lentils, with ½ c (125 ml) rice, potato, or pasta, and ⅓ c (85 ml) stir-fried vegetaables; or 1 to 1½ c (250 to 375 ml) family entrée Breast milk or ½ c (125 ml) formula in a cup
Evening snack	Breast milk or formula ¼ to ½ c (60 to 125 ml) infant cereal mixed with formula, breast milk, or water	Breast milk or formula Finger foods such as pieces of frozen fruit, cooked sweet potato, toast, vegan teething biscuits, or dry cereal flakes	Breast milk or ½ c (125 ml) formula Favorite healthy snacks

Sources of data are listed in *Becoming Vegan: Comprehensive Edition*, by Brenda Davis and Vesanto Melina (Book Publishing Company, 2014).

Key: c = cup; ml = milliliter; tbsp = tablespoon.

Nutritional analysis (for the "6 to 9 Months" column; based on larger amounts where there is a range, and on the first item where there is an option): calories: 1,170; protein: 32 g (11% of calories); fat: 64 g (48% of calories); carbohydrate: 126 g (41% of calories); dietary fiber: 11 g; calcium: 1,260 mg; iron: 18 mg; magnesium: 170 mg; phosphorus: 547 mg; potassium: 1,531 mg; selenium: 43 mcg; sodium: 201 mg; zinc: 5 mg; thiamin: 1.1 mg; riboflavin: 1.4 mg; niacin: 23.1 mg; vitamin B₆: 0.7 mg; folate: 200 mcg; pantothenic acid: 3.9 mg; vitamin B₁₂: 0.52 mcg; vitamin A: 2,317 IU (702 mcg RAE); vitamin C: 99 mg; vitamin D: 40 IU (1 mcg); vitamin E: 7.5 IU (5 mg); vitamin K: 60 mcg; omega-6 fatty acids: 9 g; omega-3 fatty acids: 1.3.

The Diet of a Good Role Model

Whether or not you're breast-feeding, your diet matters—and not just for your own health. Children take in every move made by Mom and Dad, and your habits

can lay the foundation for lifelong patterns of your children. Habits, such as eating a lot of vegetables, tend to start early in life.

Vitamin D. To one year of age, breast-fed babies need 10mcg (400 IU) of vitamin D daily as a supplement. Formula is fortified and contains sufficient vitamin D when it's the baby's main food source. From one to three years of age, the recommended intake is 15mcg (600 IU) of vitamin D.

Vitamin B$_{12}$. As mentioned, breast-feeding moms need to get enough vitamin B$_{12}$ so their breast milk will supply enough of this essential nutrient. Infant formula is fortified with vitamin B$_{12}$ and is a reliable source. As the baby takes less milk, and after weaning, provide foods or formula fortified with vitamin B$_{12}$ three times a day, or give a supplement. Recommended daily intakes are 0.5mcg from six to twelve months of age and 0.9mcg from one to three years of age.

Omega-3 fatty acids. The recommended daily intake of alpha-linolenic acid for infants six to twelve months old is 0.5 gram, and for children one to three years old, it's 0.7 gram (double to 1.4 grams when no DHA is provided). Breast-feeding moms need to get sufficient omega-3 fatty acids, since these are passed along in breast milk. If using formula, choose one with added DHA. If using a formula without DHA, one simple way to provide sufficient ALA is to give 1/4 teaspoon (1ml) of a balanced, omega-3-rich oil to babies between six and twelve months old, and then 1/2 teaspoon (2ml) of the oil to children between one and three years old. For more on omega-3 fatty acids, see chapter 4.

Toddlers and Preschoolers

When babies are standing on their own two feet and ready to head off into the world, leaving breast or bottle behind (at least some of the time), their nutrient needs change again. You can have a wonderful time exploring textures and flavors together as the baby's ability to feed himself or herself increases. However, children are often nutritionally vulnerable at this time, thanks to growth spurts and discovering the power of "No!" The key to success is to have a good dietary plan in mind while also being flexible, adjusting for your preferences and those of your child.

The Vegan Food Guide for Toddlers included in this section explains the number of servings of each food group required each day and offers guidelines on serving size. Basically, include foods from three to five of the food groups listed at every meal and from at least two food groups at snack time. Don't necessarily limit certain foods to being breakfast or supper items.

Consider possibilities such as starting your child's day with breakfast burritos or soup, or offer rice and raisin pudding at any time of day. Include iron-rich foods often, such as iron-fortified cereals.

Children have small stomachs. To keep them well nourished, provide meals or snacks every two to three hours. Have nutritious foods at the ready when hunger strikes: perhaps soy yogurt, a tray of cut-up veggies with avocado or bean dip, a fruit smoothie with hempseeds, or frozen muffins, which thaw quickly.

Though children may appear to be picky eaters, diligent detective work often proves that they are managing well and even thriving. Note their food intake, energy, and growth. They may reject much of the food on their plate at mealtime but readily eat snacks. If so, it's especially important to offer highly nutritious snacks. For example, over the course of a day, if children weighing from 25 to 33 pounds (11.5 to 15kg) consume 3 cups (750ml) of fortified soy milk, two peanut butter sandwiches, two sliced bananas, and 1/2 cup (125ml) of peas, they're getting enough calories and triple the recommended amount of protein.

VEGAN FOOD GUIDE FOR TODDLERS

Milks and formula: 2 1/2 to 3 cups (20 to 24 floz, or 600 to 750ml) total

About three 3/4- to 1-cup (6 to 8 floz, or 180 to 240ml) servings of breast milk, commercial infant formula, full-fat fortified soy milk, or a combination of these

Breads and cereals: four to six toddler-sized servings

One toddler-sized serving:
- 1/2 slice bread or a similar-sized piece of tortilla or pita bread
- 1/4 cup (60ml) cooked grain or pasta
- 1/2 cup (125ml) ready-to-eat cereal
- 1/4 cup (60ml) cooked cereal

Vegetables: two to three toddler-sized servings

One toddler-sized serving:
- 1/2 cup (125ml) salad or raw vegetable pieces
- 1/4 cup (60ml) cooked vegetables
- 1/3 cup (85ml) vegetable juice

Fruits: two to three toddler-sized servings

One toddler-sized serving:
- 1/2 to 1 fresh fruit
- 1/4 cup (60ml) cooked fruit
- 1/4 cup (60ml) fruit juice; limit to 1/2 cup (125ml) per day

Beans and alternates: two toddler-sized servings

One toddler-sized serving:

- 1/4 cup (60ml) cooked beans, peas, or lentils
- 2 ounces (60g) tofu
- 1/2 to 1 ounce (15 to 30g) veggie meat
- 1 1/2 tablespoons (22ml) nut or seed butter
- 2 tablespoons (30ml) soy yogurt

NUTRIENT NOTES

Look online or in your natural food store or pharmacy for a high-quality vegan children's multivitamin-mineral that includes adequate amounts of vitamin B_{12}, vitamin D, and iodine, along with calcium, iron, and zinc. This can give you peace of mind, especially during times when your little one seems picky, resulting in eating habits that seem unbalanced or insufficient. (Be sure to store all supplements safely away from children.)

Vitamin B $_{12}$. From age one to three years, the recommended intake is 0.9mcg per day—the amount found in 2 1/4 cups (18floz, or 550ml) of infant formula or fortified soy milk. (Check labels.)

Vitamin D. From age one until adulthood, the recommended intake is 15mcg (600 IU). Infant formula or fortified soy milk may provide vitamin D; check labels for amounts. To get enough vitamin D from sun exposure, children need to have sun on their face and forearms between 10a.m. and 2p.m.: ten to fifteen minutes for light-skinned children, and twenty minutes or more for those with darker skin. This isn't an option in winter months at latitudes above 37 degrees north, so a supplement may be necessary. Avoid excess sun exposure, and don't give more than 63mcg (2,520 IU) of supplemental vitamin D per day; excess vitamin D can be toxic.

Omega-3 fatty acids. From age one to three years, the recommended intake is 0.7 gram of alpha-linolenic acid if your child is still nursing or drinking formula. Otherwise, supplement with 1.4 grams of alpha-linolenic acid or 0.7 gram of alpha-linolenic acid plus 70mg of DHA.

Iodine. From age one to eight, the recommended intake is 90mcg. This can be obtained through a supplement, from iodized table salt (limit to 1/4tsp/1ml daily) and other iodine-rich foods, or a combination. (See section entitled "Iodine" in chapter 7).

Children to Age Twelve

Rapidly growing children have nutritional needs that are quite different from those of adults. At around age two, a toddler may weigh 27 pounds (12kg) and be 34 inches (86cm) tall. Three years later, that child might weigh 50 percent more and be 9 inches (23cm) taller. To accomplish this amazing feat of building the body, the child's diet must be rich in protein, minerals, and numerous other nutrients. The pace of growth eases slightly during the preteen years and then picks up with new force in early adolescence. In the sections that follow, we offer some meal ideas that can help ensure adequate nutrition while also transforming meal planning and preparation from a daily burden into a rewarding shared process.

Preview Passed Pages

Though children will ask for unhealthful foods and beverages, you don't have to buy them. It's best to offer more nutritious choices. For example, you can make healthy soda using sparkling water and freshly squeezed orange juice or another pure fruit juice. In place of conventional ice pops, you can make your own with ice-pop molds and a combination of fruit and either fruit juice or nondairy yogurt. Splurge on fresh berries or make a healthful fruit shake.

BREAKFAST

Eating breakfast helps children pay attention, concentrate, remember, and perform better academically. Skip the sugar-laden cereals, despite the provocative marketing ads, and create appealing and nutritious breakfasts. For a change of pace, try scrambled tofu or a smoothie with hempseeds, sunflower seeds, or a smoothie booster. Many children enjoy a "breakfast bar" similar to a salad bar; keep several types of muesli, granola, or other wholesome ready-to-eat cereals near the breakfast table, along with jars of seeds, nuts, and shredded coconut. This assortment may be popular for snacks too. Cooked cereal, fresh fruit, and fortified nondairy beverages can be added in the morning.

Planning can help ensure a peaceful start to the day, even if everyone has to be out the door early. For children who are too sleepy to eat before heading to school or day care, a grab-and-go breakfast such as a nutritious homemade muffin or a nut butter sandwich might be a good solution, providing something they can eat on the ride to school or during a morning break.

If you have time for a leisurely and companionable start, perhaps on weekends, it's fun to make pancakes together and serve them topped with fruit or fruit sauce. This activity can motivate children to become good cooks later in life. For a special breakfast that's almost instant, pop vegan frozen waffles into the toaster.

PACKED LUNCHES

Assembling lunch boxes or bag lunches can be a pleasant shared task, perhaps done the evening before. Some children prefer a familiar favorite sandwich every day. For others, a packed lunch will be more appealing if the offerings change often.

Lunch should include protein-rich foods and whole grains to help supply sustained energy through the afternoon. It may seem that a vegan diet doesn't lend itself to sandwiches, since it doesn't include meat and cheese. Fortunately, that isn't the case. The possibilities are numerous and can easily accommodate anyone's preferences. Start with a grain product, such as a baguette or crusty roll, whole-grain bread, pita bread, rice cakes, or a tortilla. Spread on some vegan buttery spread, mustard, ketchup, guacamole, olive tapenade, pickle relish, or soy mayonnaise. Add a protein, such as a tofu spread or seasoned tofu slices, nondairy cheese, falafel patties, hummus, nut or seed butter, vegetarian deli slices, a veggie burger, or refried beans. Also include a layer of vegetables, such as sprouts, lettuce, sauerkraut, shredded carrot, or sliced avocado, cucumber, bell pepper, red onion, olives, or tomato.

If your child has an insulated lunch bag, other welcome choices include nondairy yogurt and hearty salads made with beans, potatoes, pasta, or grains. Leftover pizza and pasta dishes work well too and can include gluten-free options.

DINNER

Children who aren't fond of homemade soups, cooked vegetables, or stir-fries may become more open to vegetables if they help with the preparation, perhaps bringing lettuce from the garden, washing carrots, and, when capable of handing a knife safely, chopping. Most people live on six to ten favorite meals, repeated over and over. Some time-tested favorites among children are pizza, chili, veggie burgers, falafel, tacos, burritos, and spaghetti with a pasta sauce that includes well-cooked red lentils. When made with the right ingredients, these dishes can be well-balanced nutritionally, and the leftovers are often great for packed lunches.

SNACKING

When cooking grains, pasta, and entrées, make enough that you'll have leftovers to serve as snacks. Although many children don't mind cold grains or pasta, these also can be warmed with a little tomato sauce or peanut sauce. To satisfy a sweet tooth, keep fresh fruit in a bowl on the countertop and jars of dried dates, apricots, figs, or other dried fruit handy. (Brush teeth after eating dried fruit!)

THE GOOD FOOD DAY

Table 11.5 gives examples of menus that meet the nutritional needs of children at three different weights and stages of growth. Very active children may burn more calories than the amounts supplied by these menus, in which case you can simply increase their portions or add foods to these menus. All of these menus easily meet and exceed protein recommendations. As you may note, a menu that meets recommended intakes for all nutrients leaves little room for junk food.

NUTRIENT NOTES

For children whose diets generally are good, a daily supplement isn't necessary, with the possible exceptions of vitamins B_{12} and D. However, do consider a supplement on days when food intake is less than adequate. Amounts of vitamins and minerals in supplements are more reliable than in fortified foods, so using a combination can be wise. See Table 1, Table 2 for recommended intakes.

Vitamin B $_{12}$. In addition to supplements, fortified nondairy milks provide vitamin B_{12}, as do some fortified veggie burgers and breakfast cereals.

Vitamin D. Fortified nondairy milks also provide vitamin D, but they currently don't meet the more recent, increased recommendations.

Children should get ten to fifteen minutes of sun on their faces and forearms daily (without sunscreen) to top up their vitamin D. After that, be sure they use sunscreen if they'll be outside longer. For those who live at latitudes above 37 degrees north, sunlight is insufficient for vitamin D production during the winter, so supplements can be important from October or November through March or April.

Iodine. Sufficient iodine could be obtained through a supplement, from iodized salt (limit to 1/4tsp/1ml daily), other iodine-rich food or a combination. (See section entitled "Iodine" in chapter 7).

EATING AWAY FROM HOME

Some people anticipate that a vegan diet will make life difficult for children by setting them apart. Fortunately, many parents find that this isn't such a big hurdle.

To ensure that meals away from home are nutritious, planning is essential. When traveling, check out happycow.net or vegdining.com, or do an Internetsearch to locate vegan-friendly restaurants. Breakfast can be as simple as oatmeal, cereals, fruit, toast, jam, peanut butter, and juices. Cereal can be eaten dry, or with nondairy milk or juice. Sometimes bringing one or two items from home can allow your family to enjoy school or restaurant meals without compromising dietary choices. For lunch and dinner, many restaurants include vegan options, if not as entrées then as side dishes, such as rice, baked potatoes, pasta, vegetables, or salad, which you can combine for a meal. Salad bars, whether in restaurants or markets, are often a good choice, as they include high-protein options such as peas, chickpeas, beans, and possibly tofu. In many cases, your best bet may be an ethnic restaurant, particularly Chinese, Indian, Middle Eastern, Japanese, or Thai.

Some children are naturally adventurous, and others want familiar foods when they venture out. For the less adventurous child, bring a favorite brand of crackers, individual boxed nondairy milk, mini portions of peanut butter, a favorite sandwich, or trail mix. For car travel, carry a big bottle of water to wash berries, cherry tomatoes, or peas in the pod, which you can purchase en route, plus a knife to cut fresh fruit or veggies.

TABLE 11.5. Three menus for children

44-POUND (20 kg) CHILD	PROTEIN (g)	62-POUND (28 kg) CHILD	PROTEIN (g)	80-POUND (36 kg) CHILD	PROTEIN (g)
BREAKFAST	**9 g**		**16 g**		**18 g**
1 serving fortified cereal with 2 tbsp (30 ml) hempseeds	7 g	1 c (250 ml) oatmeal with 1 tbsp (15 ml) ground flaxseeds	8 g	1 English muffin with 1 tbsp (15 ml) almond butter	9 g
1 c (250 ml) fortified nondairy milk	1 g	1 c (250 ml) fortified soy milk	7 g	Smoothie with ½ c (125 ml) blueberries, 1 banana, and 1 c (250 ml) fortified soy milk	9 g
½ cup (125 ml) calcium-fortified juice	1 g	1 banana	1 g		
LUNCH	**9 G**		**17 G**		**17 G**
¾ c (185 ml) black bean soup	5 g	1 c (250 ml) minestrone soup	7 g	Sandwich with 2 slices whole-grain bread, 2 tbsp (30 ml) peanut butter, and 1½ tbsp (22 ml) jam	15 g
3 whole wheat crackers	2 g	4 rye crackers	1 g	1 carrot	1 g
¼ c (60 ml) guacamole	1 g	1 orange or other fruit	1 g	¾ c (185 ml) orange or grape juice	1 g
½ c (125 ml) raw vegetables strips	1 g	1 c fortified soy milk	7 g		
		2 fig bars	1 g		
SUPPER	**13**		**18 G**		**22 G**
¾ c (185 ml) pasta	6 g	1 tortilla	1–3 g	1 veggie burger	8–18 g
¼ c (60 ml) vegan pesto sauce or tomato sauce with 2 tbsp (30 ml) cooked lentils	3 g	¾ c (185 ml) refried beans	10 g	1 hamburger bun	4 g
¼ c (60 ml) green peas	2 g	⅓ avocado	1 g	¼ c (60 ml) lettuce, 2 slices red onion, 2 slices tomato, and 1 tbsp (15 ml) ketchup or relish	1 g
1 c (250 ml) fortified nondairy milk	1 g	¼ c (60 ml) chopped tomato, ¼ c (60 ml) chopped lettuce, and 1 tbsp (15 ml) salsa	1 g	½ c (125 ml) baked French fries or yam fries	2 g
1 c (250 ml) raspberries	1 g	¾ c (180 ml) fortified chocolate soy milk or strawberry soy yogurt	5 g	1 c (250 ml) fortified soy milk	7 g

44-POUND (20 kg) CHILD	PROTEIN (g)	62-POUND (28 kg) CHILD	PROTEIN (g)	80-POUND (36 kg) CHILD	PROTEIN (g)
SNACKS	3 G		8 G		11 G
1 c (250 ml) fortified nondairy milk	1 g	¼ c (60 ml) raisins or currants	1 g	¼ c (60 ml) walnuts	4 g
1 banana	1 g	1 tbsp (15 ml) sesame tahini and 1 tsp (5 ml) blackstrap molasses on 1 slice toast	6 g	1 c (250 ml) fortified soy milk	7 g
¼ c (60 ml) dried apricots or 2 cookies	1 g	½ c (125 ml) fruit juice	1 g	Water	
Water		Water		Water	
Total protein	34 g	Total protein	59 g	Total protein	68 g

Sources of data are listed in *Becoming Vegan: Comprehensive Edition*, by Brenda Davis and Vesanto Melina (Book Publishing Company, 2014).

Key: c = cup; g = gram; kg = kilogram; ml = milliliter; tbsp = tablespoon; tsp = teaspoon.

If you hope to make positive changes in local school meals, an important first step may be to gather a few allies, such as vegetarian-friendly teachers, school food service personnel, or other parents. You're more likely to be successful if you approach school food service staff positively, offering encouragement, praise for their efforts, and helpful ideas and input. Whether your initial overtures are welcomed or rebuffed, you'll be contributing to a widespread movement to improve the healthfulness of school meals and include entirely vegetarian options for those who want them. Visit the Vegetarian Resource Group online (vrg.org) and look at information under "Teens, Family, and Kids" and "Food Service." Another helpful resource is the Physicians Committee for Responsible Medicine (pcrm.org). At their site, do a search for "school lunch."

Teens

Vegetarian teens tend to be significantly better nourished than their nonvegetarian peers. Studies comparing teens at Adventist schools, where diets are predominantly vegetarian, with children in public schools found that BMI was lower among vegetarians, especially girls. In addition, vegetarian girls and girls who ate more soy foods started menstruating seven months later than nonvegetarian girls, on average. Later onset of menstruation is linked to longevity and lower risk of breast cancer. A study of Australian teens also found that vegetarians were leaner and had better cholesterol levels. Heights, hemoglobin levels, and activity levels were similar in the two groups. The one disadvantage noted for the predominantly vegetarian group was lower levels of vitamin B_{12}, something that can easily be changed by taking supplements.

The teen years can be challenging—a time when kids are asserting their independence and making more of their own choices. Nutrition-related issues can become an arena for conflict, but they can also facilitate shared learning for the whole family.

Some teens become vegan within nonvegan households. Their parents may be supportive if the teen is willing to eat a nutritionally adequate vegan diet. Even more helpful is if such teens are willing to prepare entrées to complement the meals the rest of the family eats. Typically, the items needed are protein-rich beans, peas, lentils, and veggie meats.

In contrast, in some vegan families, a teenager decides to experiment with being a meat eater. It's important to let teens make their own decisions, watching over them and loving them through the process. For parents, this is a time to learn lessons about boundaries and letting go.

Here are some of the common food-related concerns that may arise during adolescence. We'll take a closer look at a few of these issues in the rest of this chapter:

- The need for increased nutrients during a major growth spurt
- Rebellion about family food guidelines
- Disinterest or being uninvolved in food preparation
- Not prioritizing good nutrition
- Distress about skin problems, premenstrual syndrome (PMS), and weight
- Development of eating disorders
- A focus on sports

NOURISHING HEALTHY SKIN

As with many aspects of appearance, skin health can be a major issue during adolescence. A surge in sex hormones can enlarge and stimulate oil glands in the skin, particularly around the nose and on the neck, chest, and back. Some people produce more oil than others, and some people's skin is less efficient at clearing away discarded cells. The result can be acne and pimples. It's important to clean the skin gently and regularly with water and mild soap, to avoid oil-based cosmetics, and to keep the skin dry. Some teens find that certain foods, such as sweets, processed foods, artificially flavored beverages, and fried foods, can result in skin reactions.

Water is an important cleanser, inside the body as well as outside. It carries away toxins that are flushed out through the kidneys. Never underestimate the effectiveness of drinking 6 to 8 cups (1.5 to 2 liters) of water daily in promoting skin health. Fruits and vegetables help keep skin clear and healthy too, in part because they contain 80 to 95 percent water by weight, and also because they contribute vitamins and phytochemicals that directly nourish the skin. Carotenoid-rich yellow, orange, red, and green vegetables and fruits give a warm glow to the skin. All of this information may help convince teenagers who are struggling with skin issues to drink more water and eat more vegetables—practices that promote health in many ways.

PREMENSTRUAL SYNDROME

Some girls experience excruciating cramps and other unpleasant symptoms at the onset of menstruation. Here are some diet-related tips that may help.

- **Eat a low-fat, high-fiber vegan diet.** A diet of whole grains, beans, vegetables, and fruits, along with a vitamin B_{12} supplement, can reduce PMS, menstrual pain, water retention, and monthly weight gain. These benefits may be related to the impact of diet on hormone levels.

- **Eat plant foods rich in B vitamins.** Research has shown that thiamin and riboflavin can reduce pain and improve mood, and that these B vitamins are best obtained from food, not supplements. Fortunately, they are plentiful in whole grains, fortified cereals, nutritional yeast, legumes, soy foods, seeds, and nuts.

- **Include beneficial oils.** Overall, a PMS-prevention diet should be moderately low in fat. However, it's helpful to include omega-3 fatty acids, such as 2 tablespoons (30ml) of ground flaxseeds or 1/4 cup (60ml) of hempseeds or walnuts each day. One study found that borage oil and evening primrose oil didn't improve PMS symptoms, despite their reputation for doing so.

- **Get enough vitamin D.** A study of college-age women showed that those with better dietary intakes of vitamin D had lower rates of PMS. This may be related to improved calcium absorption and retention, or to impacts on hormones or neurotransmitters. Sunshine also might help.
- **Avoid alcohol and sugar.** According to one study, those who experience PMS tend to consume relatively high amounts of alcohol and sugar. However, the study didn't indicate whether PMS caused the pattern of consumption or the pattern of consumption caused the PMS. Anyone troubled by PMS might try avoiding alcohol and sugar for a cycle or two to see whether it has any effect.

CALCIUM, VITAMIN D, AND BONE BUILDING

The teen years are a key time for bone mineralization and achieving the healthy bone density that's crucial for helping stave off osteoporosis later in life. Unfortunately, vegan diets can be short on calcium. Good sources include fortified juices and nondairy beverages, greens with low oxalate levels (collard greens, kale, and napa cabbage), beans, blackstrap molasses, and figs. Also some corn tortillas are also high in calcium.

Outdoor activities can help teens build bone in at least two ways: First, weight-bearing exercise helps build bone. And second, sunlight helps the body produce vitamin D, which enhances calcium absorption. Higher vitamin D levels among girls aged nine to fifteen years who participate in high-impact sports are associated with fewer stress fractures.

EATING TOGETHER

Mealtimes can offer a special occasion for adolescents to share their day with other family members. Some teens spend much of their time in their bedroom listening to music, watching television, using the computer, or talking on the phone, emerging only when famished and perhaps returning to their room to eat. It's important to give teens responsibilities that keep them involved with the rest of the family, such as setting the table for dinner, washing dishes, baking, or preparing bag lunches. It's possible to largely respect their need for private time while also requiring them to spend a half hour with the family at dinner. As a bonus, studies show that teens who have regular meals with their families eat more fruits and vegetables than teens who don't.

Pregnant and nursing moms, babies, toddlers, and children all have special nutritional needs that are more than met by a well-planned, whole-foods vegan diet.

people older than sixty-five comprise another group with unique dietary concerns and needs. With a little understanding of aging's effects on nutritional needs and a little tweaking of diet, vegan seniors can healthfully coast through the golden years.

CHAPTER 12

The Prime of Life: Vegan Nutrition for Seniors

Of Americans older than sixty-five, almost half eat at least one vegetarian meal a week. About three in one hundred never consume animal flesh, and one in one hundred is vegan. Whatever led to their dietary shift, and whether it occurred early in life or more recently, they know that a nutritious diet of plant foods is a wise choice for anyone at any age.

Seniors need fewer calories, yet their requirements for certain nutrients, such as protein, calcium, and vitamins D and vitamin B_6, increase. In other words, they have to get more bang for their nutrition buck. What they eat really has to deliver.

Fortunately, a vegan diet delivers. Studies of older vegetarians, including vegans, indicate that their intakes of many minerals and vitamins are similar to or better than those of nonvegetarians. In addition, their body weight is more likely to be in the optimal range, and they're likely to live longer.

Changes with Age

As we age, our lean muscle tissue tends to shrink while our percentage of body fat typically increases. At age sixty, women have an average of 3.5 pounds (1.6kg) less muscle than they did at twenty. Men lose even more, with 7 pounds (3.2kg) less muscle at age sixty. The shift from muscle to fat occurs for a variety of reasons: changes in hormones or in your metabolic rate, and, most importantly, reduced physical activity. Loss of muscle mass and strength can set in motion a cascade of consequences that includes worsening of diseases, increased disability, malnutrition, and even death.

Our energy expenditure decreases throughout our lifetime from the age of nineteen. Each decade a man expends 100 fewer calories daily and a woman, 70 calories fewer. Many adults gain about 1 pound (450g) or so each year if they don't adjust their menus to eliminate some calories. Around the time of menopause, women often gain an extra 10 pounds (4.5kg) and experience greater loss of muscle mass. The end result of all of these factors is that among adults older than sixty-five years of age, one in three is obese.

Just the Facts

One in eight Americans is over the age of sixty years. Since 1900, the

percentage age sixty-five and older has tripled. Among sixty-five-year-olds, **39 percent are in excellent health and have an average life expectancy of 18.8 more years. Men living to age eighty-five can expect to live 5.7 additional years and women 6.8 additional years. In 2001, there were 48,000 people in the United States who were age one hundred years or more; eight years later, this number had risen to more than 64,000.**

This slippery slide from muscle to fat and excess weight isn't the only option open to us. We can counteract it with a vegan diet, by eating a little less every decade, by focusing on more nutritious foods with a higher protein content, and by exercising. Increasing physical activity has numerous benefits, including allowing us to eat a bit more scrumptious vegan food without getting fat.

Exercise and Fitness

Lack of exercise is a primary reason for needing fewer calories as we age. Fewer than 5 percent of adults get thirty minutes of daily physical activity, and even that amount declines with age. Keeping fit is as much a key to wellness as avoiding excess calories. Regular exercise promotes physical and psychological well-being and better sleep quality. It reduces the risk of disability and vulnerability to chronic diseases such as coronary heart disease, type 2 diabetes, metabolic syndrome, stroke, hypertension, loss of cognitive function, depression, and colon, breast, endometrial, and lung cancers. Regular physical activity can keep our muscles and bones strong, our metabolic rate up, and our weight in check, and it can also help prevent falls. A Texas study of adults with an average age of seventy showed that just forty-five minutes of walking on a treadmill daily improved blood flow and built muscle.

Of course, it's important to increase an exercise program gradually. With time, seniors should aim for an hour of exercise each day and include some weight-bearing exercise to maintain strong bones, such as walking, jogging, dancing, tennis, or hiking. To keep your heart strong, add swimming, water aerobics, cycling, or kayaking. To strengthen your muscles, include weight lifting, stair climbing, or everyday activities like carrying groceries or gardening. For flexibility and balance, also include yoga, tai chi, stretching, or Pilates for flexibility and balance.

Little things also help. Work on your balance to help preserve your cognitive function and prevent falls; for example, you might try standing on one foot while in the checkout line, at the bus stop, or washing dishes. Make exercise a fun and social event by inviting friends to join you on bike rides, walks, and hikes. Running around with your grandchildren and playing with the dog also count. Experiment and create an engaging fitness program that works well for you.

Keeping fit can also save you money. A California study of 424 older adults at risk for impaired mobility and diminished ability to walk safely and independently estimated that an eight-month to one-year physical activity program cost only $1,309 while preventing disability-related costs of $28,206 for the year. The program involved thirty minutes of activity a day in the gym or at home and included stretching.

Getting Enough Nutrients

As we age and ideally eat fewer calories and exercise more, we need to make sure we still get the protein, minerals, vitamins, and fiber that we need. In the following sections, we'll provide recommendations on how you can do just that.

PROTEIN

Many seniors, vegan or not, don't meet their protein needs, and this nutrient deserves special consideration. Protein requirements for seniors are at least as high as those for younger people, perhaps slightly higher. There are currently no separate dietary reference intakes for seniors, but many experts suggest 1 or 1.1g of protein per kilogram (2.2lb) of body weight daily as a goal. That works out to about 61 grams per day for a 135-pound (61kg) person, and 75 grams for a 165-pound (75kg) person, which translates to 15 to 20 grams of protein at each meal plus a couple of protein snacks.

Vegan protein has been shown to be more than sufficient in maintaining the muscle mass of seniors, even if they get slightly less protein than nonvegetarians. In a study of men ages sixty to seventy who were doing resistance training, researchers found that a soy-rich diet was as effective as one that emphasized beef for improving muscle strength and power, without the negative effects on cholesterol associated with beef consumption.

A vegan diet may be an advantage because excess protein from meat, poultry, and fish can worsen the decline in kidney function that some seniors experience. Adding protein powders based on soy, peas, pumpkin seeds, or rice to smoothies can be a simple way to increase protein intake. (For more on vegan sources of protein, see chapter 3 and table 11.3.)

IRON

Iron-deficiency anemia is common in seniors no matter what their diet. Low iron levels can be caused by a variety of conditions, including chronic bleeding in the gastrointestinal tract, dental problems, diminished sense of taste and smell, poor appetite, challenges in obtaining food or making meals, and poverty. Anemia can also result from chronic inflammation, chronic kidney disease, or insufficient dietary iron. Complications of anemia in the elderly include greater risk of mortality, cardiovascular disease, cognitive dysfunction, falls, fractures, longer hospitalizations, and reduced bone density.

Seniors don't need more iron than younger people. Senior women actually need less iron than women in their childbearing years, who lose iron during menstruation. The recommended intake for older vegan women and men is 14.4mg per day, a level that isn't difficult to reach, as many plant foods are rich in iron. In fact, vegetarians and vegans tend to have higher iron intakes than nonvegetarians. Plus, their higher vitamin C intake from fruits and vegetables enhances absorption of iron.

Foods rich in iron also tend to be excellent sources of protein and zinc. These include soy foods, hummus, peas, lentils, beans, fortified breakfast cereals, meat analogs, and whole grains. Dried apricots, raisins, dark chocolate, and blackstrap molasses are also good sources of iron. (For more information on iron see chapter 7.)

ZINC

A deficiency in zinc can result in poor wound healing, reduced immune function, and dermatitis in the elderly. Lack of zinc also affects our ability to taste, which can have an effect on appetite. Zinc deficiency can result from poor absorption of this mineral, physical stress, trauma, muscle wasting, and use of certain medications. Fortunately, deficiency problems seem to resolve once people get enough zinc: taste returns, dermatitis improves, and wounds heal more quickly. Zinc supplements can help, but they can interfere with the absorption of other minerals, so getting zinc from food or as part of a multi-vitamin-mineral supplement is preferable.

Foods high in zinc include oats, whole-grain products, fortified breakfast cereals, cashews, beans, peas, lentils, fortified meat analogs, soy foods, seeds, and seed butters. Pine nuts, pecans, wheat germ, and fresh and sun-dried tomatoes also are good sources of zinc. (For more information on zinc, see chapter 7.)

CALCIUM AND VITAMIN D

To maintain strong bones, we need a combination of nutrients—especially calcium, vitamin D, and protein—and we need more of these nutrients as we age.

The recommended intake for calcium increases from 1,000 to 1,200mg per day for people older than fifty. Some experts suggest it should be increased to 1,500mg per day after age sixty-five, since our ability to absorb calcium diminishes as we get older. Many adults find it challenging to obtain that much calcium from food. In that case, it's helpful to eat more foods fortified with calcium and take an optional supplement.

Vitamin D, which is required for the absorption of calcium, plays a role in regulating bone mass. It also plays an essential role in immune function and dental health. In addition, low levels of vitamin D are linked with excess weight gain in women sixty-five and older.

At age seventy, the recommended intake for vitamin D goes from 15mcg (600 IU) to 20mcg (800 IU). Many experts recommend more. Seniors with daily intakes of about 20mcg (800 IU), along with 1,000 to 1,200mg of calcium, have less risk of falling and fractures than those who get less. Maintaining an adequate level of vitamin D may even help you live longer.

As we age, vitamin D production in the skin, liver, and kidney becomes less efficient. At seventy, vitamin D production is only 25 percent of what it was at age twenty-five. Seniors may want to have their vitamin D level checked periodically to determine whether they should be taking supplements.

Other nutrients also help keep our bones strong. One key nutrient is vitamin K, found in leafy green vegetables. Adding just 2 tablespoons (30ml) of kale to a smoothie or eating 1 cup (250ml) of romaine lettuce, 2 cups (500ml) of cabbage, or 1/2 cup (125ml) of broccoli a day will help maintain the complex protein-mineral structure of your bones.

The 1,600-calorie menu in chapter 14 provides approximately 2,000mg of calcium (depending on one's choice of calcium-set tofu) and the 2,000-calorie menu in chapter 14 provides about 1,300mg of calcium. (For more details on osteoporosis and bone health, see the section "Osteoporosis,".)

VITAMIN B^12

Vitamin B_{12} keeps nerves in good repair and helps rid the body of a troublesome by-product of metabolism called homocysteine. High homocysteine levels in the blood increase the likelihood of depression, heart attack, and stroke and may heighten the risk of dementia. Vitamin B_{12} is needed for a healthy nervous system; confusion, disorientation, and memory loss can be symptoms of a shortage of this vitamin. In such cases, if the deficiency is recognized and reversed soon enough, these symptoms often go away.

Other signs of deficiency include fatigue, depression, irritability, mood swings, restlessness, apathy, insomnia, and perhaps poor hearing. Lack of vitamin B_{12} is linked to megaloblastic anemia and DNA damage that can increase susceptibility to cancer. In vegetarians whose vitamin B_{12} levels are below normal, supplementation has been shown to improve arterial function and reduce the risk of atherosclerosis.

Our ability to absorb B_{12} often decreases as we age due to decreases in stomach acid and other factors. A deficiency of this vitamin can also result from intestinal surgery, thyroid problems, use of nitrous oxide during medical procedures, or use of laxatives, antacids, or alcohol.

The recommended daily intake of vitamin B_{12} for adults is 2.4mcg per day. Although you might think vegan seniors are especially at risk for deficiency, most vegans are accustomed to using supplements and foods fortified with B_{12} and continue to do so as they get older. The form of vitamin B_{12} in fortified foods is readily absorbed, even by those with diminished stomach acid. As a result, vegan seniors are able to get plenty of absorbable B_{12}. (For more details on vitamin B_{12}, see chapter 6.)

ANTIOXIDANTS

Vitamins A, C, and E and the mineral selenium provide powerful protection against free radical damage. Antioxidants are linked to a reduced risk of heart disease, cataracts, macular degeneration, various forms of cancer, and even wrinkles. The high concentrations of antioxidants in vegetables and fruits give vegans a considerable advantage. With all of the carotenoid-rich yellow, orange, red, and green plant foods in their diets, vegetarians have a significantly reduced risk of developing cataracts, and vegans have even less risk. In one study, nonvegetarians who changed to a low-fat vegan diet for fourteen or twenty-two weeks markedly improved their intakes of vitamins A and C (along with folate, magnesium, potassium, and fiber). Vitamin E intakes were better than those of people on nonvegetarian diets, although they were still slightly low, which is to be expected if a diet is low in fat. Including some higher-fat foods, such as avocado, seeds, nuts, and olives or olive oil, can help ensure adequate vitamin E intake.

Older people may have dental problems that cause them to shy away from fresh vegetables and fruits. However, soft cooked fruits, cooked vegetables, and freshly squeezed or bottled juices can take the place of foods that are more difficult to chew while still delivering plenty of protective nutrients. Baked sweet potatoes and winter squash are comforting, easy to eat, and rich in vitamin A, as are fresh or frozen mangoes and papaya. You may think of vitamin C primarily in relation to orange juice or citrus fruit, but you can get your recommended intake for the day from 1 cup (250ml) of cooked potato plus 1/2 cup (125ml) of cooked broccoli. And when it comes to selenium, you can get an adequate amount just by eating a big Brazil nut every other day. (For more details about vitamins A, C, and E, see chapter 6. For more information on selenium, see chapter 7.)

VITAMIN B^6 (PYRIDOXINE)

One vitamin that people need slightly more of as they age is vitamin B_6. This vitamin, which is abundant in many fruits, is involved in amino acid metabolism and building hemoglobin. That's just one of several good reasons to be sure to eat four servings of fruit per day, as recommended in chapter 14. There are plenty of other vegan sources of vitamin B_6, including avocado, fortified breakfast cereals, legumes, nutritional yeast, nuts, seeds, spinach, and whole grains. (For more information on vitamin B_6, see section entitled "Vitamin B_6 (Pyridoxine)")

FIBER, FLUIDS, AND INTESTINAL HEALTH

Dietary fiber comes from plant foods, so a vegan diet is a great help in avoiding constipation and staying regular. The fiber in legumes, whole grains, vegetables, and fruits keeps waste and toxins moving on and out through the intestine and helps maintain a good mix of intestinal bacteria and stable blood sugar levels. Because vegans typically consume plenty of fiber, they are advised to avoid adding wheat bran to foods, since it can compromise mineral absorption. And as healthful as whole, unprocessed plant foods are, seniors who are frail or have poor appetites may benefit from including some refined grains in the diet to help increase calorie intake.

Many seniors are susceptible to dehydration. The sense of thirst may become less acute as we get older, and infections and certain medications can also affect hydration. In addition, the kidneys become less adept at concentrating urine as people age, resulting in more frequent trips to the bathroom. Unfortunately, fear of incontinence leads some older people to drink less water and other fluids. However, it's important to keep beverages handy and sip on them often, emphasizing beverages that are calorie-free or low in added sugars, such as water, fortified nondairy milks, and herbal teas. Another way to increase hydration is by eating more fruits and vegetables; many are more than 90 percent water.

Raw Food for Seniors

The exciting world of raw vegan foods has a lot to offer seniors, particularly in terms of blended vegetable soups. See the books *Becoming Raw,* by B. Davis and V. Melina (Book Publishing Company, 2010), or the *Raw Food Revolution Diet,* by C. Soria, B. Davis, and V. Melina (Book Publishing Company, 2008) for a number of delicious and nutrient-rich soups, sauces, and pâtés

based on pureed vegetables, seeds, and nuts.

Planning Senior Meals

For planning meals and menus, The Vegan Plate is a helpful guide. For many people, the minimum servings from each food group will provide enough calories. In general, emphasize legumes and vegetables for a diet rich in protein and a wide variety of vitamins and minerals. Fruit is important for its potassium content. Seniors often find that three servings from the grains group are sufficient, and this approach tends to be ideal for those who want to lose weight. Nuts, seeds, and their butters provide important minerals, and the fat they contain promotes absorption of protective phytochemicals, minerals, and fat-soluble vitamins.

Although seniors need a highly nutritious diet, certain practical factors interfere with this. Chewing, swallowing, and digesting food and absorbing nutrients may be impaired for a variety of reasons. Poor oral health, loss of teeth, ill-fitting dentures, and other dental problems can make chewing difficult. Changes in the stomach and intestinal lining can affect digestion and nutrient absorption. Fortunately, a vegan diet has advantages in these regards.

Even without intending to be vegan, some elderly people are motivated to switch from meat to tofu because tofu is easier to chew and swallow. Tofu can easily be incorporated into fruit smoothies, providing a tasty and easily consumed source of protein, iron, zinc, calcium, and numerous other nutrients. If the smoothie includes mango, orange juice, or strawberries, it will also be an excellent source of vitamins A and C. Seasoned or marinated tofu can also be the centerpiece of lunch and dinner menus.

As mentioned, despite how healthful whole grains are, for some seniors products made with refined grains, such as enriched white bread or rolls, couscous, and white rice may be a good choice because they're easier to chew. Plus, most vegan diets provide so much fiber in vegetables, fruits, legumes, nuts, and seeds that using some refined products is nutritionally acceptable, especially for seniors. That said, some whole grains are easy to chew and swallow, such as quinoa and oatmeal.

By the age of seventy, people have just 30 percent of the taste buds they had as young adults. Zinc helps maintain that sensation of taste, so seniors should be sure to consume foods that are rich in zinc, such as cashews, seeds, nut and seed butters, legumes, soy foods, and whole grains. A huge downside to loss of taste and smell is that people often pile on salt to make food more flavorful. However, excess sodium can increase the risk of hypertension and contribute to heart disease, stroke, and kidney disease. If a diminished sense of taste is an issue, flavor foods with herbs, spices, lemon juice, and other low-sodium seasonings.

Maintain Your Brain

Older adults with higher intakes of antioxidants from foods are likely to have less cognitive decline and less degenerative disease. In addition to eating antioxidant-rich foods, getting sufficient omega-3 fatty acids, exercising your body and mind, and taking supplemental vitamin B$_{12}$ and DHA (docosahexaenoic acid) can help protect brain function. (For more information on omega-3 fatty acids, see chapter 4.)

EASY MEALS

Loss of appetite can be related to sensory loss, poor health, diminished cognitive status or isolation. You may have enjoyed food preparation when you could shop for interesting ingredients or when you were cooking for others but lost interest after becoming more homebound or cooking for only one. Perhaps physical disabilities, loss of mobility, or lack of transportation make it a real challenge to put together a meal. Poor eyesight can make it hard to read package directions, and limited hand strength or coordination can make opening packages a challenge. To help with these challenges, here are some meal ideas and kitchen tips that can help you put together simple, easy to chew, affordable, appealing meals that also deliver good nutrition.

BREAKFAST

- Bagel, toast, or soft bread with nut butter, sesame tahini, or blackstrap molasses, accompanied by fresh fruit
- Hot cereal or fortified ready-to-eat cereal with fruit, nuts, seeds, and fortified nondairy milk
- Scrambled tofu with sautéed onions, garlic, spinach, mushrooms, peppers, or other vegetables, seasoned with nutritional yeast, turmeric, or other seasonings, accompanied by rye toast and fresh fruit or juice
- Smoothie made with fresh or frozen blueberries, banana, hempseeds, and tofu or protein powder

LUNCH AND DINNER

- Baked potato with steamed broccoli and chickpeas, drizzled with Liquid Gold Dressing and sprinkled with toasted sunflower or pumpkin seeds
- Baked yam with black beans and steamed kale

- Baked tofu with barbecue sauce, green salad, and steamed yam
- Canned low-sodium soup with beans, peas, or lentils, with added chopped greens of your choice
- Canned low-sodium baked beans or chili atop baked sweet potato, with a spinach salad
- Veggie burger with baked potato wedges and green beans
- Vegan pizza and green salad
- Tacos made with soft tortillas, refried beans, avocado, lettuce, and salsa
- Hummus, crackers, and raw vegetables
- Flavored rice mix with veggies, peas, beans, or edamame
- Soup with dip and raw vegetables sticks or crackers
- Marinated three-bean salad and soup
- Pasta with prepared sauce and lentils
- Pasta with prepared sauce, greens, and chickpeas
- Peanut butter or nut butter and banana sandwich
- Quinoa with chopped veggies and lima beans
- Vegetable stir-fry with seasoned or baked tofu on brown rice
- Sandwich of avocado and tomato slices and vegan meat (optional) on wholegrain bread

PREP TIPS

- Add cashews to vegetable soups and blend for a creamy texture. (Blended cashews thicken when heated.)
- Add cubes of tofu to soups to enhance nutrition; for a creamy texture, blend the tofu into the soup.
- Bake a variety of root vegetables at the same time, for example, potatoes and yams. You could also bake tofu with barbecue sauce, peanut sauce, or another sauce at the same time. Then you can quickly put together tasty meals based on these ingredients for days.
- Mix crumbled tofu with vegan mayonnaise and your favorite seasonings for a sandwich filling.
- Dried beans are economical, and soaking them for a few hours and then discarding the soaking water before cooking will reduce flatulence. Cook beans in quantity and freeze them in smaller portions. If using canned beans, be sure to rinse them well to remove some of the sodium, or just buy a lowsodium variety.
- Eat ripe soft fruits such as papayas, peaches, nectarines, mangoes, pears, bananas, melons, kiwifruit, and berries.
- Bake or stew fruit.
- Grate harder fruits, such as apples, for salads.

- Substitute quinoa for rice or other whole grains in a variety of dishes. It's higher in protein and minerals than other grains and cooks in only fifteen minutes. Be sure to rinse the quinoa before cooking.
- Invest in a good juicer. Fresh juices are an excellent way to get lots of nutrients that are easily absorbed.
- To prevent spoilage, keep bread in the freezer. Remove a slice or two at a time for toast or a sandwich.
- Keep some canned fruits and vegetables in the pantry for easy snacks and side dishes or for adding to recipes.
- Make large batches of hearty soups or stews and freeze in smaller portions.
- Mild curry paste adds a superb blend of flavors to cooked lentils and beans.
- Order Chinese take-out, such as vegetables, tofu, and rice, and get enough for leftovers.
- Red lentils, which take just fifteen to twenty minutes to cook, are a great source of iron, protein, and zinc. They can be added to tomato sauce, other sauces, and soups.
- See the 1,600-, 2,000-, and 2,500-calorie menus in chapter 14 and adapt these to your preferences.
- Slice kale into thin strips or chop it in a food processor, then add it to salads.

- Well-cooked vegetables may be easier to eat: try soft-cooked squash, yams, sweet potatoes, zucchini, eggplant, potatoes, and other veggies.

Other Challenges

Declining health and other age-related challenges can have an impact on how well nourished an elderly person is. One issue is medications that can affect nutrient status. For example, proton pump inhibitors, which are prescribed for peptic ulcers and gastroesophageal reflux disease, are linked with deficiencies of calcium and other nutrients, and also with certain infections.

Digestive difficulties, swallowing problems, hypertension, and other disease conditions can all require dietary modifications. Unfortunately, discussion of these issues is beyond the scope of this book. However, we can recommend a few resources. A helpful book for those with diabetes or metabolic syndrome is *Defeating Diabetes,* by B. Davis and T. Barnard, MD (Book Publishing Company, 2003). And, because 52 percent of people older than sixty-five have some form of arthritis, you may be interested to know that a raw vegan diet has proven helpful for some people with rheumatoid arthritis and some with fibromyalgia. (For more on rheumatoid arthritis.) You might also be interested in *Bravo: Health-Promoting Meals from the TrueNorth Kitchen,* by R. Bravo, the skilled chef at TrueNorth Health

Center in California, a clinic that provides highly effective treatment for type 2 diabetes, hypertension, and rheumatoid arthritis using fasting and a vegan diet free of sugar, oil, and salt.

For healthy, delicious, and easy recipes, see the companion volume to this book, *Cooking Vegan*, by V. Melina and J. Forest (Book Publishing Company, 2012).

Senior Resources

Though our focus in this book is nutrition, other lifestyle factors also are key to good health in the senior years: regular exercise, loving relationships, a positive attitude, and a great sense of humor. Though these topics are outside of the nutrition realm, we'd like to share a few suggestions.

VEGETARIAN ASSOCIATIONS

More and more communities have lively vegetarian associations with members ranging from newborns to those dancing through the doors in their nineties. Those in wheelchairs are, of course, also welcome. If you're Internet-savvy, look for a local group by doing a search using the name of your town, state, or region plus the word "vegetarian" or "vegan." If you're less familiar with computers or need a little help, ask at your local library.

Vegetarian associations usually organize potluck dinners, meetings, and restaurant get-togethers on a regular basis, and sometimes put together food fairs and annual festivals. You may find these events a great place to meet like-minded people, begin new friendships, learn about cooking classes, and get involved as a volunteer. Vegetarian associations tend to be open to new ideas for outreach, including the creation of seniors support groups or local social networking.

From the comfort of your home, using a computer you can explore Meetups (meetup.com)—groups based on shared interests, such as vegan food or animalrights—and then see if you want to meet someone or a group in person. Internetdating may also be a reasonable way to meet potential partners or friends. A search using the words "vegan online dating" will quickly show you numerous vegan-friendly websites to explore.

TRAVEL TIP

Two websites that can help you find excellent vegan fare whether you are going to Paris, Prague, Portland, or Perth are happycow.net and vegdining.com. Clickon the continent you plan to visit, narrow your search down to the city, and thenprint the restaurants there that suit your fancy. Happycow also offers an app for mobile phones.

COMMUNITY SUPPORT

If you are housebound or have difficulty getting around or preparing meals, many supermarkets and some natural foods stores offer grocery delivery services. These can include delicious vegan items from the deli department. Food delivery programs such as Meals on Wheels often have vegetarian but not vegan options, although new services offering plant-based meals are beginning to make their mark. The Vegetarian Resource Group (vrg.org) has created afour-week menu cycle specifically for Meals on Wheels that is vegan and vegetarian. Encourage your local Meals on Wheels to participate in this program.

Through state and tribal agencies, the Senior Farmers' Market Nutrition Program provides low-income seniors (over age sixty) with coupons that can be exchanged for eligible fruits, vegetables, and fresh herbs at farmers' markets, roadside stands, and community-supported agriculture programs. The US Department of Health and Human Services Administration on Aging provides funding for nutrition education and home-delivered meals to low-income seniors through the Older Americans Act and the US Department of Agriculture's SNAP program, among others. These may include vegan menu items. In some areas, other meal programs are available that allow older people to meet in a central location to enjoy a meal in the company of others, often with transportation to the site being provided.

About 29 percent of older adults live alone, and some of these seniors would prefer to have a greater sense of community while continuing to have their own home. One approach that successfully addresses the problem of isolation while retaining the best aspects of independent living is cohousing. Cohousing is a type of collaborative housing in which residents actively participate in the design and operation of their own neighborhoods. Members often share meatless meals as more vegetarians and vegans join their communities. One book on this topic is *Senior Cohousing: A Community Approach to Independent Living,* by C. Durrett (New Society Publishers, 2009). Online information can be found at cohousing.org.

FOOD IN CARE FACILITIES

For those in search of a suitable care home for a vegan or vegetarian, whether yourself or a loved one, consider checking into those run by Seventh-day Adventists. These health-oriented folks have expertise in providing nutritious, delicious, and varied vegetarian meals. A local Seventh-day Adventist church can probably help you find a facility.

For short-term care, be aware that Seventh-day Adventist hospital cafeterias provide vegetarian and vegan meals. And in Portland,

Oregon, great progress has been made in creating a hospital restaurant that is entirely vegan, the Living Well Bistro.

You may be pleasantly surprised to find that some nursing homes and assisted living facilities are willing and able to accommodate a vegan or vegetarian senior, especially if you help the busy workers figure out practical solutions to the challenge of providing suitable entrées along with their main menu. One resource on quantity cooking at care facilities is *Vegan in Volume: Vegan Quantity Recipes for Every Occasion,* by N. Berkoff (Vegetarian Resource Group, 2000).

VEGAN AND VEGETARIAN DIET SPECIALISTS

Dietetic associations in the United States, Canada, the United Kingdom, Europe, and Australia list dietitians who specialize in vegetarian and vegan nutrition and nutritional aspects of disease. They can be contacted through the association's website. The Academy of Nutrition and Dietetics has a strong vegetarian dietary practice group (vegetariannutrition.net) with a link for "Find an RD" (registered dietitian) as well as numerous online resources.

Keeping fit is of tremendous value at any age. Whether you're a long-distance runner, an endurance athlete, or just someone who likes to go to the gym a few

times a week, a vegan diet can see you through your active lifestyle. Learn how, in chapter 13.

CHAPTER 13

The Fit Vegan

Exercise generates energy and vitality. it improves brain function, boosts mood, reduces stress, strengthens bones, enhances metabolism and the production of hormones, supports immune function, and reduces the risk of chronic diseases, such as diabetes, heart disease, and cancer.

Fit vegans are among the most persuasive ambassadors of a vegan lifestyle. Without saying a single word, they tell the world that it isn't necessary to eat chickens, pigs, or cows to be fit—to run fast, jump high, or be strong. Their contributions are immeasurable because, without this reassurance, many people wouldn't give a vegan lifestyle a second thought. A fit vegan will essentially silence the naysayers.

You don't have to be an elite athlete to serve as an example; just make exercise a priority in your daily life. It doesn't matter so much what type of exercise you choose, as long as you do something. As your fitness level improves, so will your health. Those around you will notice.

In this chapter, we'll consider the ins and outs of exercise for everyone, from sedentary individuals to elite, competitive athletes. We'll examine the benefits of exercise, review the research regarding vegan fitness, provide guidelines regarding exercise for nonathletes, and then dive into the world of competitive sports and how vegans can maximize their athletic performance.

The Endless Benefits of Exercise

Being fit allows us to live life to its fullest. Fitness dramatically improves health and gives us the freedom to pursue all of our goals.

Exercise isn't a luxury or self-indulgence. It is a necessity, just like eating, sleeping, and breathing. The human body is built to move. If you hope to achieve optimal health, exercise isn't an option; it's an imperative. If you're at all skeptical, consider the top ten benefits of exercise:

1. **Exercise reduces the risk of death and disease.** Recent research puts inactivity on par with smoking and obesity as a leading cause of death. Inactivity increases sick days, doctor's visits, hospitalizations, and use of medications. Even moderate physical activity substantially reduces the risk of heart disease, stroke, high blood pressure, type

2 diabetes, metabolic syndrome, osteoporosis, several forms of cancer, and many other medical conditions. Exercise increases insulin sensitivity, reduces bad cholesterol (LDL), boosts good cholesterol (HDL), lowers blood pressure, and improves gastrointestinal function, balance, coordination, and lung function.

2. **Exercise boosts immunity.** People who exercise regularly don't get sick as often as those who are inactive. (However, high-intensity exercise can increase the risk of infection. The theory is that the body is so busy trying to repair tissue damage caused by extreme exercise that it's less able to defend against attackers.)

3. **Exercise suppresses inflammation.** Chronic inflammation increases insulin resistance, atherosclerosis, nerve degeneration, and tumor growth. Regular moderate exercise reduces inflammation. Precisely how physical activity accomplishes this task isn't known, but exercise does increase levels of antiinflammatory compounds in the body. It also reduces visceral fat (fat in and around vital organs), decreasing the release of proinflammatory molecules.

4. **Exercise sharpens the mind.** Physical activity, particularly aerobic exercise, may be among the most powerful protectors of the brain and nervous system. Exercise increases oxygenation and blood flow to brain tissue, boosts chemicals associated with improved cognition, and enhances growth factors responsible for the production and preservation of nerve cells. It can also augment cognitive function in seniors and reduce the risk of developing dementia and Alzheimer's disease.

5. **Exercise increases happiness.** Physical activity promotes the release of endorphins, brain chemicals that act as natural antidepressants and pain relievers—and that give people the famous runner's high. Levels of endorphins and other beneficial brain chemicals remain elevated for several days following exercise, increasing happiness and decreasing stress. Exercise may also be an effective treatment for depression.

6. **Exercise improves your sex life.** Regular physical activity stimulates blood flow, reduces the risk of erectile dysfunction, improves endurance, and boosts energy. It also incites hormonal changes that increase libido, promote relaxation, and reduce

performance anxiety. Of course, being fit also boosts self-confidence and sex appeal.

7. **Exercise helps control weight.** Exercise burns calories, boosts metabolism, and promotes energy balance. Of course, this varies with the duration and intensity of physical activity. Even without an exercise program, you can increase your level of physical activity simply by taking the stairs instead of the elevator, walking more briskly, or doing simple household chores more vigorously.

8. **Exercise improves sleep.** Exercise can promote falling asleep more quickly and sleeping more deeply. While this may be because exercise is tiring, being physically active also enhances mood, reduces anxiety, and increases serotonin production—all of which promote good sleep. One caveat: For some people, exercising late in the evening or close to bedtime can be stimulating and interfere with sleep.

9. **Exercise enhances energy and endurance.** Physical activity strengthens muscles, builds bones, makes the heart work more efficiently, boosts lung capacity, and increases balance and coordination. It ensures that sufficient oxygen and nutrients are delivered to cells throughout the body.

Being fit makes everything easier: shopping, housecleaning, gardening, playing with your children or grandchildren, walking with a friend or neighbor, and so much more.

10. **Exercise improves appearance and well-being.** Regardless of a person's age, gender, and physical ability, exercise tones muscles, reduces cellulite, and enhances complexion and skin health. Exercise also improves posture, strength, energy, and self-esteem. A fit body is a huge confidence booster. Fitness also decreases anxiety, making life more enjoyable.

Getting Fit and Staying Fit

With so many obvious benefits to exercise, it seems strange that an estimated 60 percent of Americans don't do it. While it's tempting to chalk that up to laziness, inactivity is more likely about missed opportunities, the lack of social support systems, time constraints, conveniences, fears, and insecurities. If you don't exercise regularly, now is the time to make it a real priority. It doesn't matter how old you are, how coordinated you are, or how busy you are, you have the potential to get fit. In the following sections, we'll give you the information you need to get started.

TYPES OF EXERCISE

You may wonder what type of exercise is best. The answer is simple: the type of exercise you'll do consistently. Choose activities that are reasonably accessible to you and that you enjoy. You want exercise to be something you look forward to. If you have a family, select some activities that you can all enjoy together.

While all forms of exercise afford health benefits, there are three main types of exercise: aerobic activity, resistance training, and flexibility exercises. A well-rounded exercise program that features all three types is ideal for optimum fitness.

Aerobic activity. Aerobic, or cardio, activity is any physical activity that utilizes your large muscle groups to get your heart and lungs working harder than they do when you're sedentary. This type of exercise is especially important for endurance, circulation, and heart health. Examples include jogging, brisk walking, bicycling, swimming, skating, climbing stairs, cross-country skiing, and jumping rope.

Resistance training. Resistance or strength training is any physical activity that builds, strengthens, firms, and tones your muscles. This type of exercise helps improve bone density, balance, and coordination. Examples include push-ups, lunges, pull-ups, and any exercise that uses free weights or a weight machine.

Flexibility exercises. Flexibility exercises are activities that improve your range of motion and lengthen your muscles. They can help reduce stiffness, aches, and pains. Examples include yoga, Pilates, and stretching routines.

HOW MUCH TO EXERCISE

Any amount of exercise is better than none. However, to enjoy the maximum benefits, you need to work your way up to thirty to sixty minutes a day. The following exercise guidelines are adapted from the US government's Physical Activity Guidelines for Americans.

Children and adolescents: Children and adolescents need one hour or more of exercise per day. At least three days a week should include vigorous activity, and at least three days should include strength training.

Adults (ages eighteen to sixty-four): Adults should get 2.5 to 5 hours per week of moderate intensity activity, or 1.25 to 2.5 hours of vigorous exercise. At least two days should include strength training for all muscle groups.

Older adults (ages sixty-five and older): Follow the guidelines for adults if possible; if not, just be as active as your abilities allow. Include exercises that maintain or improve balance and do some resistance training with light weights.

Disabled: Those who are disabled should follow the guidelines for their age group as much as their disability permits.

Pregnancy and postpartum: Healthy pregnant women who haven't been doing vigorous exercise should get at least 2.5 hours of moderately intense aerobic exercise per week. Women who regularly engage in vigorous aerobic activity can continue during pregnancy if this is approved by their health care provider.

CREATING AN EXERCISE PROGRAM

To maintain a high level of fitness, it's best to exercise daily or almost daily. If you can't imagine setting aside thirty to sixty minutes a day for exercise, start by taking ten minutes and build from there. If you gradually increase the duration, frequency, and intensity of your workouts, your fitness goals will seem easier to achieve, and you'll also reduce your chances of injury. Table 13.1 provides a sample weekly fitness plan that meets the preferred guidelines for a healthy adult. Of course, you can substitute activities of your choice.

TABLE 13.1. Sample weekly fitness schedule

DAY	ACTIVITY	DURATION	TYPE OF EXERCISE
Monday	Jog or brisk walk	30 to 60 minutes	Aerobic
	Stretch	10 minutes	Flexibility
Tuesday	Bike ride	30 minutes	Aerobic
	Free weights	20 minutes	Resistance
	Stretch	10 minutes	Flexibility
Wednesday	Yoga	60 minutes	Resistance and flexibility
Thursday	Swim	30 minutes	Aerobic
	Free weights	20 minutes	Resistance
	Stretch	10 minutes	Flexibility
Friday	Yoga	60 minutes	Resistance and flexibility
Saturday	Jog or brisk walk	30 to 60 minutes	Aerobic
	Stretch	10 minutes	Flexibility
Sunday	Rest day		

WHEN TO EXERCISE

When to exercise depends entirely on your body clock, your schedule, and your personal preferences. There's no universally applicable "best" time. If you wake up bright-eyed and bushy-tailed, you may enjoy exercising early in the day. If you aren't a morning person, it may be best for you to exercise in the late afternoon or early evening. Some evidence indicates that endurance and strength are at their peak in the late afternoon when body temperature is high and muscles are warm, so exercising at this time may reduce the risk of injury.

If you can't exercise when you most feel like it because of work or family commitments or other schedule issues, know that your body clock is adjustable and a different time may eventually work well for you. If your schedule is so busy that you can't spare thirty to sixty minutes for exercise, you may find that you're able to manage shorter blocks of ten to twenty minutes two or three times a day.

The Vegan Athlete

Whether you aspire to be a world-class competitor or are a recreational athlete aiming to improve your performance, rest assured that a varied and well-planned vegan diet can provide all of the nutrients you need to meet your goals. Some people insist that vegan diets provide a competitive edge, particularly when it comes to endurance sports, while others argue that they put athletes at a disadvantage, especially when it comes to strength. Despite these strong opinions, studies suggest that plant-based diets are neither particularly beneficial nor detrimental to athletic performance. Of course, well-planned vegan diets are associated with a reduction in risk for chronic diseases, and that may translate into health advantages in the long term.

The bottom line is, vegan diets can and do support optimal performance in athletes when they are well designed. Consider just a small sampling of the world-class athletes who are vegan:

- **Patrik Baboumian.** Strongman; European champion in powerlifting, setting two world records in the 125 to 140kg (275 to 310 pound) category. Winner of the German loglift championships; record holder for fronthold and keg lift.

- **Brendan Brazier.** Professional Ironman triathlete; winner of the Canadian 50-kilometer (31-mile) ultramarathon in 2003 and 2006.
- **Mac Danzig.** American mixed martial artist (MMA), with titles including MMA national amateur MMA champion, Gladiator Challenge lightweight champion, International Fighting Championships lightweight champion, five-time King of the Cage world lightweight champion, and *The Ultimate Fighter* season six winner.
- **Steph Davis.** Rock climber; only woman to have free-soloed at the 5.11+ grade; featured in an extreme sport film climbing the Mineral Canyon in Utah, and appeared on the March 2013 cover of *Climbing* magazine.
- **Ruth Heidrich.** Triathlete champion; winner of more than nine hundred gold medals for marathons, ultramarathons, other running events, and triathlons; set three world fitness records in her age group; named one of the top ten fittest women in North America in 1999 at the age of sixty-four (others were in their twenties and thirties).
- **Scott Jurek.** American ultramarathon champion; winner of multiple elite ultrarunning titles, including the US record for twenty-four-

hour distance on all surfaces—165.7 miles (266.7km), equal to 6.5 marathons in one day; the 153-mile (246km) Spartathlon; the 100.5-mile (161.7km) Hardrock 100; the 135-mile (217km) Badwater Ultramarathon; the Miwok 100K; and the 100-mile (161km) Western States Endurance Run, which he won seven times in a row; also named one of the top runners of the decade by the *Washington Times*; deemed a "hero of running" by *Runner's World*; named ultrarunner of the year three times by *Ultrarunning Magazine*.

- **Georges Laraque.** Retired Canadian professional NHL hockey player; at 6 feet 3 inches (1.9 meters) and 260 pounds (118kg), one of the toughest guys in the league.
- **Fiona Oakes.** Marathon runner and firefighter; winner of several international marathons; personal best marathon time of 2 hours and 28 minutes.
- **John Salley.** Retired professional basketball player; first player in NBA history to win a championship with three different franchises.

Fueling Peak Performance for Athletes

There are four main factors that drive athletic performance: genetics, training, diet, and drive. While there isn't much you can do about genetics, the other factors are largely up to you. Each of these variables can be exploited to provide a competitive edge. Diet alone can't guarantee athletic success, but enriching the fuel that sustains your physical activity will improve your efficiency. This can make a critical difference when a win or loss is determined by a split second. Of course, a deficient diet can undermine even the most consistent and determined athletic effort. The key to fueling peak performance is consuming a healthful balance of all the necessary nutrients and meeting your energy needs.

ENERGY TO BURN

There are two main sources of energy that fuel muscles: carbohydrates and fat. These fuels are readily available in the bloodstream from the foods you consume and from your body stores. Glucose, or blood sugar, is stored as glycogen and provides about 5 percent of your stored energy reserves. The lion's share of your stored fuel is fat, and most people have enough to last for many hours or even days of exercise.

The fuel of choice for your muscles depends on the type, intensity, and duration of the activity and your fitness level. During the first few minutes of exercise, the body relies almost exclusively on carbohydrates for energy. As exercise continues, more fats are used. Within about twenty or thirty minutes of activity, the body uses about half carbohydrates and half fats. If you continue with low- to moderate-intensity exercise, you'll use mostly fat for fuel. If you continue with high-intensity exercise, you'll use mostly carbs because your body can't metabolize fat fast enough to provide all the energy needed for more demanding activities.

THE AEROBIC AND ANAEROBIC SYSTEMS

Any exercise that uses large muscle groups over an extended period of time is an aerobic, or cardio, activity. Examples include running, swimming, biking, cross-country skiing, rowing, hiking, and canoeing. Aerobic refers to forms of exercise that train the heart, lungs, and cardiovascular system to process and deliver oxygen more quickly and efficiently to every part of the body. As a result, a fit person can exercise longer and more vigorously and recovers more quickly at the end of an aerobic session.

When your heart and lungs can't provide your muscles with sufficient oxygen for aerobic activities, your body switches to anaerobic metabolism to generate energy. During anaerobic metabolism, the body uses only glucose, not fat as fuel. The anaerobic system prevails in the first two or three minutes of exercise or when activity is so intense that the body's intake of oxygen can't keep up with energy demands. This occurs in speed sports, such as sprinting and other quick track events, short-distance swim races, basketball, hockey, volleyball, football, baseball, lacrosse, and speed skating. It also occurs in power sports involving sudden intense movements, such as weight lifting, bodybuilding, field events (throwing and jumping disciplines), and wrestling.

MEETING ENERGY NEEDS OF ACTIVE VEGANS

Energy needs vary depending on body size, weight, composition, metabolism, gender, age, and the amount and type of physical activity, and generally range between 2,000 and 6,000 calories a day. For casual fitness buffs who exercise a few times a week, calorie needs increase only slightly, if at all. Elite endurance athletes, on the other hand, such as ultramarathoner Scott Jurek, may need to eat 5,000 to 8,000 calories per day.

Getting enough calories is essential for optimal physical performance. The best indicators of adequate energy intake are body weight and composition. Eating more than you need increases body fat, which can compromise performance and endurance and cause injuries. If you don't eat enough calories, your body will use muscle protein for fuel, which can reduce muscle mass and endurance. Eating too little can also lower your metabolic rate, reduce the amount of energy available for exercise, and compromise your nutritional, immune, and endocrine status. This is of particular concern for women (see "The Female Athlete Triad,"). In young athletes, insufficient energy intake can hinder growth and development.

It's entirely possible to take in a lot of calories on a vegan diet (see chapter 14 for sample high-calorie menus.) However, plant foods tend to be high in fiber and lower in calories, so it's important that vegan athletes with increased energy needs include plenty of energy-dense vegan options. You may find it easier to meet your energy needs by eating more frequent meals and snacks, and during heavy training, you may need to take advantage of every eating opportunity, including large snacks before bed. Great choices include smoothies, sandwiches, whole-grain cereal, grain and bean salads, stir-fries, healthful baked goods, bean soups and stews, seasoned tofu, nori rolls, avocados, trail mix, toast with nut butter, vegan power bars, nondairy yogurt with fruit and granola, and pasta dishes. If you find it difficult to consume enough calories, incorporating more foods in liquid form, such as smoothies, and some refined foods, such as pasta, may be helpful. You may need to introduce higher-fiber foods, such as legumes, gradually to minimize gastrointestinal discomfort. In addition, you may find it helpful to moderate your intake of very high fiber foods, as they are filling and may reduce the volume of food you are able to consume.

CARBOHYDRATES

Carbohydrates, discussed in detail in chapter 5, provide the primary fuel for active vegans and vegan athletes. Large intakes of carbs are associated with an improved capacity for exercise and larger stores of glycogen. Vegans may be at an advantage here, since both quantity and quality of carbohydrates tend to be high in plant-based diets. If you rely on whole plant foods (whole grains, vegetables, fruits, legumes, nuts, and seeds) as your primary sources of carbohydrates, they will also provide a healthful complement of protein, fat, vitamins, minerals, and phytochemicals—all of which contribute to peak performance.

The Female Athlete Triad

The female athlete triad is a syndrome that can arise in women who participate in sports that emphasize leanness. It's characterized by disordered eating, lack of menstruation, and osteoporosis and is more common in athletes involved in endurance sports, such as distance running, and aesthetic sports, such as dancing, gymnastics, swimming, and figure skating.

Those thought to be at greatest risk are athletes who restrict calories, limit the types of foods they eat, exercise for prolonged periods, or are vegetarian. The reason vegetarian diets are associated with increased risk may be that women often choose a vegetarian diet as a means of restricting calories. In addition, vegetarian diets that are very high in fiber and low in fat may promote fecal excretion of estrogens, reducing estrogen levels in the body.

Vegan female athletes need to be sure to eat sufficient calories, protein, iron, and zinc. Very lowcalorie diets—less than 1,500 calories per day—pose the greatest risk. In some cases, reducing fiber by replacing some legumes with tofu, some whole grains with refined grains, and some fruits and vegetables with fresh juices may be helpful.

Recommended carbohydrate intakes for athletes range from approximately 5 to 12 grams per kilogram (2.2lb) of body weight per day (g/kg/d). The amount depends on training needs. Table 13.2 provides guidelines suitable for all athletes. Table 13.3 lists a variety of foods or food combinations providing 50 grams of carbohydrates. The options that include refined foods may be more suitable as part of a pre-event meal (discussed in detail a bit later in the chapter).

TABLE 13.2. Carbohydrate needs for athletes

RECOMMENDED CARBOHYDRATE INTAKE (g/kg OF BODY WEIGHT)	ACTIVITY LEVEL
5–7 g/kg per day	Medium-duration, low-intensity training (60–90 minutes/day)
7–12 g/kg per day	Medium- to long-duration endurance training (1–3 hours/day)
10–12 g/kg per day	Extreme endurance training (4+ hours/day)

Source of data: International Olympic Committee, "IOC Consensus Statement on Sports Nutrition 2003" (2003), www.sfsn.ethz.ch/PDF/ IOC_Conseus2003.pdf.

TABLE 13.3. Vegan foods providing 50 grams of carbohydrate

FOOD	PORTION SIZE
Peanut butter and banana sandwich	2 slices bread, 2 tbsp (30 ml) peanut butter, 1 small banana (or ½ large)
Fruit smoothie	1 banana, 1 c (250 ml) soy milk, 1 scoop protein powder,* 1 c (250 ml) strawberries
Pea, lentil, or bean soup and bread	1¼ c (310 ml) pea, lentil, or bean soup, 1 large slice rye or other bread
Cereal, blueberries, and soy milk	1 oz (30 g) cold cereal, ¾ c (185 ml) blueberries, 1 c (250 ml) soy milk
Almond yogurt with apple and granola	1 c (250 ml) yogurt, 1 apple, ¼ c (60 ml) granola
Muffin with almond butter and orange juice	1 nutritious muffin, 1 tbsp (15 ml) almond butter, ½ c (125 ml) fresh orange juice
Power bar	1 commercial vegan power bar*
Pita bread and hummus	1 pita bread, ½ c (125 ml) hummus*
Brown rice with tofu and vegetables	¾ c (185 ml) rice with 2 c (500 ml) vegetables and 2 oz (60 g) tofu

Source of data: US Department of Agriculture, Agricultural Research Service, *USDA National Nutrient Database for Standard Reference*, Release 25 (2012), ndb.nal.usda.gov.

Key: c = cup; g = gram; ml = milliliter; oz = ounce; tbsp = tablespoon.

*Check labels for product-specific information.

FAT

In addition to being an important energy source, dietary fat provides essential fatty acids and is a carrier of fat-soluble vitamins (A, D, E, and K) and protective phytochemicals. After you meet your carbohydrate and protein needs, the remainder of your calories should come from healthy fat. For athletes, that usually translates to 20 to 35 percent of calories from fat.

Reducing fat intake below 20 percent won't enhance your athletic performance and isn't generally recommended. If you eat less than 15 percent of calories from fat, you may not have enough energy when you need it during training. In addition, for women this may cause exercise-related amenorrhea (ceasing of menstruation).

On the other hand, try not to exceed 35 percent of calories from fat, as this could result in insufficient intake of carbs and protein.

Vegan athletes should rely primarily on whole plant foods for fat because they also provide protein, carbs, and valuable vitamins, minerals, and phytochemicals. Excellent choices include nuts and seeds (and nut and seed butters, milks, and the like), avocados, olives, and soy foods. And although concentrated oils lack many of the essential nutrients provided by high-fat whole foods, these products can help athletes with high calorie requirements meet their energy needs; just be sure to select high-quality oils.

PROTEIN

A common notion among athletes, coaches, and trainers is that protein is the most vital nutrient, and the more the better. Some athletes hesitate to make the switch to a vegan diet because they've always heard that plants don't provide enough protein. Although athletes do need more protein, they can get plenty from a well-designed vegan diet.

Protein plays only a very small role as a fuel source for exercise. However, adequate protein is critical for maintenance of lean body tissue and exercise performance. Current research and recommendations by sports nutrition authorities indicate that 1g/kg/d is the minimum intake for vegan athletes. Endurance athletes should try to get 1.3 to 1.5g/kg/d, and those who focus on strength activities should aim for 1.3 to 1.9g/kg/d while building muscle.

The vegan athletes at greatest risk for inadequate protein intake are those who restrict their calories or eat fewer concentrated protein sources, such as legumes, tofu, tempeh, and veggie meats. It's important to consume good sources of protein at each meal. Vegans who have trouble eating enough protein may find it helpful to add vegan protein powder to smoothies. Table 13.4 lists foods that provide approximately 10 grams of protein per serving. Table 13.5 provides suggestions for boosting protein content of meals by replacing low-protein foods with higher-protein options. (For more ideas on how to boost protein consumption, see table 10.3, and table 11.3.)

TABLE 13.4. Vegan foods providing 10 grams of protein

FOOD	SERVING SIZE
Almonds	⅓ c (85 ml)
Black bean soup	⅔ c (160 ml)
Deli slices*	3 slices
Firm tofu	4 oz (120 g)
Hempseeds	3 tbsp (45 ml)
Hummus	½ c (125 ml)
Peanuts	⅓ c (85 ml)
Peas, raw	1¼ c (310 ml)
Power bar*	1
Pumpkin seeds	¼ c (60 ml)
Veggie burger (patty only)*	½–1

Sources of data: US Department of Agriculture, Agricultural Research Service, *USDA National Nutrient Database for Standard Reference, Release 25* (2012), ndb.nal.usda.gov. Manitoba Harvest, "Nutrients: Hemp Hearts" (2012, healing-source.com/about_HempHearts_b.htm#NUTRIENTS.

Key: c = cup; g = gram; ml = milliliter; oz = ounce; tbsp = tablespoon.

*Check labels for product-specific information.

TABLE 13.5. Suggestions for increasing the protein content of meals

INSTEAD OF:	CHOOSE:	PROTEIN GAINED (APPROX.)
BREAKFAST		
1½ c (375 ml) cornflakes, 1 c (250 ml) rice milk	1 c (250 ml) granola, 1 c (250 ml) soy milk	19 g
3 pancakes, 2 tbsp (30 ml) maple syrup	3 pancakes, 3 vegan sausages, ½ c (125 ml) cooked blueberries	14 g
LUNCH		
1½ c (375 ml) vegetable soup, 2 slices whole wheat toast with 2 tsp (10 ml) margarine	1½ c (375 ml) lentil soup, 2 slices whole wheat toast with 2 tbsp (30 ml) peanut butter	23 g
3 c (750 ml) green salad, 2 tbsp (30 ml) Italian dressing, 2 slices garlic bread	3 c green salad, 4 oz (120 g) grilled tofu, 2 tbsp (30 ml) tahini dressing, 2 slices multigrain Italian bread	13 g
DINNER		
2 c (500 ml) pasta, 1 c (250 ml) marinara sauce	2 c (500 ml) pasta, 1 c (250 ml) red lentil sauce	8 g
3 c (750 ml) vegetable curry, 1 c (250 ml) brown rice	3 c (750 ml) chickpea and vegetable curry, 1 c (250 ml) quinoa	15 g
SNACK		
2 c (500 ml) green smoothie with banana, blueberries, kale, and water	2 c (500 ml) green smoothie with banana, blueberries, kale, hemp protein powder, and water	20 g
2 oz (60 g) pretzels or popcorn	1 vegan power bar	6–14 g*

Sources of data: US Department of Agriculture, Agricultural Research Service, *USDA National Nutrient Database for Standard Reference*, Release 25 (2012), ndb.nal.usda.gov. Manitoba Harvest, "Nutrients: Hemp Hearts" (2012, healing-source.com/about_HempHearts_b.htm#NUTRIENTS.

Key: c = cup; g = gram; ml = milliliter; oz = ounce; tbsp = tablespoon; tsp = teaspoon.

*Check labels for product-specific information.

Vitamins and Minerals for Vegan Athletes

Not surprisingly, athletes' needs for vitamins and minerals are often higher than those of inactive people because these micronutrients play key roles in the body's use of fuel, carbs, fats, and protein. Vitamins and minerals are also important for immune function, production of hemoglobin, minimizing oxidative damage to the body, and the synthesis, maintenance, and repair of muscle and bone tissue. In addition, mineral status can have profound effects on performance.

Many people assume that athletes need to take vitamin and mineral supplements, but most athletes get enough vitamins and minerals from dietary sources as long as they eat enough food to ensure they have sufficient energy. This is also true for vegan athletes, with the exception of vitamin B_{12} and possibly riboflavin, vitamin D, iron, zinc, calcium, magnesium, and electrolytes.

Although not essential for all athletes, multivitamin-mineral supplements may be useful, especially for those who restrict energy intake or are dieting, have poorly planned diets or eating disorders, are pregnant or breast-feeding, or are recovering from injury. Otherwise, single-nutrient supplements can be used to address specific medical or nutritional challenges, such as iron deficiency. (For more details on specific vitamins and food sources, see chapter 6, and for minerals see chapter 7.)

VITAMIN B^12

Because B_{12} is lacking in whole plant foods, all vegans, including athletes, must rely on fortified foods or supplements to ensure adequate intake of this nutrient. Some athletes take B_{12} shots in an effort to boost oxygen delivery to tissues and enhance performance. While B_{12} shots can be highly effective for vegan athletes who have a deficiency, there's no evidence that athletes with good B$_{12}$ status benefit from them.

RIBOFLAVIN

The need for riboflavin increases with training due to its role in energy production. While most vegan diets provide ample riboflavin, vegan athletes who restrict caloric intake may not get enough, so it's important to include sufficient reliable sources of this nutrient, such as nutritional yeast, almonds, leafy greens, broccoli, asparagus, mushrooms, and fortified cereals.

VITAMIN D

In addition to its critical role in calcium absorption and bone health, vitamin D is directly involved in the formation and maintenance of the nervous system and skeletal muscles. Vegan athletes who consume few fortified foods, train indoors, or live in northern latitudes can probably benefit from a vitamin D supplement. Although the RDA for vitamin D is just 15mcg (600 IU) for adults ages nineteen to forty-nine years, a growing number of experts suggests a daily intake of at least 25mcg (1,000 IU) daily.

IRON

Insufficient iron is the most common mineral deficiency among athletes, especially female endurance athletes. Iron is required for the transport and handling of oxygen and for enzymes involved in energy production. High-impact exercise and intense endurance activity can cause iron losses, reducing the blood's ability to carry oxygen and resulting in muscle fatigue and impaired performance.

Endurance athletes' iron requirements are increased by about 70 percent. This is especially true for distance runners. For this reason, vegan athletes and long-distance runners should aim for an iron intake above 32mg per day for women and 14mg per day for men. All female endurance athletes need to keep tabs on their iron status.

Vegan athletes, especially women of menstruating age and endurance athletes, should eat plenty of iron-rich plant foods and iron-fortified foods, along with foods rich in vitamin C. If you're iron deficient, you may require an iron supplement. However, it's important to know your iron status before you take supplements, because excessive iron can be dangerous.

ZINC

Zinc is involved in energy production and immune function and helps heal muscle injuries. A deficiency of zinc can reduce muscle strength, cardiorespiratory function, endurance, metabolic rate, and protein use, adversely affecting performance. Insufficient zinc can also lead to weight loss, decreased endurance, increased risk of osteoporosis, and anorexia.

Intense exercise can accelerate loss of zinc. Very high-carb, low-protein, lowfat diets also elevate the likelihood of zinc deficiency, particularly in female and endurance athletes. Because vegans tend to have lower zinc intakes and reduced zinc absorption, their risk for zinc deficiency may be somewhat higher.

Vegan athletes may need as much as 50 percent more than the RDA to maintain adequate zinc levels. This would mean an intake of about 16.5mg for men and 12mg for women. The best plant sources of zinc include legumes, tofu, nuts, seeds, whole grains, and wheat germ. It's best to avoid single-nutrient zinc supplements, since they often exceed the tolerable upper limit of 40mg, potentially resulting in nutritional imbalances. If intakes are low, a multi-vitamin-mineral supplement providing an extra 5 to 10mg is usually sufficient to ensure needs are met.

CALCIUM

Calcium is critical for muscle contractions, transmission of nerve impulses, and numerous other body functions. It's also essential for bone health, and poor calcium status is linked to reduced bone density and stress fractures. Some vegan athletes may be at increased risk, particularly females who don't consume enough calories, have eating disorders, or are postmenopausal or not having periods.

Vegan athletes should meet the RDA for calcium (1,000 to 1,300mg daily). Female athletes who are at risk for osteoporosis should aim for 1,500mg per day. To accomplish this, most vegans need to incorporate some fortified foods, such as nondairy beverages, and eat plenty of calcium-rich plant foods. If you can't meet the recommended intake with food, take a supplement.

MAGNESIUM

Magnesium has a profound effect on muscle function. Evidence suggests that even marginal magnesium deficiency diminishes performance and can cause muscle cramps.

Intense endurance activities can increase magnesium requirements by 10 to 20 percent due to losses in urine and sweat. Athletes who restrict calories are at increased risk of deficiency. Vegans generally consume enough magnesium, from nuts, legumes, greens, and whole grains. If you aren't meeting daily recommended intakes (320mg for women; 420mg for men), add magnesium-rich foods to your diet. Some individuals may benefit from taking a magnesium supplement.

ELECTROLYTES

Electrolytes are electrically charged minerals in our body fluids that regulate hydration, nerve and muscle function, blood pH, blood pressure, and the repair of damaged tissues. These include sodium, potassium, chloride, calcium, and magnesium.

The amounts of potassium, sodium, and chloride athletes need vary widely among athletes and depend largely on fluid losses. Vegans who eat plenty of fruit and legumes get plenty of potassium. But like all athletes, they can quickly become depleted of sodium and chloride during intense endurance sports, and insufficient levels of these nutrients can seriously impair performance. Endurance athletes commonly require significantly more sodium and chloride than the upper limit for daily intake, which is 2,300mg for sodium and 3,600mg for chloride. For endurance events lasting more than two hours, use beverages that contain sodium and potassium (for details, see the section "Event Food and Fluid," a bit later in this chapter).

Eating to Excel

Compared to the general population, athletes require more energy to fuel their exercise and more fluids to compensate for losses through sweat. It's important to select meals, snacks, and beverages and the timing of consumption according to the intensity and duration of the activity and the individual needs of the athlete. Hydration is especially important, as a loss of more than 2 percent of body mass via fluids can adversely affect performance, especially in warm climates and at high altitudes. Dehydration is also associated with heat exhaustion and heat stroke. The foods and fluids you consume before, during, and after events or training sessions can make or break your performance.

PRE-EVENT FOOD AND FLUID

The purpose of a pre-event meal is to provide sufficient fuel to sustain yourself during the event. The trick is to eat just enough to maximize performance while avoiding undigested food in your stomach. Timing is everything. The closer you get to an event, the smaller your meal should be. Liquid meals may be more convenient and tolerable within one hour of an event, especially if you tend to experiences nausea, cramps, or vomiting after eating solid food.

Consuming a meal that provides 200 to 300 grams of carbohydrate three to four hours prior to an event has been shown to enhance performance (see table 13.3 for examples of foods providing 50g of carbohydrates). The high carbohydrate content will boost energy. The meal also should be relatively low in fat and fiber to help hasten digestion. Choose foods that you tolerate well. If you're prone to reflux, avoid caffeine, chocolate, fatty or fried foods, and carbonated beverages, which make things worse. If you frequently experience diarrhea, you may need to reduce fiber intake for about twenty-four to thirty-six hours prior to an event.

Generally, an athlete's store of glycogen in the muscles is sufficient for events that last sixty to ninety minutes. You can boost your stores twenty-four hours before the event by eating carbohydrate-rich meals and decreasing your activity level. During events longer than ninety minutes, athletes may experience extreme fatigue, hitting the wall when glycogen becomes depleted. To avoid this, thirty-six to forty-eight hours before the event, start exercising less and eating a high-carb diet, consuming about 10g/kg/d.

Drink 1 1/2 to 3 cups (375 to 750ml) of water or a sport beverage at least four hours before training or before the event. The smaller amount is recommended for smaller people; larger people should drink in the higher range. In events that last longer than one hour and offer little opportunity for hydration, drink fifteen minutes before the start of the event.

EVENT FOOD AND FLUID

Most active individuals don't need special food or beverages for less than one hour of exercise or training. However, there is some evidence that sports drinks providing 6 to 8 percent carbohydrates—14 to 18 grams of carbohydrate per cup (250ml)—benefit performance in intense endurance events lasting less than one hour. The additional carbohydrates help maintain blood sugar levels and can be particularly useful if the event or activity takes place in the early morning on an empty stomach. Fluids providing more than 8 percent carbohydrates (such as soda) can slow digestion and aren't recommended.

For events or activities lasting more than one hour, most athletes should eat foods containing carbohydrates at a rate of about 30 to 60 grams of carbohydrate per hour during the event. If the event lasts three hours or longer, it might be a good idea to up that to 90 grams of carbs per hour. Eating carbs every fifteen to twenty minutes, rather than all at once, is best. Eating carbs during exercise is particularly important for athletes who didn't carbo-load prior to the event, who haven't eaten a meal in three to four hours, or who have been restricting calories to lose weight.

In addition to a fuel supply, athletes need to remain hydrated. Sometimes athletes become dehydrated because their sweat rate exceeds their ability to absorb fluids from the stomach. Common signs of dehydration include muscle cramps and fatigue, low blood pressure, dizziness, and headache. And while most cases of dehydration are the result of fluid loss exceeding fluid intake, some athletes may begin an event in a dehydrated state because they have too little time between events to rehydrate or are limiting foods and fluids in an effort to make a weight class for competition.

There are two ways to replenish carbohydrates, fuel, and electrolytes during endurance events. First, you can consume water and solid foods, such as energy bars. Although this approach is very effective, it isn't always convenient during competition. The second approach is to consume beverages that provide fluid, energy, and electrolytes, such as sports drinks. Choose a beverage that provides 6 to 8 percent carbohydrates and 125 to 175mg of sodium per cup (250ml). With heavy sweating, more sodium may be required. Potassium status is less affected by sweating than sodium status is, so a potassium-rich diet may be sufficient to maintain levels during events. However, some authorities do suggest using sports beverages with potassium, particularly during endurance events.

Sports Drinks: All They're Cracked Up to Be?

The value of sports drinks is hotly debated within the scientific and athletic communities. Amid the confusion, one thing is very clear: sports drinks are not only useless for most consumers, they are a health scourge. The last thing the average consumer or recreational athlete needs is an infusion of calories, sugar, and salt. While use of sports drinks for serious endurance athletes is certainly more justified, water and solid food are more nutritious options for fuel and hydration.

For athletes who prefer to avoid solid food during training and events, coconut water and juices are great alternatives, and a combination of the two provides an excellent balance of carbohydrates and electrolytes. Coconut water with added fruit juice is significantly higher in carbohydrates than plain coconut water. Vegetable juices, such as carrot juice, beet juice, and green juices are also reasonable choices. Because beet juice is high in nitrates, it may enhance performance by reducing the amount of oxygen needed during exercise. However, beets aren't the only nitrate-rich vegetable. Arugula, bok choy, carrots, celery, collard greens, radishes, rhubarb, spinach, and Swiss chard also provide hefty doses. Happy juicing!

POST-EVENT FOOD AND FLUID

After an event or training session, you need to rehydrate your body, restore glycogen, and repair lean body tissue. Food and fluid needs depend on the intensity and duration of the event or training session and the timing of the next event. If you're participating in more than one event in a day, the time between events is critical. If you do a single event, the post-event protocol is less significant.

Ideally, you should start replenishing glycogen within thirty minutes of an event. Generally, eating 55 to 80 grams of carbs for a 120-pound (54kg) person or 70 to 110 grams for a 160-pound (73kg) person right after the event, and again 2.5 and 4.5 hours later is recommended, especially if you'll be participating in another event. This type of refueling isn't as important if you'll have rest days before your next event or training day.

Some authorities suggest consuming a 3-to-1 ratio of carbohydrates to protein to ensure sufficient protein for muscle tissue synthesis and repair. This means 100 grams of carbohydrates would be accompanied by 33 grams of protein. (See table 3.3, for amounts of protein in foods.) Other experts simply suggest eating 15 to 25 grams of protein after workouts or events in addition to carbohydrates.

After an event or training session, athletes also need to replace fluids and sodium lost in perspiration. Generally, try to drink 6 cups (1.5L) of fluid for every 2.2 pounds of body weight (1kg) lost.

Putting It All Together

The keys to peak performance, regardless of dietary pattern, are to stay well hydrated and eat sufficient quantities of a wide variety of nutrient-dense whole foods. The information and menus in chapter 14 will assist you in making healthful food choices at various levels of caloric intake. The menus are appropriate for active vegans, including competitive athletes. For most athletes, the 2,500- to 2,800-calorie or 4,000-calorie menu will be most suitable, although for athletes requiring fewer calories or trying to lose weight, the lower-calorie menus provide sufficient protein and should be nutritionally adequate.

Table 13.6 lists suggested numbers of servings from each food group at various levels of caloric intake. Feel free to vary the number of servings to suit your eating style, being sure to get at least the minimum number of servings from each group recommended in chapter 14. Select calcium-rich foods in each category to meet the recommended intake of six to eight servings of calorierich foods. "Other choices" refers to foods such as added fats or added sugars and other foods that don't fit into any of the food groups. If you don't use these foods, select a greater number of servings from whatever food group you wish to roughly equal the number of calories designated for "Other choices."

PRACTICAL TIPS

Here are some tips that will help you make the most of your choices in each food group as you plan your fitness diet.

Vegetables. If you have difficulty eating the recommended number of servings from this group, try to include vegetables at lunch as well as dinner, and use a mixture of raw and cooked vegetables (cooking condenses vegetables and makes it easier to eat larger amounts). Keep cut-up, ready-to-eat vegetables handy for snacks. Juicing vegetables also greatly reduces their bulkiness, making it easier to eat more. Try making dehydrated vegetable chips for crunch appeal. Kale, zucchini, and sweet potatoes work especially well. You can find recipes for these on the Internet.

Fruits. To increase fruit consumption, add fruit to breakfast cereal, bring a few pieces of fruit to enjoy as snacks at work or school, add fruit to smoothies, and make fruit-based desserts. Fresh fruit juices are another option. Avocado can be added to smoothies.

Legumes. The protein powerhouses of the plant kingdom, beans and products made from beans, are important for athletes. If you have difficulty eating enough servings, get creative. Use white beans in dips and pâtés, add cooked red lentils to spaghetti sauce, and include sprouted peas in salads. Experiment with ethnic cuisines, and use a wide variety of products made from beans, such as hummus, tofu, tempeh, and vegan meats.

TABLE 13.6. Suggested servings from food groups at various caloric intakes

FOOD GROUP (AVERAGE CALORIES*)	SERVING SIZE	2,000 CAL	2,500 CAL	3,000 CAL	4,000 CAL	5,000 CAL
Vegetables (30 calories)	½ c (125 ml) raw or cooked vegetables or vegetable juice 1 c (250 ml) raw leafy vegetables	6	8	9	10	12
Fruits (60 calories)	½ c (125 ml) fruit or fruit juice ¼ c (60 ml) dried fruit 1 medium fruit	4	5	6	7	8
Legumes (125 calories)	½ c (125 ml) tofu, tempeh, or cooked beans, peas, or lentils 1 c (250 ml) raw peas or sprouted lentils or peas ¼ c (60 ml) peanuts 2 tbsp (30 ml) peanut butter 2 oz (60 g) vegan meat	3	4	5	7	9
Grains (90 calories)	½ c (125 ml) cooked cereal, pasta, or whole grains 1 slice bread ½ c (125 ml) raw corn or sprouted quinoa, buckwheat, or other grain 1 oz (30 g) ready-to-eat cereal	8	10	12	14	16
Nuts and seeds (200 calories)	¼ c (60 ml) nuts and seeds 2 tbsp (30 ml) nut or seed butter	2	2	3	4	6
Other choices (80 calories)	2 tsp (10 ml) oil 2 tbsp (30 ml) maple syrup ½ oz (15 g) dark chocolate	1	2	3	4	5

Source of data: US Department of Agriculture, Agricultural Research Service, *USDA National Nutrient Database for Standard Reference*, Release 25 (2012), ndb.nal.usda.gov.

*Calorie estimates are based on an average of several choices, and individual items can vary considerably from these estimates. Please note:
- Starchy vegetables provide at least double the calories of other vegetables.
- The energy content of legumes varies widely. See table 3.3 for more precise calorie counts. Peanuts and peanut butter contain about 200 calories per serving (similar to nuts and seeds).
- Whole grains are heavier and slightly higher in calories than bread.

Key: c = cup; g = gram; mg = milliliter; oz = ounce; tbsp = tablespoon; tsp = teaspoon.

Grains. Eating the suggested amount of grains to increase your calories can seem daunting. But one serving is only 1/2 cup (125ml) of grains or 1 slice of bread. It's easy for big eaters to get six servings of grains in one meal—for example, 2 cups (500ml) of rice plus a whole-grain roll, or 2 cups (250ml) of pasta plus 2 slices of garlic bread will provide six servings. Likewise, 2 cups (500ml) of oatmeal with 2 slices of toast provides six servings. If you prefer to limit your intake of grains, eat more servings from all of the other groups.

Nuts and seeds. Nuts, seeds, and their butters are valuable nutrition allies for vegan athletes. Include them with most meals, and be sure omega-3 selections are part of the mix. Sprinkle nuts and seeds on salads and cereals, and use nut or seed butters on crackers, toast, celery, and in salad dressings. Nut-based cheeses, spreads, yogurts, and other dairy replacements are a great addition to the diet.

Other choices. The foods in this category are fats and oils, concentrated sweeteners such as maple syrup and blackstrap molasses, chocolate, and other sweet treats. While it isn't necessary to eat these foods, most people do, so it's important to include them in your calorie count. Plus, these foods can help boost calories if you have very high energy needs, while also adding flavor and variety to your diet.

We are nearing the end of our tour through the land of vegan nutrition. You've learned what a nourishing, health-supporting vegan diet should include. Now you just need to know how to put all of that information together into tasty menus that are designed specifically for you. Well, just turn the page and—voilà!—chapter 14, The Vegan Food Guide.

CHAPTER 14

The Vegan Food Guide

You may wonder how you can take all of the information in this book and boil it down into healthful daily meals for you and your family. Take heart. You are likely to discover that, as a vegan, your options actually increase as you become more familiar with the broad spectrum of plant foods. Although these choices are also available to nonvegetarians, we humans tend to not look outside of our comfort zone. When you shift your gaze in a new direction, entire worlds open up, in this case, new cuisines, new flavors, new textures, new aromas, and new food experiences. How exciting is that?

This chapter takes into account each essential nutrient and weaves all of them together into a plan that meets recommended intakes, combining information from the rest of the book into a simple guide for daily food intake with the goal of glowing, optimal health. We call our planning tool The Vegan Plate. We provide several sample menus, each for a day's worth of delicious vegan food.

The **Vegan Plate** features five food groups (listed in the first column of table 14.1). The next column gives examples of foods in each group and serving size. The next column presents calcium-rich foods from each of these groups: foods that provide 100 to 150mg calcium per serving. Be sure to choose six to eight servings of these foods daily. The right-hand column includes notes on how to optimize nutrition with each food group. This information is followed by a brief recap of sources of a few nutrients of special interest in vegan diets: omega-3 fatty acids, vitamins B$_{12}$ and D, and iodine.

It isn't essential to achieve the minimum intake of every food group every single day, though this could be your goal over time. Eating patterns can vary greatly and still meet recommended intakes on average over the course of a few days.

This guide is very versatile, applying equally to those who want a well-designed menu for weight loss, people whose energy requirements have decreased with age, those on raw foods diet, and athletes with high energy requirements. It may seem to recommend a lot of servings, but the amounts eaten at a meal can vary considerably from one person to another, and we usually eat more than one serving from a particular food group at a meal. For example, I cup (250ml) of soy milk, fruit, oatmeal, pasta, or rice actually counts as two servings.

Following this guide means that most of your calories will come from wholesome, nutrient-packed foods. Although you might occasionally indulge in foods high in sugar or fat, there isn't a lot of room for such items in any diet that meets recommended intakes of nutrients, whether or not the diet is vegan.

The Vegan Plate

"The Vegan Plate" diagram shown below is coordinated to match table 14.1. Here's how to use the information: Vegetables, shown to take up just over one-quarter of your plate in the diagram, should come from the listings in table 14.1; legumes, shown to take up just under a quarter of your plate, should come from that section of the table; and so on.

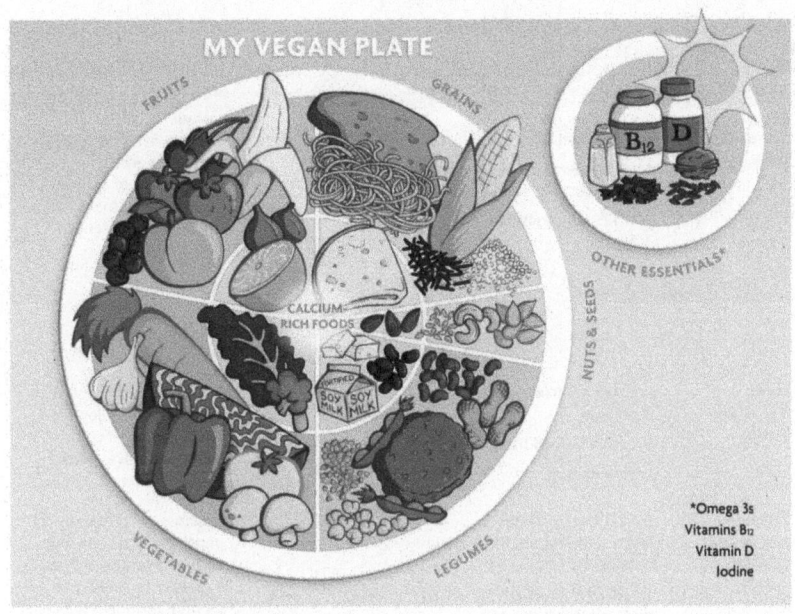

TABLE 14.1. Food groups and serving sizes

FOOD GROUP AND SERVINGS PER DAY	FOODS IN THIS GROUP WITH SERVING SIZE	CALCIUM-RICH FOODS WITH SERVING SIZE	NOTES
Vegetables: 5 or more servings	½ c (125 ml) raw or cooked vegetables 1 c (250 ml) raw leafy vegetables ½ c (125 ml) vegetable juice	1 c (250 ml) cooked bok choy, broccoli, collard greens, kale, mustard greens, napa cabbage, or okra 2 c (500 ml) raw bok choy, broccoli, collard greens, kale, or napa cabbage ½ c (125 ml) calcium-fortified tomato or vegetable juice	Include at least 2 daily servings of calcium-rich greens. Choose from the full rainbow of colorful vegetables: purple, blue, green, yellow, orange, red, and white.
Fruits: 4 or more servings	½ c (125 ml) fruit or fruit juice ¼ c (60 ml) dried fruit 1 medium fruit	½ c (125 ml) calcium-fortified fruit juice ¼ c (60 ml) dried figs 2 oranges	Fruits are excellent sources of potassium. Enjoy the full spectrum of colorful fruits, and make them your sweet treats.
Legumes: 3 or more servings	½ c (125 ml) cooked beans, peas, lentils, tofu, or tempeh 1 c (250 ml) raw peas or sprouted lentils or peas ¼ c (60 ml) peanuts 2 tbsp (30 ml) peanut butter 1 oz (30 g) vegan meat	1 c (250 ml) black or white beans ½ c (125 ml) fortified soy milk or soy yogurt ½ c (125 ml) calcium-set tofu (look for calcium on the ingredient list), cooked soybeans, or soy nuts	Legumes are great sources of protein, iron, and zinc with an average of 7 to 9 grams of protein per serving. Include a selection from this group at most meals.
Grains: 3 or more servings	½ c (125 ml) cooked cereal, pasta, quinoa, rice, or other grain 1 oz (30 g) bread ½ c (125 ml) raw corn or sprouted quinoa, buckwheat, or other grain 1 oz (30 g) cold cereal	1 oz (30 g) calcium-fortified cereal or bread 1 calcium-fortified tortilla	Select whole grains as often as possible. Adjust the number of grain servings to suit your energy needs; some need many more servings. Some fortified cereals and tortillas are particularly high in calcium.
Nuts and seeds: 1 or more servings	¼ c (60 ml) nuts or seeds 2 tbsp (30 ml) nut or seed butter	¼ c (60 ml) almonds 2 tbsp (30 ml) almond butter or sesame tahini	Seeds and nuts contribute copper, selenium, other minerals, vitamin E, and fat; choose some that are rich in omega-3s.

Sources of data are listed in *Becoming Vegan: Comprehensive Edition,* by Brenda Davis and Vesanto Melina (Book Publishing Company, 2014).

Key: c = cup; g = gram; mg = milliliter; oz = ounce; tbsp = tablespoon.

Other Essentials

Here are recommendations on a few essential nutrients of interest to vegans: omega-3 fatty acids, vitamins B_{12} and D, and iodine. For more on omega-3s, see chapter 4; for more on vitamins B$_{12}$ and D, see chapter 6; for more on iodine, see chapter 7.

Omega-3 fatty acids. Include at least one of the following:

- 2 tablespoons (30ml) of ground flaxseeds or chia seeds
- 1/4 cup (60ml) of hempseeds
- 1/3 cup (85ml) of walnuts
- 1 1/2 teaspoons (7ml) of flaxseed oil
- 1 1/2 tablespoons (22ml) of hempseed oil
- 2 1/2 tablespoons (37ml) of canola oil

Taking a supplement of 200 to 300mg of vegan DHA two to three times per week may be beneficial for some individuals (such as during pregnancy or for those with diabetes). A supplement that combines DHA with EPA can also be used.

Vitamin B$_{12}$. Include one of the following:

- A daily supplement that provides at least 25mcg of vitamin B$_{12}$
- Twice a week, a supplement that provides at least 1,000mcg of vitamin B$_{12}$
- Three servings daily of foods fortified with vitamin B$_{12}$, such as nondairy milks, vegan meats, or breakfast cereals, totaling at least 4mcg of vitamin B$_{12}$ for the day (2/3 of the Daily Value [DV] on food labels). For one of those servings, you can substitute 2 teaspoons

(10ml) of Red Star Vegetarian Support Formula nutritional yeast flakes.

Vitamin D. Get vitamin D in the following ways:

- Expose your face and forearms to warm sunshine for fifteen minutes every day between 10a.m. and 2p.m. if you have light-colored skin, twenty minutes if you're dark-skinned, and thirty minutes if you're a senior.

- If you can't get enough sun exposure—for instance, during winter, especially in northern latitudes—take a supplement or eat fortified foods. The recommended daily vitamin D intake for adults is 15mcg (600 IU) to age seventy and 20mcg (800 IU) after seventy. Amounts of vitamin D as high as 100mcg (4,000 IU) are considered safe.

Iodine. Include one of the following:

- A multivitamin-mineral supplement that provides 150mcg of iodine

- About 3/8 teaspoon (2ml) of iodized salt. Note that sea salt generally isn't iodized; if it is, this will be declared on the label.

Practical Pointers

In addition to the preceding tips, a few simple dietary approaches will help ensure optimum nutrition and well-being:

- **Eat a wide variety of foods from each food group.** Variety helps ensure you consume sufficient quantities of a broad range of nutrients, phytochemicals, and fiber. It also makes meals much more interesting.

- **Fill at least half of your plate with vegetables and fruits.**

- **Be moderate in your intake of concentrated fats, oils, and added sugars.** These foods are generally rich in calories but poor sources of nutrients. Excessive intakes of fat and sugar will crowd out foods that offer valuable nutrients. It's better to use whole foods such as seeds, nuts, avocados, and olives as your sources of fat, and fruits as your source of sugar, rather than extracted oils and sugars.

- **Watch your sodium intake.** Using ready-to-eat processed foods can make life easier, but relying excessively on canned, frozen, and other processed foods can result in excessively high sodium intakes.

- **Aim for an hour of physical activity each day.** Activity is central to energy balance and overall health. It also helps maintain muscle strength, bone density, balance, and mental well-being.

- **Drink enough water to stay hydrated.** Fluids such as water, herbal teas, and vegetable juices can help maintain good health and prevent kidney stones and urinary tract infections. Let thirst be your guide.

Sample Menus

Following are four sample menus with varying amounts of calories. Each has been planned for specific body types or activity levels. Select the one that meets your needs as an example of a meal plan to follow, with variations, on a daily basis.

You'll find a few other sample menus in chapter 11:

- A menu for pregnant or breast-feeding women, with 2,135 calories daily and 97g of protein
- Three menus for infants of different ages
- Three menus for children of different weights There also is a
- table showing suggested daily food servings for weight gain,
- vegan food guide for toddlers,
- list of easy meals, complete with prep tips,
- table of ways to increase the protein content of meals, and
- list of suggested servings from food groups at various caloric intakes.

The other four menus focus on family meals with children's favorites, simple dishes, raw foods, and holidays and celebrations. Each menu is presented at three calorie levels: 1,600 calories, 2,000 calories, and 2,500 calories.

In the menus that follow, food groups are indicated by the following letters:

   C = calcium-rich foods
   F = fruits
   G = grains
   L = legumes
   N = nuts and seeds
   n-3 = sources of omega-3s
   V = vegetables

After each menu, we total how many foods from each group it includes and provide a nutritional analysis for the day.

Menus for Every Taste

For more menus, see the companion volume to this book, *Cooking Vegan,* by V. Melina and J. Forest (Book Publishing Company, 2012). It includes a dozen menus with delicious recipes to support each. Eight of the menus are based on cuisines from around the world: North American, Asian Fusion, East Indian, French, Italian, Japanese, Mexican, and Middle Eastern. The other four menus focus on family meals with children's favorites, simple dishes, raw foods, and holidays and celebrations. Each menu is presented at three calorie levels: 1,600 calories, 2,000 calories, and 2,500 calories. The more than 150 recipes include nutritional analyses.

In this book you also will find a chapter on making friends with new ingredients, including healthful oils, sweeteners, thickeners, nondairy milks, soyfoods, and herbs and spices, along with specific directions for cooking grains and legumes. You will learn how to substitute vegan for nonvegan items in recipes and will have a helpful shopping list and kitchen equipment list. If you don't feel adept in the kitchen, the chef tips are designed to make your culinary experiences more pleasurable and productive.

1,600-CALORIE SAMPLE MENU

This high-protein menu is suitable for small or elderly people or people who want to lose weight. To reduce the amount of protein, replace soy milk with other fortified nondairy beverages.

BREAKFAST

1/2 cup (125ml) cooked cereal or 1 ounce (30g) dry cereal 1G

1/2 cup (125ml) raspberries or other fruit 1F

1/2 cup (125ml) fortified soy milk	1L, 1C

LUNCH

Soup of 1 cup (250ml) cooked lentils plus 1 cup (250ml) cooked vegetables (onion, carrot, celery)	2L, 2V
4 rye wafers or rice crackers	1G
2 cups (500ml) raw vegetables (peppers, cherry tomatoes, cucumber, carrots)	2V
1 1/2 cups (375ml) watermelon or other fruit	3F

SUPPER

Stir-fry of 2 cups (500ml) green vegetables (broccoli, napa cabbage)	2V, 1C
with 1/2 cup (125ml) cubed calcium-set tofu	1L, 1C
and 1 teaspoon (5ml) sesame oil, 1 teaspoon (5ml) tamari	-
1/2 cup (125ml) cooked whole grain, such as brown rice, millet, or quinoa	1G
1/2 cup (125ml) fortified soy milk	1L, 1C

SNACK

Chocolate shake of 1 banana, 1/2 cup (125ml) blueberries,	2F
with 1 cup (250ml) fortified chocolate soy milk, 1/4 cup (60ml) hempseeds	2L, 2C, 1N, 1N-3

Total servings of food groups: Total grains 3; vegetables 6; fruits 6; legumes 7; nuts and seeds 1; calcium-rich foods 6; omega-3s 1

Vitamin B$_{12}$ is supplied by three servings of fortified soy milk.

Vitamin D is supplied by fortified soy milk; add sunshine or a supplement.

Nutritional analysis: calories: 1,597; protein: 80g (19% of calories); fat: 43g (23% of calories); carbohydrate: 241g (58% of calories); dietary fiber: 52g; calcium: 1,964mg; iron: 22mg; magnesium: 680mg; phosphorus: 1,583mg; potassium: 4,700mg; sodium: 826mg; zinc: 14mg; thiamin: 1.7mg; riboflavin: 10.9mg; niacin: 23mg; vitamin B$_6$: 2.2mg; folate: 904mcg; pantothenic acid: 5.3mg; vitamin B$_{12}$: 5.4mcg; vitamin A: 1,438mcg RAE (4,746 IU); vitamin C: 283mg; vitamin D: 10mcg (400 IU); vitamin E: 13mg (19.5 IU); omega-6 fatty acids: 13.8g; omega-3 fatty acids: 9.7g

2,000-CALORIE SAMPLE MENU

This menu provides enough protein for adults (including recreational athletes) weighing 168 pounds (76kg) at a suitable level of 1 gram of protein per kilogram (2.2lb) of body weight. Almond milk is a source of vitamin E. Blackstrap molasses and sesame tahini are a tasty combination on toast, and both are good sources of calcium. Dark chocolate is not only tasty; it's also high in iron.

BREAKFAST	
2 slices toast (2 ounces/60g total)	2G
with 2 tablespoon (30ml) sesame tahini and I table-spoon (15ml) blackstrap molasses	IN, 2C
I cup (250ml) calcium-fortified orange juice	2F, 2C

LUNCH	
Taco: I tortilla and I cup (250ml) black beans, pinto beans, or refried beans	IG, 2L, IC
with I tomato, I cup (250ml) lettuce, 1/4 avocado, and salsa	3V
1/2 cup (125ml) fortified almond milk	IC

SUPPER	
1/2 cup (125ml) cooked whole grain, such as brown rice or quinoa, or I whole-grain roll (I ounce/30g)	IG
4 cups (IL) salad of kale, romaine lettuce, and napa cabbage	4V
with 2 tablespoons (30ml) Liquid Gold Dressing (page 105)	IN-3
1/2 cup (125ml) cubed tempeh with lemon and ginger or BBQ sauce	IL

SNACKS	
1/4 cup (60ml) dried figs and I orange	2F, IC
1/4 cup (60ml) pumpkin seeds	IN
1/2 cup (125ml) fortified almond milk	IC
I ounce (30g) dark chocolate	-

Total servings of food groups: grains 4; vegetables 7; fruits 4; legumes 3; nuts and seeds 2; calcium-rich foods 8; omega-3s 1

Vitamin B_{12} is supplied by nutritional yeast in Liquid Gold Dressing and fortified nondairy milk.

Vitamin D is supplied by fortified juice and almond milk; add sunshine or a supplement.

Nutritional analysis: calories: 1,958; protein: 76g (15% of calories); fat: 76g (32% of calories); carbohydrate: 268g (53% of calories); dietary fiber: 48g; calcium: 1,294mg; iron: 22mg; magnesium: 808mg; phosphorus: 1,867mg; potassium: 4,847mg; sodium: 1,100mg; zinc: 12mg; thiamin: 3.2mg; riboflavin: 2.2mg; niacin: 23mg; vitamin B_6: 2.9mg; folate: 826mcg; pantothenic acid: 5mg; vitamin B_{12}: 5.6mcg; vitamin A: 1,313mcg RAE (4,333 IU); vitamin C: 294mg; vitamin D: 5mcg (200 IU); vitamin E: 15mg (22.5 IU); omega-6 fatty acids: 20.9g; omega-3 fatty acids: 5.8g

2,500- TO 2,800-CALORIE SAMPLE MENU

This menu provides 2,500 calories and meets the recommended intakes for adults. To increase the calories to 2,800, add a bit more food, such as a piece of fruit and two cookies. Using the Vega One nutritional shake rather than seeds boosts levels of most nutrients well above the recommended intake. Convenience foods such as vegan meats and canned baked beans or chili can be high in sodium, so check labels—or use homemade versions, which are typically lower in sodium.

BREAKFAST	
1 bagel with 2 tablespoons (30ml) peanut butter; or 1 cup (250ml) whole-grain cereal with nuts	2G, 1L
Fruit smoothie: 1 scoop (35.9g) Vega One nutritional shake or 1/4 cup (60ml) sunflower seeds or hempseeds	1L, 4C
with 1 cup (250ml) calcium-fortified juice (or nondairy milk)	2F, 2C
and 1/2 banana and 1/2 cup (125ml) strawberries	2F

LUNCH	
1 1/2 sandwiches: 3 slices whole-grain bread (3 ounces/90g)	3G
with 3 slices vegan turkey	1.5L
and 1 tomato and 1 cup (250ml) lettuce	2V
and 1 tablespoon (15ml) vegan mayo	-

SUPPER	
1 cup (250ml) baked beans or vegetarian chili	2L
1 cup (250ml) baked squash or yam	2V
1 cup (250ml) steamed broccoli	2V, 1C
1 baked potato with 2 tablespoons (30ml) Earth Balance buttery spread	1V

SNACKS	
I cup (250ml) trail mix: 1.3 cup (85ml) walnuts, 1.3 cup (85ml) raisins, 1.3 cup (85ml) dried apricots	IN, 2F, IN-3
I cup (250ml) calcium-fortified nondairy milk	2C

Total servings of food groups: grains 5, vegetables 7, fruits 6, legumes 5.5, nuts and seeds 1, calcium foods 9, omega-3s 1

Vitamin B_{12} is supplied by the Vega One nutritional shake and fortified vegan meat, or add a supplement.

Vitamin D is supplied by fortified juice and nondairy milk and the Vega One nutritional shake; add sunshine or a supplement.

Nutritional analysis: calories: 2,501; protein: 97g (15% of calories); fat: 75g (25% of calories); carbohydrate: 395g (60% of calories); dietary fiber: 59g; calcium: 1,858mg; iron: 30mg; magnesium: 772mg; phosphorus: 1,793mg; potassium: 6,841mg; sodium: 2,200mg; zinc: 24mg; thiamin: 2.9mg; riboflavin: 2.2mg; niacin: 34mg; vitamin B_6: 4mg; folate: 898mcg; pantothenic acid: 11mg; vitamin B [12]: 4.2mcg; vitamin A: 988mcg RAE (3,260 IU); vitamin C: 409mg; vitamin D: 55mcg (2,200 IU); vitamin E: 27mg (40.5 IU); omega-6 fatty acids: 20g; omega-3 fatty acids: 5.6g

4,000-CALORIE SAMPLE MENU

This menu contains plenty of protein without substantial reliance on soy. Other protein-rich options are scrambled tofu for breakfast or soy-based veggie burgers.

BREAKFAST

2 cups (500ml) granola; or 4 pancakes or waffles with maple syrup	4G
2 oranges or other fruit	2F, 1C
2 cups (500ml) fortified almond milk or other nondairy milk	4C

LUNCH

Burgers: 2 whole wheat hamburger buns	4G
with 2 fortified black bean burgers	1G, 1L
and sliced tomato, red onion, chopped lettuce, and spreads	2V
1 1/2 cups (375ml) potato salad	3V
1/2 cup (125ml) mango, or 1 apple or other fruit	1F

SUPPER

Stir-fry of 1 cup (250ml) chickpeas and 1.3 cup (85ml) cashews	2L, 1.5N
with 2 cups (500ml) greens (such as broccoli, okra, napa cabbage)	4V, 2C
and 1 cup (250ml) carrots or peppers	2V
and 1 teaspoon (5ml) sesame oil, 1 teaspoon (5ml) tamari	-

2 cups (500ml) noodles or rice	4G
1 tablespoon (15ml) olive oil	-

SNACKS	
1/2 cup (125ml) hummus	1L
8 crackers	1G
1 peach or other fruit	1F
1 cup (250ml) fortified almond milk or other nondairy milk (or juice)	2C
1/2 cup (125ml) walnuts	1N, 1N-3
1 power bar (68g) or dessert	

Total servings of food groups: grains 14; vegetables 11, fruits 4, legumes 4; nuts and seeds 2.5, calcium foods 9, omega-3s 1

Vitamin B_{12} is supplied by the fortified nondairy milk and veggie burger, or a add supplement.

Vitamin D is supplied by fortified nondairy milk; add sunshine or a supplement.

Nutritional analysis: calories: 4,002; protein: 128g (13% of calories); fat: 152g (32% of calories); carbohydrate: 584g (55% of calories); dietary fiber: 88g; calcium: 1,826mg; iron: 37mg; magnesium: 910mg; phosphorus: 2,589mg; potassium: 6,258mg; sodium: 2,300mg; zinc: 23mg; thiamin: 7.4mg; riboflavin: 2.5mg; niacin: 38mg; vitamin B_6: 3.9mg; folate: 1,646mcg; pantothenic acid: 16mg; vitamin B_{12}: 3.8mcg;

vitamin A: 1,844mcg RAE (6,085 IU); vitamin C: 425mg; vitamin D: 8mcg (317 IU); vitamin E: 52mg (78 IU); omega-6 fatty acids: 33g; omega-3 fatty acids: 6g vitamin A, 1,844mcg RAE (6,085 IU); vitamin C; 425mg; vitamin D; 8mcg (317 IU); vitamin E 52mg (78 IU); omega-6 fatty acids: 33g; omega-3 fatty acids 6g

APPENDIX

Recommended Intakes of Vitamins and Minerals

The Dietary Reference Intakes (DRIs) are a comprehensive set of reference values that indicate recommended daily intakes for vitamins, minerals, and other nutrients for healthy populations. The DRIs have been established by American and Canadian scientists through a review process overseen by the US National Academies, which is an independent, nongovernmental body, and they reflect the current state of scientific knowledge with respect to nutrient requirements. They can be used for assessing and planning diets.

The recommended dietary allowance (RDA) is the average daily dietary intake of a nutrient that is sufficient to meet the requirement of most (97 to 98 percent) healthy persons. This number can be used as a goal for individuals and is likely to exceed the recommended intake for most people within that age or gender group. These are shown in bold type.

Adequate intake (AI) is the intake level suggested when an RDA cannot be determined due to insufficient data. The AI is more of a good guess or estimate of the amount needed to promote health. In the tables, these are shown in regular rather than bold type.

These and tolerable upper intake level (UL) are available through the Institute of Medicine of the National Academies online at iom.edu/Activi ties/Nutrition/SummaryDRIs/~/media/Files/Activity %20Files/Nutrition/DRIs/New%20Material/5DRI%2 0Values%20SummaryTables%2014.pdf or by scanning the QR code below. Alternate measures sometimes used (such as international units, or IU) can also be found at this website. For additional details and reports see the website io m.edu. The UL is the highest daily intake of a nutrient, consumed on a continuing basis, that is considered safe, in other words likely to pose no risks of adverse health effects for most individuals.

In table A.1, "Vit" refers to vitamin. For further details on vitamins and essential minerals, see chapters 6 and 7 and the websites lpi.orego nstate.edu/infocenter/vitamins.html and lpi.oregon state.edu/infocenter/minerals.html.

US National Academies DRIs

TABLE A.1. Dietary Reference Intakes for Vitamins

AGE / LIFE STAGE	VIT A mcg	VIT C mg	VIT D mcg	VIT E mg	VIT K mcg	THIAMIN mg	RIBOFLAVIN mg	NIACIN mg	VIT B_6 mg	FOLATE mcg	VIT B_{12} mcg	PANTOTHENIC ACID mg	BIOTIN mcg	CHOLINE mg
INFANTS														
0–6 months	400	40	10	4	2.0	0.2	0.3	2	0.1	65	0.4	1.7	5	125
7–12 months	500	50	10	5	2.5	0.3	0.4	4	0.3	80	0.5	1.8	6	150
CHILDREN														
1–3 years	300	15	15	6	30	0.5	0.5	6	0.5	150	0.9	2	8	200
4–8 years	400	25	15	7	55	0.6	0.6	8	0.6	200	1.2	3	12	250
MALES														
9–13 years	600	45	15	11	60	0.9	0.9	12	1.0	300	1.8	4	20	375
14–18 years	900	75	15	15	75	1.2	1.3	16	1.3	400	2.4	5	25	550
19–30 years	900	90	15	15	120	1.2	1.3	16	1.3	400	2.4	5	30	550
31–50 years	900	90	15	15	120	1.2	1.3	16	1.3	400	2.4	5	30	550
51–70 years	900	90	10	15	120	1.2	1.3	16	1.7	400	2.4	5	30	550
>70 years	900	90	20	15	120	1.2	1.3	16	1.7	400	2.4	5	30	550
FEMALES														
9–13 years	600	45	15	11	60	0.9	0.9	12	1.0	300	1.8	4	20	375
14–18 years	700	65	15	15	75	1.0	1.0	14	1.2	400	2.4	5	25	400
19–30 years	700	75	15	15	90	1.1	1.1	14	1.3	400	2.4	5	30	425
31–50 years	700	75	15	15	90	1.1	1.1	14	1.3	400	2.4	5	30	425
51–70 years	700	75	15	15	90	1.1	1.1	14	1.5	400	2.4	5	30	425
>70 years	700	75	20	15	90	1.1	1.1	14	1.5	400	2.4	5	30	425
PREGNANCY														
14–18 years	750	80	15	15	75	1.4	1.4	18	1.9	600	2.6	6	30	450
19–30 years	770	85	15	15	90	1.4	1.4	18	1.9	600	2.6	6	30	450
31–50 years	770	85	15	15	90	1.4	1.4	18	1.9	600	2.6	6	30	450
LACTATION														
14–18 years	1,200	115	15	19	75	1.4	1.6	17	2	500	2.8	7	35	550
19–30 years	1,300	120	15	19	90	1.4	1.6	17	2	500	2.8	7	35	550
31–50 years	1,300	120	15	19	90	1.4	1.6	17	2	500	2.8	7	35	550

Key: g = gram; mcg = microgram; mg = milligram

TABLE A.2. Dietary Reference Intakes for Minerals

LIFE STAGE / AGE	CALCIUM mg	CHROMIUM mcg	COPPER mcg	FLUORIDE mg	IODINE mcg	IRON mg	MAGNESIUM mg	MANGANESE mg	MOLYBDENUM mcg	PHOSPHORUS mg	SELENIUM mcg	ZINC mg	POTASSIUM g	SODIUM g	CHLORIDE g
INFANTS															
0–6 months	200	0.2	200	0.01	110	0.27	30	0.003	2	100	15	2	0.4	0.12	0.18
7–12 months	260	5.5	220	0.5	130	11	75	0.6	3	275	20	3	0.7	0.37	0.57
CHILDREN															
1–3 years	700	11	340	0.7	90	7	80	1.2	17	460	20	3	3.0	1.0	1.5
4–8 years	1,000	15	440	1	90	10	130	1.5	22	500	30	5	3.8	1.2	1.9
MALES															
9–13 years	1,300	25	700	2	120	8	240	1.9	34	1,250	40	8	4.5	1.5	2.3
14–18 years	1,300	35	890	3	150	11	410	2.2	43	1,250	55	11	4.7	1.5	2.3
19–30 years	1,000	35	900	4	150	8	400	2.3	45	700	55	11	4.7	1.5	2.3
31–50 years	1,000	35	900	4	150	8	420	2.3	45	700	55	11	4.7	1.5	2.3
51–70 years	1,000	30	900	4	150	8	420	2.3	45	700	55	11	4.7	1.3	2.0
> 70 years	1,200	30	900	4	150	8	420	2.3	45	700	55	11	4.7	1.2	1.8
FEMALES															
9–13 years	1,300	21	700	2	120	8	240	1.6	34	1,250	40	8	4.5	1.5	2.3
14–18 years	1,300	24	890	3	150	15	360	1.6	43	1,250	55	9	4.7	1.5	2.3
19–30 years	1,000	25	900	3	150	18	310	1.8	45	700	55	8	4.7	1.5	2.3
31–50 years	1,000	25	900	3	150	18	320	1.8	45	700	55	8	4.7	1.5	2.3
51–70 years	1,200	20	900	3	150	8	320	1.8	45	700	55	8	4.7	1.3	2.0
> 70 years	1,200	20	900	3	150	8	320	1.8	45	700	55	8	4.7	1.2	1.8
PREGNANCY															
14–18 years	1,300	29	1,000	3	220	27	400	2.0	50	1,250	60	13	4.7	1.5	2.3
19–30 years	1,000	30	1,000	3	220	27	350	2.0	50	700	60	11	4.7	1.5	2.3
31–50 years	1,000	30	1,000	3	220	27	360	2.0	50	700	60	11	4.7	1.5	2.3
LACTATION															
14–18 years	1,300	44	1,300	3	290	10	360	2.6	50	1,250	70	14	5.1	1.5	2.3
19–30 years	1,000	45	1,300	3	290	9	310	2.6	50	700	70	12	5.1	1.5	2.3
31–50 years	1,000	45	1,300	3	290	9	320	2.6	50	700	70	12	5.1	1.5	2.3

Key: g = gram; mcg = microgram; mg = milligram

RESOURCES

NUTRITION BOOKS

Becoming Raw. Brenda Davis and Vesanto Melina, Book Publishing Company, 2010.

Becoming Vegan: Comprehensive Edition. The Complete Reference to Plant-Based Nutrition. Brenda Davis and Vesanto Melina, Book Publishing Company, 2014.

The Complete Idiot's Guide to Plant-Based Nutrition. Julieanna Hever, Alpha Books, 2011.

Cooking Vegan. Vesanto Melina and Joseph Forest, Book Publishing Company, 2012. (Companion volume to **Becoming Vegan.** Published in Canada as **Cooking Vegetarian.** Joseph Forest and Vesanto Melina, Harper Collins, 2011.)

Defeating Diabetes. Brenda Davis and Tom Barnard, Book Publishing Company, 2000.

The Dietitian's Guide to Vegetarian Diets. Reed Mangels, Virginia Messina, and Mark Messina, Jones and Bartlett Learning, 2011.

The Everything Vegan Pregnancy Book. Reed Mangels, Adams Media, 2011.

Food Allergies: Health and Healing. Jo Stepaniak, Vesanto Melina, and Dina Aronson, Books Alive, 2010.

Food Allergy Survival Guide. Vesanto Melina, Jo Stepaniak, and Dina Aronson, Healthy Living Publications, 2004.

The Plant-Powered Diet. Sharon Palmer, The Experiment, 2012.

Raising Vegetarian Children. Jo Stepaniak and Vesanto Melina, McGraw-Hill, 2003.

Raw Food Revolution Diet. Cherie Soria, Brenda Davis, and Vesanto Melina, Book Publishing Company, 2008.

Vegan for Her: The Women's Guide to Being Healthy and Fit on a Plant-Based Diet. Ginny Messina and J.L. Fields, Da Capo Lifelong Books, 2013.

Vegan for Life. Jack Norris and Virginia Messina, Da Capo Lifelong Books, 2011.

NUTRITION WEBSITES

Brenda Davis. brendadavisrd.com

Dietary Reference Intakes. fnic.nal.usda.gov/dietary-guidance/dietary-reference-intakes

Linus Pauling Institute's Micronutrient Information Center. lpi.oregonstate.edu/infocenter

Nutrition Facts. nutritionfacts.org

Physicians Committee for Responsible Medicine. pcrm.org

USDA National Nutrient Database for Standard Reference. ndb.nal.usda.gov

The Plant-Based Dietitian. plantbaseddietitian.com

Vegan Health. veganhealth.org

The Vegan RD. theveganrd.com

Vegetarian Diets Position of the Academy of Nutrition and Dietetics. eatright.org/About/Content.aspx?id=8357

Vegetarian Nutrition Dietetic Practice Group of the Academy of Nutrition and Dietetics. vegetariannutrition.net/faq

Vesanto Melina. nutrispeak.com

VEGAN AND VEGETARIAN WEBSITES

American Vegan Society. americanvegan.org

The Compassionate Cook. compassionateco ok.com

Happy Cow. happycow.net

International Vegetarian Union. ivu.org

North American Vegetarian Society. navs-online.org

One Green Planet. onegreenplanet.org

Vegan Outreach. veganoutreach.org

Vegan Society. vegansociety.com

VegDining. vegdining.com

Vegetarian Resource Group. vrg.org

Vegetarian Summerfest. vegetariansummerfe st.org

VegNews. vegnews.com

VegSource. vegsource.com

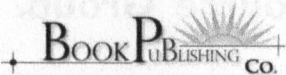
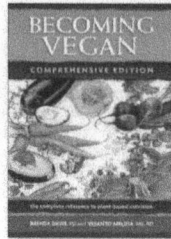
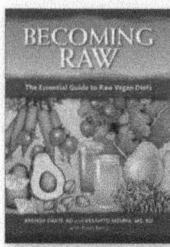
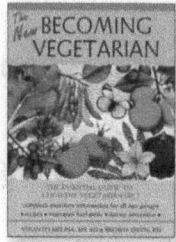
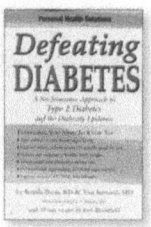
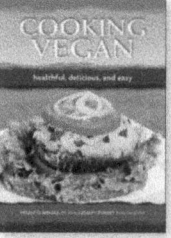
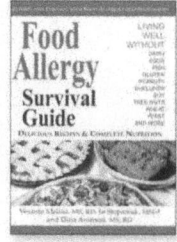
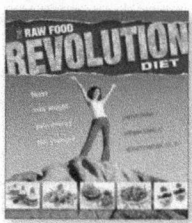

Back Cover Material

Whether you're considering going vegan for your health, out of concern for the environment, or to avoid contributing to the suffering of animals, *Becoming Vegan: Express Edition* has all the information you need in order to provide nutritious vegan meals for yourself, your family, and your friends.

Internationally acclaimed vegan dietitians Brenda Davis and Vesanto Melina present the latest findings on the following:

- **using plant foods to protect against cancer, heart disease, and other chronic illnesses**
- **obtaining essential protein without meat, eggs, or dairy products**
- **maintaining a healthy weight and discovering the keys to fitness**
- **designing balanced vegan diets for infants, children, and seniors**
- **incorporating "good" fats and learning where to find them**
- **meeting calcium needs without dairy products**
- **understanding the importance of vitamin B$_{12}$**
- **ensuring a healthy vegan pregnancy and ample nutrition for breast-feeding**

Completely revised, this seminal classic offers fresh insights into the implications of becoming vegan—for individuals, for animals, and for our fragile planet. It includes new information on the health benefits of vegan diets and a blueprint for clean eating. This streamlined "express" version is extensive yet easily understandable for anyone who wants to construct an optimal plant-based diet.

Registered dietitian BRENDA DAVIS is a leader in her field and an esteemed, popular speaker. She is a past chairperson of the Vegetarian Nutrition Dietetic Practice Group of the Academy of Nutrition and Dietetics (formerly the American Dietetic Association) and coauthor of more than seven books, including *Defeating Diabetes*. Brenda is the 2007 inductee into the Vegetarian Hall of Fame.

VESANTO MELINA, a registered dietitian and a sought-after speaker and consultant, has taught nutrition at the University of British Columbia and Bastyr University in Seattle. She coauthored the joint position paper on vegetarian diets for the Academy of Nutrition and Dietetics and Dietitians of Canada and is currently a consultant to the government of British Columbia.

***

"There's no other book as informative and comprehensive as Becoming Vegan; it's a treasure trove of facts and helpful hints

and it's sure to put you on the path of health and healing."

KATHY FRESTON, *New York Times* bestselling author of *The Lean, Veganist,* and *The Quantum Wellness Cleanse*

Health professionals and nutrition enthusiasts: Be sure to look for Becoming Vegan: Comprehensive Edition. *Expanding on the more compact "express" version, this indispensable reference sets the standard on vegan nutrition and contains additional topics, in-depth analyses, and full citations of scientific studies.*

A

Abramowitz, Rubin, *4*
Academy of Nutrition and Dietetics, *397, 489*
acesulfame K, *201*
addictive substances, avoiding, *363, 394*
Adequate Intake (AI),
  for fiber, *177, 179*
  omega-3 fatty acids, *141*
Adventist Health Study-1, *51*
Adventist Health Study-2, *51, 72, 74*
Adventist Mortality Study, *56*
aerobic exercise, *45, 496, 498, 505, 507*
age issues,
  see children; infants; seniors,
agribusiness, *9*
ahimsa, defined, *4*

air quality, food industry and, *38, 40*
alcohol consumption,
  avoiding, *363*
  avoiding, during pregnancy, *416*
  chronic disease and, *54*
  osteoporosis and, *95*
  toxicity of, *168*
allergies, to foods, *302, 304, 306, 432, 434*
allium vegetables, *293*
alpha-linolenic acid (ALA), *137, 139, 141, 416*
alpha-tocopherol (vitamin E), *223, 225, 230, 232*
American Academy of Pediatrics, *423, 427, 430*
American Association for the Advancement of Science, *47*
American Heart Association, *158*

American Institute for Cancer Research, 72
American Vegan Society, 4
amino acids, 64, 112, 114, 116
anaerobic metabolism, 505, 507
angina, 68
animal rights issues, 7, 28, 31
antibiotics, given to animals, 12, 19, 26
antioxidants,
  cancer and, 79
  cardiovascular disease and, 65
  for seniors, 473, 475
  vitamin A as, 223, 225, 228
  vitamin C as, 223, 225, 228, 230
  vitamin E as, 223, 225, 230, 232
apple shape body type, 84, 328, 332
aquaculture, 26, 28
Aronson, D., 306
arteries,
  see cardiovascular disease (CVD),
arthritis, rheumatoid, 103
artificial sweeteners, avoiding, 354, 357
ascorbic acid (vitamin C), 223, 225, 228, 230
aspartame, 201
avocados, 155, 158, 382

B
Baboumian, Patrik, 502
'bad fats', 132
bags, reusable, 42
Barnard, T., 484
beef cattle, 19, 21
beriberi, preventing, 234
Berkoff, N., 489
beta-carotene (vitamin A), 95, 223, 225, 228, 425
beverages,
  see fluids,
bifidobacteria, 300, 302
biotin (vitamin B7), 241
blackstrap molasses, 197, 199
blood clots, 64, 65
blood pressure, 61
blood sugar,

see glycemic index (GI); sugar; type 2 diabetes,

body frame, underweight and, *370*

body mass index (BMI),
  blood pressure and, *61*
  overweight and, *323, 328*
  pregnancy and, *402*
  underweight and, *365, 368, 370*

body shape, *84, 328, 332*

bone health,
  see osteoporosis brain health,
  dementia and, *101*
  exercise for, *494*
  seniors and, *480*

Bravo: Health-Promoting Meals form the TrueNorth Kitchen (Bravo), *484*

Bravo, R., *484*

Brazier, Brendan, *502*

breakfast, for children, *448*

breast cancer, *72, 79*

breast-feeding,

see lactation,

British Vegetarian Society, *2*

broiler chickens, *14, 16*

Burkitt, Denis, *173*

BusinessWeek, *45*

C

caffeine,
  avoiding, during pregnancy, *416, 418*
  osteoporosis and, *95*

calciferol (vitamin D), *215, 216, 219, 221, 223*

calcium,
  benefits of, *95, 97, 262, 264, 266, 268*
  for exercise, *518*
  for lactation, *427*
  osteoporosis and, *88, 90, 95, 97, 262, 264, 266, 268* (see also osteoporosis),
  for pregnancy, *412*
  for seniors, *470, 473*
  for teens, *460*

calories,
  from carbohydrates, *118, 168, 169, 384*

energy-dense foods
for weight gain, *376,
378, 380, 382, 384*
energy imbalance and
weight, *332, 334*
(see also overweight;
underweight),
exercise and, *507, 523,
525, 529*
from fat, *118, 130, 145,
148, 151, 153*
menus for different
caloric intake levels,
542, 544, 546, 549
in Paleo diet,
pregnancy and, *405*
from protein, *118, 128,
168*
cancer,
deaths from, *69*
diet and lifestyle, *69, 72*
generally, *69*
overweight and, *325*
prevention tips for, *79,
81*
raw vegan diet and, *74,
76*
soy and, *79, 128*
treatments for, *76, 79*

vegan diet for
prevention of, *72, 74*
capture fisheries, *24, 26*
carbohydrates, *165, 168,
169, 171, 173, 175, 177, 179,
182, 184, 186, 188, 189, 192,
194, 197, 199, 201, 205, 206*
calories from, *118, 168,
169, 384*
fiber and, *173, 175, 177,
179, 182, 184, 186*
food for exercise, *505,
507, 509, 523, 525*
glycemic index (GI)
and, *201, 205, 206*
grains and, *188, 189, 192*
importance of, *165, 168*
refined, *171, 173*
sugar and, *194, 197, 199,
201*
types of, *168, 169, 171*
carbon compounds, in
manure, *35, 38*
cardiovascular disease
(CVD),
abnormal blood
coagulation and, *64, 65*
cholesterol and, *56, 58,
61, 65, 68, 128, 134*

emerging risk factors, 65

fiber for cardiovascular health, 177

generally, 56

high blood pressure and, 61

homocysteine and, 64

inflammation and, 64

overweight and, 325

triglycerides and, 61

vegan diet for, 65, 68, 69

care facilities, vegan food in, 487, 489

carnitine, 114, 116

cataracts, 101

cattle, food industry and, 19, 21, 24, 38

celiac disease, 192

Centers for Disease Control and Prevention, 336, 365

chemical contaminants, avoiding, 306, 309

chia seeds, 155

chickens, food industry and, 14, 16

children,

to age twelve, 446, 448, 450, 452, 455

dietary fat needed by, 151

exercise for, 498

infants, 108, 110, 210, 212, 215, 216, 423, 425, 427, 430, 432, 434, 437, 438, 442

omega-3 fatty acids for infants, 143

protein for, 108, 110

teens, 455, 458, 460, 461, 498

toddlers and preschoolers, 442, 443, 446

cholesterol,

cardiovascular disease and, 56, 58, 61, 65, 68

high-density lipoprotein (HDL), 58

low-density lipoprotein (LDL), 58, 65, 68, 128

oxidized cholesterol (oxycholesterol), 61

sterols, 134

triglycerides, 61

very low-density lipoprotein (VLDL), *61*

choline, *246*

chromium, *279*

clear-cutting, *26*

coagulants, vitamin K and, *246, 248*

cobalamin,

    see vitamin B12,

coconut oil, *158, 161, 163*

coconut sugar, *199*

colorectal cancer, *72, 74, 76*

community support, vegan food and, *487, 489*

'complete' protein, *116, 118*

complex carbohydrates, *168, 169, 171*

composting, *42*

concentrated animal feeding operations (CAFOs), *9*

Context Marketing, *45, 47*

conventional vegan diet, defined, *311*

Cooking Vegan (Melina, Forest), *128, 484, 540*

copper, *279*

cravings, overcoming, *345*

C-reactive protein (CRP), *64*

cruciferous vegetables, *293*

'cruelty-free' meat, problem of, *28, 31*

cyanocobalamin,

    see vitamin B,

D

dairy alternatives, for weight gain, *382*

dairy industry,

    calcium and, *88*

    cows, *21, 24*

    formula for infants, *430, 432*

Danzig, Mac, *502*

date sugar, *199*

Davis, B., *484*

Davis, Steph, *502*

Defeating Diabetes (Davis, Barnard), *484*

deforestation, *38*

dehydrocholesterol, *219*

dementia, *101*

desertification, *38*

diabetes,
see type 2 diabetes,
Dietary Guidelines
Advisory Committee
(2010), *54*
Dietary Reference
Intakes (DRIs),
dietary vegans, defined,
7
dietetic associations, *489*
Diet for a New America
(Robbins), *4*
dieting, problem of, *336,*
338
digestion,
enzymes and, *293*
improving, *347*
of protein, *110, 112*
Dinshah, H. Jay, *4*
diverticular disease, *101,*
103
docosahexaenoic acid
(DHA), *137, 139, 143, 416*

E
Earth, resources of, *31,*
33, 35, 38, 40, 42
eating disorders, *372*
eicosapentaenoic acid
(EPA), *137, 139, 143, 416*
electrolytes, *521, 523, 525*
Ellis, Frey, *4*
energy,
B vitamins and, *234,*
237, 239, 241, 243, 246
energy-dense foods
for weight gain, *378,*
380, 382, 384
overweight as energy
imbalance, *332, 334*
seniors and, *463, 466*
England, veganism in, *2*
enrichment, *173*
environmental issues,
air quality, *38, 40*
cancer and, *69*
global warming, *33, 35*
land use, *38*
overweight and, *334,*
336
resource depletion,
31, 33
water, *35, 38*
enzymes, *293*
EPIC-Oxford, *51, 56, 74,*
101, 368
esophageal cancer, *72*

Esselstyn, Caldwell, *68*

essential fatty acids, *137, 139, 141, 143*

  see also omega-3 fatty acids,

estrogen, *76*

ethnicity,

  cancer and, *69, 79*

  diabetes and, *86*

  fat intake and, *145, 151*

  protein complementing and, *116, 118*

  protein digestibility of different diets, *110*

European Prospective, Investigation into Cancer and Nutrition (EPIC), *51*

  see also EPIC-Oxford,

exercise, *491, 494, 496, 498, 500, 502, 505, 507, 509, 510, 512, 514, 516, 518, 521, 523, 525, 528, 529*

  achieving fitness, *496, 498, 500*

  benefits of, *491, 494, 496*

  for bone health, *93*

  dietary fat needed for, *145*

  eating habits and, *521, 523, 525, 528*

  food and activity diaries, *340, 342, 392*

  lack of, *54*

  nutrients for, *505, 507, 509, 510, 512, 514, 516, 518, 521*

  overweight and, *336*

  during pregnancy, *418*

  as priority, *361, 363*

  protein for, *110*

  recommendations, *538*

  for seniors, *466, 468*

  tips for, *528, 529*

  vegan athletes, *500, 502*

  for weight gain, *392, 394, 395*

eye health, *101*

F

factory farms, *9, 35*

  see also food industry,

Fasano, Alessio, *192*

fast and easy vegan diet, defined, *311*

fat (body),

see also overweight;
underweight,
body mass index
(BMI), *61, 323, 328, 365,
368, 370, 402*
body shape, *84, 328, 332*
diabetes and, *84*
of seniors, *463*
waist to hip ratio, *328,
332*
fat (dietary), *130, 132, 134,
137, 139, 141, 143, 145, 148,
151, 153, 155, 158, 161, 163*
benefits of, *88*
calories from, *118, 130,
145, 148, 151, 153*
cardiovascular disease
and, *58*
cholesterol and lipids,
56, 58, 61, 65, 68, 128, 134
composition of, in
selected foods, *158, 161*
energy-dense foods
for weight gain, *378,
380, 382, 384*
exercise and, *505, 510*
fatty acids, defined,
132, 134

fatty acids, essential,
137, 139, 141, 143
good versus bad, *132*
importance of, *130, 163*
limiting, *357*
low-fat vegan diet, *148,
151, 311, 312*
requirements for, *143,
145, 148, 151, 153*
sources of, *153, 155, 158,
161, 163, 354*
female athlete triad, *509*
fiber,
Adequate Intake for,
177, 179
benefits of, *175, 177*
cancer and, *72, 74, 81*
cardiovascular disease
and, *58, 61, 65, 68*
diabetes and, *86*
diverticular disease
and, *101*
gas from, *179, 182, 184*
generally, *173, 175*
high-fiber diet, *184, 186*
for seniors, *475, 478*
sources of, *184*
types of, *175*
'finishing' facilities, *19*

fish,
  food industry and, *24,
  26, 28*
  pescatarians, *74*
flexibility exercises, *498*
flexitarians, defined, *47*
fluids,
  for exercise, *521, 523,
  525, 528*
  for lactation, *430*
  recommendations, *538*
  for seniors, *475, 478*
  water, *35, 38, 357, 359, 458*
  for weight gain, *378*
folate (vitamin B9, folic
acid),
  benefits of, *243, 246*
  for lactation, *243*
  for pregnancy, *414, 416*
food addiction,
overcoming, *345*
Food Allergy Survival
Guide, The (Melina,
Aronson, Stepaniak), *306*
food and activity diaries,
340, 342, 392
food industry,
  agribusiness and, *9*
  cattle, *19, 21, 24*

chickens, *14, 16*
'cruelty-free', *28, 31*
fish, *24, 26, 28*
flesh food and dairy
product industries as
linked, *4*
pigs, *9, 12, 14*
food preparation,
  mineral absorption
  and, *259*
  phytochemicals and,
  295
  protein and
  digestibility, *110, 112*
  raw vegan diet and
  cancer, *74, 76*
food sensitivities, *302,
304, 306, 432, 434*
Forest, J., *128, 484, 540*
formula feeding, *430, 432*
4,000-calorie sample
menu, *544*
fowl, food industry and,
14, 16
free radicals, *72*
fructose, *199, 201*
fruitarian diet, defined,
311

G

gallbladder,
   gallstones, *103*
   overweight and, *325*
gamma-linolenic acid
(GLA), *137, 139, 143*
gas, from fiber, *179, 182,
184*
gender,
   see also lactation;
   pregnancy; vitamins;
   individual types of
   cancer,
   body shape and, *328*
   exercise and, *509*
   osteoporosis and, *90*
   premenstrual
   syndrome, *458, 460*
   soy and, *128*
   underweight and, *370*
genetic engineering, of
animals, *16, 24, 28*
genetics,
   cancer and, *69*
   diabetes and, *86*
   underweight and, *370*
gillnetting, *26*
global warming, food
industry and, *33, 35*

glucose,
   diabetes and, *84, 86*
   (see also glycemic
   index (GI); type 2
   diabetes),
   exercise and, *363, 505*
   generally, *81, 84, 86, 88*
   glycogen, *241, 523*
   sweeteners, *197*
gluten, *192*
glycemic index (GI),
   generally, *201*
   GI and glycemic load
   (GL) of selected
   foods, *201, 205*
   limitations, *205, 206*
goals, setting, *338, 342*
'good fats', *132*
gout, *325*
grains,
   for exercise, *529*
   generally, *188, 189*
   gluten in, *192*
   limiting, *352*
   whole-grain hierarchy,
   189
greenhouse gas
emissions, *33, 35*

H

happiness, exercise and, *494*

Harris Interactive poll, *45*

Hawken, Paul, *31*

heart attack, *64, 65*
    see also cardiovascular
      disease (CVD),

Heidrich, Ruth, *502*

Helicobacter pylori, *158*

Helio, *300*

hempseeds, *155*

herbs, *354*

high-density lipoprotein
(HDL), *58, 148*

high-fat diet, *151, 153*

high-fiber diet, *184, 186*

high-sensitivity
C-reactive protein
(hs-CRP), *64*

histadine, *112*

homocysteine, *64, 243*

hormones,
    balancing, *350, 368*
    given to animals, *12, 19,
    24*
    skin of teens and, *458*

Humane Slaughter Act,
16

hydrogenated oils, *357*

hypertension, *61*

hypothyroidism, *334*

I

infants, *423, 425, 427, 430,
432, 434, 437, 438, 442*
    breast feeding, *423, 425,
    427, 430*
    food allergies in, *432,
    434*
    formula feeding, *430,
    432*
    menus for, *438, 442*
    protein requirements
    and, *108, 110*
    scientific evidence
    about vegan diet
    during pregnancy, *397,
    399*
    (see also pregnancy),
    solid foods for, *434,
    437, 438*

inflammation,
    cardiovascular disease
    and, *64*
    controlling, *345*

exercise for, *494*

insoluble fiber, *173*

insulin, *84, 361, 363*

    see also type 2 diabetes,

intestinal health,

    bacteria for, *76*

    fiber and, *175, 177, 182, 184*

    leaky gut, *304, 306, 347*

    prebiotics and probiotics, *298, 300, 302*

    for seniors, *475, 478*

inulin, *300*

iodine,

    benefits of, *276, 277*

    children to age twelve, *452*

    for pregnancy, *412*

    recommendations, *536*

    for toddlers and preschoolers, *446*

iron,

    benefits of, *268, 271, 273*

    for exercise, *516, 518*

    infants and, *434, 437, 438*

    for lactation, *427*

    for pregnancy, *409*

    for seniors, *468, 470*

isoflavones, *79, 128*

isoleucine, *112*

J

juicing, *76, 228*

Jurek, Scott, *502*

K

ketones, *168*

Keys, Ancel, *151*

kidney disease, *103*

L

lactation,

    formula feeding compared to, *430, 432*

    generally, *423, 425*

    nutrients for, *210, 212, 215, 216, 243, 425, 427, 430*

    resources for, *432*

lactobaccilus, *300, 302*

lacto-ovo vegetarian diet, *65*

land use, food industry and, *38*

Laraque, Georges, *502*

lauric acid, *161*

layers (chickens), *16*

leaky gut syndrome, *304, 306, 347*

legumes,
benefits of, *350, 352*
for exercise, *528, 529*
fiber from, *182, 184*
leucine, *112*
Lifestyle Heart Trial, *68*
linoleic acid (LA), *137, 139, 141*
Liquid Gold Dressing (recipe), *216*
liver detoxification, *225*
livestock industry, *19, 21, 24, 38*
Livestock's Long Shadow (United Nations Food and Agriculture Organization), *33*
Living Planet Report 2010 (World Wildlife Fund), *35*
Living Well (Fasano), *192*
longevity, *466*
longlining, *26*
low-density lipoprotein (LDL), *58, 65, 68, 128*
low-fat vegan diet, defined, *148, 151, 311, 312*
lunch, for children, *450*
lung cancer, *72*

lysine, *112, 114*

M

macrobiotic diet,
defined, *312*
pregnancy and, *399*
macronutrients,
balancing, *118*
carbohydrates as, *165, 168*
fat as, *130*
protein as, *108*
magnesium, *279, 518, 521*
malnutrition, *49*
manganese, *279, 281*
manure, *35, 38*
marijuana, *416*
meal planning,
away from home, *452, 455*
for children to age twelve, *448, 450, 452, 455*
for exercise, *521, 523, 525, 528, 529*
family time and, *460, 461*
for infants, *438, 442*
meal frequency, *376, 378*

menus for different caloric intake levels, *359, 542, 544, 546, 549*
  for pregnancy, *418, 421, 423*
  as priority, *359, 361, 388, 390, 392*
  for seniors, *478, 480, 482, 484*
Mediterranean diet, *151, 158, 312*
Melina, V., *128, 306, 484, 540*
menaquinone (vitamin K), *246, 248*
metablism, boosting, *350*
metabolic markers,
  for cancer, *76*
  for diabetes, *86*
metabolic syndrome, *84, 86, 177*
methane, *33*
methionine, *64, 112*
micronutrient deficiency, *49*
minerals, *257, 259, 262, 264, 266, 268, 271, 273, 276, 277, 279, 281, 282, 289*
  absorption of, *259, 262*

calcium, *88, 90, 95, 97, 262, 264, 266, 268, 412, 427, 460, 470, 473, 518*
chromium, *279*
copper, *279*
for exercise, *514, 516, 518, 521*
generally, *257, 259*
iodine, *276, 277, 412, 446, 452, 536*
iron, *268, 271, 273, 409, 427, 434, 437, 438, 468, 470, 516, 518*
magnesium, *279, 518, 521*
manganese, *279, 281*
phosphorus, *93, 95, 281*
potassium, *281*
for pregnancy, *404, 409, 412, 414*
recommended intakes,
selenium, *281*
for seniors, *468, 470*
sodium, *95, 281, 282, 538*
in vegan foods, *282, 289*
zinc, *273, 412, 427, 470, 518*
molasses, *197, 199*
monosodium glutamate (MSG), *304*

monounsaturated fats, *132, 134*

morning sickness, *404, 405*

muscle mass, reduced, *368*

N

National Restaurant Association, *45*

neotame, *201*

niacin (vitamin B3), *237, 239*

Nimmo, Catherine, *4*

nitrous oxide, *33*

noncaloric sweeteners, *201*

nonviscous fiber, *173*

Nurses' Health Study, *88, 248*

nutrient-dense vegan diet, defined, *312*

nutrients,
   see fat (dietary); fiber; minerals; protein; vitamins,

nutritional yeast, *215*

Nutrition Security Institute, *38*

nuts,
   exercise and, *529*
   fat in, *153, 155*
   omega-3 fatty acids in, *137*
   weight gain and, *380*

O

Oakes, Fiona, *502*

oats, gluten and, *192*

obesity, defined, *328*
   see also overweight,

oligosaccharides, *182, 300*

olives, *158*

omega-3 fatty acids,
   for cardiovascular health, *65*
   for infants, *442*
   for lactation, *430*
   for pregnancy, *416*
   recommendations, *536*
   sources of, *137, 139, 141, 143*
   for toddlers and preschoolers, *446*

omega-6 fatty acids, *137, 139, 141, 143*

organic foods,
   advantages of, *40*

Ornish, Dean, *68*

osteoporosis,
  bone health and, *90, 93, 460*
  calcium and, *88, 90, 95, 97, 262, 264, 266, 268*
  preventing, *99*
  protein and, *97, 99*
  risk factors and, *93, 95*
  underweight and, *368*
  vitamin D and, *97*
overnutrition, *49*
overweight, *323, 325, 328, 332, 334, 336, 338, 340, 342, 345, 347, 350, 352, 354, 357, 359, 361, 363*
  adopting vegan diet for health, *350, 352, 354, 357, 359, 361*
  body mass index (BMI) and, *323, 328*
  body shape and, *84, 328, 332*
  defined, *328*
  as energy imbalance, *332, 334*
  environmental factors of, *334, 336*
  exercise and, *494, 496*
  healthy lifestyle habits for, *340, 361, 363*
  physiological factors of, *334*
  pregnancy and, *405*
  problems of, *323, 325, 342, 345, 347, 350*
  weight loss and, *336, 338, 340, 342, 359*
oxalates, *262*
oxidized cholesterol (oxycholesterol), *61*

P

packaging, *40, 42*
Paleo diet, vegan diet compared to,
pantothenic acid (vitamin B5), *239, 425*
pear shape body type, *328, 332*
pellagra, preventing, *237*
percent fat, *65*
pescatarians, *74*
phenylalanine, *112*
phosphorus, *93, 95, 281*
phylloquinone (vitamin K), *246, 248*

physical exams, need for, 340

phytate, 259

phytochemicals, 65, 293, 295, 298

phytosterols, 134, 298

pigs, food industry and, 9, 12, 14

platelet aggregation, 64, 65

polycystic ovarian syndrome, 325

polyunsaturated fats, 134, 137

portion size, 532, 538

positive thinking, weight and, 338, 340

potassium, 281

'Power Vegan' (BusinessWeek), 45

prebiotics, 298, 300, 302

pregnancy, 397, 399, 402, 404, 405, 406, 409, 412, 414, 416, 418, 421, 423

   see also children; infants; lactation, exercise during, 418, 498

   folate (vitamin B, 21

folic acid) for, 243

   meal planning for, 418, 421, 423

   nutrients needed during, 402, 404, 405, 406, 409, 412, 414, 416

   preparing for, 402

   resources for, 432

   scientific evidence on vegan nutrition for, 397, 399

   substances to avoid during, 416, 418

   vitamins for, 210, 212, 215, 216, 243

premenstrual syndrome, 458, 460

preschoolers, vegan foods for, 442, 443, 446

probiotics, 298, 300, 302

processed foods, limiting, 354, 538

prostate cancer, 72

protein, 106, 108, 110, 112, 114, 116, 118, 128

   amino acids and, 64, 112, 114, 116

   for bone health, 95

calories from, *118, 128, 168*

complementing, *116, 118*

defined, *108*

digestibility of, *110, 112*

for exercise, *512, 514*

importance of, *106, 128*

for lactation, *427*

osteoporosis and, *97, 99*

for pregnancy, *406, 409*

requirements for, *108, 110*

for seniors, *468*

from soy, *128*

for weight gain, *384, 385*

Protein Power Smoothie (recipe), *388*

pure vegetarians, defined, *7*

purse seining, *26*

pyridoxine (vitamin B6), *239, 241, 475*

Pythagoras, *2*

R

raw vegan diet,
    cancer and, *74, 76*

defined, *312, 314*

lysine and, *116*

for seniors, *478*

Reader's Digest, *47*

rebaudioside A, *201*

recipes,
    Liquid Gold Dressing, *216*
    Protein Power Smoothie, *388*

recombinant bovine growth hormone (rBGH), *24*

recommended dietary allowances (RDA),
    omega-3 fatty acids, *139*
    protein, *108, 110*

refined carbohydrates, *168, 169, 171, 188, 189*

renal failure, *103*

resistance training, *394, 498*

resource depletion, food industry and, *31, 33*

resources, lists of, *432, 484, 487, 489*

retinol,
    see vitamin A,

rheumatoid arthritis, *103*
riboflavin (vitamin B2), *237, 516*
rickets, preventing, *215, 216*
Robbins, John, *4*

S

saccharin, *201*
Salley, John, *502*
saturated fats, *58, 134*
school-aged children, vegan foods for, *446, 448, 450, 452, 455*
scurvy, preventing, *230*
seasonal foods, advantages of, *40*
seeds,
    for dietary fat, *155*
    for exercise, *529*
    omega-3 fatty acids in, *137*
    for weight gain, *380*
selenium, *281*
seniors, *463, 466, 468, 470, 473, 475, 478, 480, 482, 484, 487, 489*
    brain health of, *480*
    challenges of, *484*

    exercise for, *466, 468, 498*
    meals for, *478, 480, 482, 484*
    nutrients for, *468, 470, 473, 475, 478*
    physical changes of, *463, 466*
    protein requirements and, *110*
    raw vegan diet for, *478*
    resources for, *484, 487, 489*
    vitamin B12 for, *212*
    vitamin D for, *216*
S-equol, *79*
serum ferritin, *268*
Seven Countries Study, *151*
Seventh-Day Adventists,
    care facilities of, *489*
    studies, *51, 56, 72, 74*
sex life, exercise and, *494*
simple carbohydrates, *168, 169, 171*
1,600-calorie sample menu, *542*
skin, of teens, *458*

slaughterhouses, *12, 14, 16, 19, 21, 24*
   see also food industry,
sleep,
   apnea, *325*
   exercise and, *496*
   importance of, *363, 395*
smoothies, *385, 388*
snacks,
   avoiding, *357*
   for children, *448, 450*
   fruit as dessert, *352, 354*
   healthful, *384*
soaking, for digestibility, *110*
sodium, *95, 281, 282, 538*
soluble fiber, *173*
soy, *79, 128*
spices, *354*
sports drinks, *525*
sprouting, *192, 295, 298*
Staphylococcus aureus, *19*
starch-based vegan diet, defined, *314*
starches, *168, 169, 171*
Stepaniak, J., *306*
sterols, *134, 298*
stevia, *201*

'stickers', *12, 14*
stomach cancer, *72*
stools, cancer and, *76*
stress management, *363, 394*
subcutaneous fat, *84*
sucralose, *201*
sucrose, *194*
sugar,
   alternatives to, *197, 199, 201, 354, 357*
   excessive amounts of, *194, 197*
   fructose and, *199, 201*
   fruit as dessert, *352, 354*
   generally, *194*
   prebiotics, *300*
   simple carbohydrates, *168, 169, 171*
   sources of, *199*
sugar alcohols, *201*
sulfites, *304*
sun,
   benefits of, *361*
   vitamin D and, *219, 221*
supplements,
   see minerals; vitamins,

T

The Farm (Summertown, Tennessee), *399, 434*

taste sense, seniors and, *478, 480*

teens,
  see also children,
  exercise for, *498*
  vegan foods for, *455, 458, 460, 461*

thiamin (vitamin B1), *234, 237*

threonine, *112*

thyroid, *276, 334*

tobacco,
  avoiding, *363*
  avoiding, during pregnancy, *416*
  chronic disease and, *54*

toddlers, vegan foods for, *442, 443, 446*

tofu,
  for seniors, *478*
  for weight gain, *380, 382*

toxins, avoiding, *347*

trans-fatty acids, *58, 134*

transportation, impact on environment, *33, 42*

travel, vegan food for, *487*

treats,
  see snacks,

triglycerides, *61*

tryptophan, *112, 114*

2,000-calorie sample menu, *544*

2,500- to 2,800-calorie sample menu, *544*

type 1 diabetes, *84*

type 2 diabetes, *4*
  blood sugar and exercise, *363, 505*
  defined, *81, 84, 86*
  fiber and, *177*
  metabolic markers of, *86*
  overweight and, *325*
  preventing, *88*
  seniors and, *484*
  treating, *86, 88*

'ugly fats', *132*

U

underweight, *365, 368, 370, 372, 375, 376, 378, 380, 382, 384, 385, 388, 390, 392, 394, 395*
  causes of, *370, 372, 375*

healthy lifestyle habits
for, *392, 394, 395*
pregnancy and, *405*
problems of, *365, 368,
370*
weight gain for, *375,
376, 378, 380, 382, 384, 385,
388, 390, 392*
United Nations Food
and Agriculture
Organization (FAO), *35*
unrefined carbohydrates,
168, 169, 171, 173
U.S. Environmental
Protection Agency
(EPA), *35*

V
valine, *112*
veal calves, *21, 24*
vegan diet, *49, 51, 54, 56,
58, 61, 64, 65, 68, 69, 72, 74, 76,
79, 81, 84, 86, 88, 90, 93, 95, 97,
99, 101, 103, 104, 291, 293, 295,
298, 300, 302, 304, 306, 309,
311, 312, 314, 321*
   see also
   carbohydrates;
   children; fat (dietary);

lactation; minerals;
overweight;
pregnancy; protein;
seniors; underweight;
vegan ethics; vitamins,
benefits of, *49, 291, 293*
cancer prevention
and, *69, 72, 74, 76, 79, 81*
cardiovascular disease
prevention and, *56, 58,
61, 64, 65, 68, 69*
cataract prevention
and, *101*
chemical
contaminants,
avoiding, *306, 309*
choosing, *309, 311, 312,
314*
clean, green food
choices, *314*
definitions, *2, 4, 7, 47*
dementia prevention
and, *101*
diverticular disease
prevention and, *101, 103*
enzymes in, *293*
food sensitivities, *302,
304, 306*

gallstone prevention and, *103*

as lifestyle, *4, 7*

as mainstream, *42, 45, 47*

occasional indulgence with, *321*

osteoporosis prevention and, *88, 90, 93, 95, 97, 99*

Paleo diet compared to,

phytochemicals in, *293, 295, 298*

phytosterols in, *298*

prebiotics and probiotics in, *298, 300, 302*

rheumatoid arthritis prevention and, *103*

scientific evidence on, *51, 54, 56, 104*

transitioning to, *314*

type 2 diabetes prevention and, *81, 84, 86, 88*

for weight problems, *350, 352, 354, 357, 359, 361*

(see also overweight; underweight),

vegan ethics, *2, 4, 7, 9, 12, 14, 16, 19, 21, 24, 26, 28, 31, 33, 35, 38, 40, 42, 45, 47*

animal rights issues and, *7, 28, 31*

Earth's resources and, *31, 33, 35, 38, 40*

food industry and, *9, 12, 14, 16, 19, 21, 24, 26, 28*

origin of, *2, 4*

perspective and, *7, 9*

planet-friendly habits for, *40, 42*

vegan as mainstream, *42, 45, 47*

vegan lifestyle and, *4, 7*

Vegan Food Guide, *531, 532, 536, 538, 540, 542, 544, 546, 549*

food groups and serving sizes, *532*

menus, *538, 540, 542, 544, 546, 549*

minerals, *536*

omega-3 fatty acids, *536*

practical pointers, *538*

Vegan Plate, *531, 532*

vitamins, *536*

Vegan in Volume: Vegan Quantity Recipes for Every Occasion (Berkoff), *489*

'veganized' treats, *321, 336*

vegetarian, defined, *2, 4*

Vegetarian Resource Group (VRG), *45*

very low-density lipoprotein (VLDL), *61*

visceral fat, *84*

viscous fiber, *173*

vitamin A, *95, 425*

vitamin B12,

benefits of, *208, 210, 212, 215*

cardiovascular health and, *64*

for children to age twelve, *452*

diabetes and, *88*

for exercise, *516*

for infants, *442*

for lactation, *210, 212, 425, 427*

during pregnancy, *414*

recommendations, *536*

for seniors, *473*

for toddlers and preschoolers, *446*

vitamin D,

for cardiovascular health, *65*

for children to age twelve, *452*

for exercise, *516*

for infants, *442*

for lactation, *215, 216, 427*

osteoporosis and, *97*

during pregnancy, *414*

recommendations, *536*

for seniors, *470, 473*

for teens, *460*

for toddlers and preschoolers, *446*

vitamins, *208, 210, 212, 215, 216, 219, 221, 223, 225, 228, 230, 232, 234, 237, 239, 241, 243, 246, 248, 255*

A, *95, 223, 225, 228, 425*

B, *28, 49, 88, 101, 208, 210, 212, 215, 414, 425, 427, 442, 446, 452, 473, 516, 536*

B vitamins (other than B12), *234, 237, 239, 241, 243, 246, 414, 416*
C, *223, 225, 228, 230*
D, *65, 97, 215, 216, 219, 221, 223, 414, 427, 442, 446, 452, 460, 470, 473, 516, 536*
E, *223, 225, 230, 232*
for exercise, *514, 516, 518, 521*
K, *246, 248*
during pregnancy, *402, 404*
recommended intakes, for seniors, *470, 473, 475*
in vegan foods, *248, 255*

W
waist to hip ratio, *328, 332*
waste, reducing, *42*
water,
see also fluids,
benefits of, *357, 359*
food industry and, *35, 38*
for healthy skin, *458*
Watson, Donald, *4*
weight,
see also overweight; underweight,
body mass index (BMI), *61, 323, 328, 365, 368, 370, 402*
diabetes and, *84*
fiber and, *177*
nutrition and, *51*
weight gain, for underweight, *375, 376, 378, 380, 382, 384, 385, 388, 390, 392*
weight gain, in pregnancy, *405*
weight loss, *336, 338, 340, 342, 359*
white flour,
see refined carbohydrates,
whole foods fat from, *132*
whole-foods,
vegan diet, defined, *314*
whole-grain hierarchy, *189*
(see also grains),
'Why Whales Are People Too' (Reader's Digest), *47*

World Cancer Research
Fund, *72*
World Health
Organization, *54, 197, 365,
423*
World Wildlife Fund, *35*

Z

zinc,
   benefits of, *273*
   for exercise, *518*
   for lactation, *427*
   for pregnancy, *412*
   for seniors, *470*

www.ingramcontent.com/pod-product-compliance
Ingram Content Group UK Ltd.
Pitfield, Milton Keynes, MK11 3LW, UK
UKHW021946301224
3893UKWH00037BB/804